THE SCIENTIFIC BASIS OF TOXICITY ASSESSMENT

DEVELOPMENTS IN TOXICOLOGY AND
ENVIRONMENTAL SCIENCE

Volume 6

THE SCIENTIFIC BASIS OF TOXICITY ASSESSMENT

Proceedings of the Symposium on The Scientific Basis of Toxicity Assessment held in Gatlinburg, Tennessee, U.S.A., 15-19 April, 1979.

Editor

HANSPETER R. WITSCHI

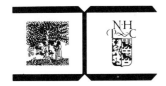

1980

ELSEVIER/NORTH-HOLLAND BIOMEDICAL PRESS
AMSTERDAM • NEW YORK • OXFORD

ISBN for this volume: 0-444-80200-2
ISBN for the series: 0-444-80013-1

Published by:
Elsevier/North-Holland Biomedical Press
335 Jan van Galenstraat, P.O. Box 211
Amsterdam, The Netherlands

Sole distributors for the USA and Canada:
Elsevier North-Holland Inc.
52 Vanderbilt Avenue
New York, N.Y. 10017

Library of Congress Cataloging in Publication Data

Symposium on the Scientific Basis of Toxicity
    Assessment, Gatlinburg, Tenn., 1979.
    The scientific basis of toxicity assessment.

    (Developments in toxicology and environmental
science ; v. 6)
    Includes bibliographies and indexes.
    1. Toxicity testing--Congresses. 2. Toxicology--
Congresses. I. Witschi, Hanspeter. II. Title.
III. Series.
RA1199.S95 1979   615.9'05   79-28108
ISBN 0-4444-80200-2

Printed in The Netherlands

PREFACE

For more than 30 years the Biology Division of the Oak Ridge National Laboratory has sponsored an annual spring conference. Each of these symposia has covered an area in which significant and exciting new research was being done and which promised that even more knowledge of fundamental biological processes would be developed in the near future.

In April 1979 the theme of the conference was "The Scientific Basis of Toxicity Assessment." During the last few years, the science of toxicology has received much attention. There is an ever growing awareness that toxic hazards in our daily environment may be a threat to our well-being It is the goal of toxicology, as a predictive science, to understand such hazards. Only then will we be able to deal successfully with both the real and the imaginary hazards we face today and in all likelihood will continue to face in the future if we hope to maintain and to improve the quality of life. Research in toxicology will never guarantee us absolute safety. However, sound and responsible toxicology will help to make intelligent decisions and will assist us in weighing risks against benefits in the assessment of our increasingly complex chemical environment.

In order for toxicology to be a truly predictive science, we need to explore and to understand how chemicals affect the structural and functional integrity of living organisms. Knowledge has to be acquired at each level of biological organization and the powerful tools of modern research must be fully exploited.

The scope of the present meeting was deliberately a broad one. The problems and issues in toxicology were defined first. A discussion followed which explored new avenues on how to detect and how to predict untoward interactions of chemicals with living systems. The pathways of chemicals through the environment, within animals and single cells, and their interaction with critical target molecules were described with selected examples, and the role of metabolism of foreign compounds in producing toxicity was explored. Of equal importance was to learn how the organism reacts toward a chemical insult. Finally, three most basic questions were discussed: how do we best use the information we generate in experiments with animals to predict hazard for man, what can toxicology learn from the closely related discipline of radiation biology, and where has the basic approach to toxicological problems met with success. The papers in this volume hopefully will give us some indication how close we have come to our goals and will help to identify directions of future research.

At this point it is a pleasure to thank all my colleagues who helped to plan this meeting: Dr. Robert A. Neal, Vanderbilt University, Nashville; Dr. J. E. Gibson, Chemical Industry Institute of Toxicology, Research Triangle Park; Drs. S. I. Auerbach and C. W. Gehrs, Environmental Sciences Division, ORNL, and, from the Biology Division, Drs. R. J. M. Fry, R. F. Kimball, S. Mitra, J. K. Selkirk and T. J. Slaga. The success of even the best planned meeting depends upon enthusiastic speakers and a receptive audience; we were fortunate to have both. Particular thanks go to the then Director of the Biology Division, Dr. J. B. Storer, and to the Associate Director for Biomedical Sciences of ORNL, Dr. C. E. Richmond, for their continuing support.

The meeting was sponsored by the Biology Division of the Oak Ridge National Laboratory (operated by the Union Carbide Corporation for the Department of Energy). Travel for speakers and chairpersons was supported by a grant from the National Institute of Environmental Health Sciences.

Finally, I would like to acknowledge the most competent and unfailingly enthusiastic help of Mrs. Mary Jane Loop, without whose experience and cheerfulness the meeting never would have gone as smoothly as it did.

Hanspeter Witschi

CONTENTS

viii

© 1980 Elsevier/North-Holland Biomedical Press
The Scientific Basis of Toxicity Assessment
H. Witschi, editor.

SYMPOSIUM ON THE SCIENTIFIC BASIS OF TOXICITY ASSESSMENT:
OPENING REMARKS

CHESTER R. RICHMOND
Oak Ridge National Laboratory, Oak Ridge, Tennessee 37830

It is my pleasure to welcome you to Gatlinburg and the 32nd Annual Research
Conference of the Oak Ridge National Laboratory's Biology Division. The topic of this
conference, The Scientific Basis for Toxicity Assessment, is in my opinion both timely
and especially important.

I am pleased to see among the registered participants representatives of various federal
agencies (at the risk of the sin of omission, I will mention NCI, DOE, EPA, NSF, NIEHS,
FDA, and TVA), numerous universities, research institutes, industrial organizations, state
health organizations and members of the technical information community. The composition of this particular group reflects society's broad interest in the production, distribution,
utilization and disposal of materials which at some time in their life cycle may cause more
detriment than benefit to man. The materials may interact directly with living systems
or indirectly via complicated and only partly understood mechanisms. People are
bombarded each day with news about toxic and hazardous materials in the fire detectors
within their homes, their work places, their outside environment, their food, the air they
breathe, and even in the materials their children sleep in. I am not certain how they
(the general taxpaying public) will respond to information concerning transformation,
promoting agents, metabolic degradation products, and cocarcinogens. Many will be
more convinced that the situation is getting worse, fewer may selectively tune out the
daily news of the toxic material of the day or month as they become oversaturated, and
a few might appreciate that more knowledge is being accumulated about this extremely
complicated process of how materials, whether precursors or derivatives, either alone or
in various combinations, ultimately affect man. I say ultimately, since years or even
decades may be involved between exposure and effect. Obviously, much time and
money must be spent to do the job even for the most important materials (once we decide
what they are).

Some will ask if it is an impossible task; that is, to test product after product using
only one or several relatively simple tests (if we can once agree on the test).

2

Some will say that the work is not scientifically rewarding or challenging and they lose interest. Others may find the questions challenging and delve even deeper into the underlying mechanism of how toxic materials interact with living material.

Some will also point out that compared to the early nineteen hundreds infant mortality has been reduced and life span is greater. So why all the fuss and concern, especially since life in general is easier.

The comedians, both amateur and professional, will continue to thrive on this subject as they suggest such things as bans on materials that are known to be hazardous to rats.

What are the problems? How do we develop dosimetric schemes to relate exposure to effect as has been done in the field of radiation? Should we develop dosimetric schemes and models or should we be content with learning relationships between exposure and effect? Should we place more effort on understanding underlying mechanisms? How do we extrapolate data from one or more species to man? What commitment of resources should be made nationally? To what level of risk should society be protected from a given material for a given benefit?

I sometimes think that our society has little real feeling for our understanding of the vast commitment of resources required to "protect" them from toxic materials. I am not certain that the responsible federal agencies fully understand what they will receive from their investment of public funds in this area.

Those of you who count yourselves among the scientific community need to continually seek to understand underlying mechanisms of toxicity as we go about our screening and testing activities, for this is probably the only certain way to ultimately reduce the time and therefore money required to obtain necessary data and information.

Those of you who represent government agencies must combine efforts and learn to communicate more efficiently with each other and interact more often. Research dollars can be stretched through multiple agency planning and support. Although there have been some recent efforts in this regard, there is still much room for improvement. And, please, do not regulate promoting agents or even suggest doing so at this time.

Those of you in industry are moving ahead and committing more resources to this question of toxicity assessment. I personally believe there is much room for more inter-action between private industry and the large national research and development laboratories. And I would like to see more efforts in this area.

Let me now in closing come to what I see is the real bottom line. That is, what constitutes a reasonable or a de minimus risk? Each regulatory agency approaches a problem from its perspective and Congressional mandates. We seem to be continually embroiled in debates, even as to the definition of toxic materials or hazardous materials or carcinogens, even years after regulatory legislation has passed. We know much more in the relative sense about some classes of materials than others and we must develop some way of determining how safe is safe for one class of materials, so that attention can be directed to other classes where our ignorance is greater. Otherwise we will be misplacing resources that are already spread too thin. We need some mechanism to look across the regulatory agencies to see how they treat risk assessment (hopefully without creating a new agency). No risk is the greatest risk of all and in the real world no risk is not actually achievable. Also the scientists at the work bench need this kind of guidance as they work within their own specialty areas.

Again, it is my pleasure to welcome you to our 32nd Annual Research Conference. I join John Storer in hoping that all of us will profit from a lively and stimulating exchange of ideas on how to explore and understand mechanisms of toxicity. On behalf of the Oak Ridge National Laboratory, I welcome you to this symposium, to Gatlinburg, and to the Great Smoky Mountains.

THE PROBLEMS AND ISSUES IN TOXICOLOGY
Chairman: Michael S. Rose

© 1980 Elsevier/North-Holland Biomedical Press
The Scientific Basis of Toxicity Assessment
H. Witschi, editor.

THE PROBLEMS AND ISSUES IN TOXICOLOGY: INTRODUCTION

M. S. ROSE

ICI Central Toxicology Laboratory, Alderley Park, Macclesfield, Cheshire,
United Kingdom SK10 4TJ

Toxicology is ultimately concerned with the evaluation of the hazards associated with the use of chemicals. Most working toxicologists will accept that there is no such thing as a totally safe chemical. The oxygen we breathe is extremely toxic to man and experimental animals when the concentration is raised fivefold. Equally, if the concentration is lowered fivefold there is a toxic response. I think this example illustrates the nature of the problem facing toxicologists. Clearly, we cannot "regulate" the use of oxygen, and we know from a few million years epidemiology that there is a safe level of exposure.

Modern society has come to depend upon the use of a large number of chemicals in industry and agriculture. One of our jobs as toxicologists is to define the conditions under which these can be used safely. In order to do this, we carry out studies in experimental animals and then extrapolate these results to man. However, it is clear that different species or even strains of animals can respond differently to the same chemical. This raises the question "which response gives us an indication of the likely response to man?". There are large gaps in our knowledge, not least our understanding of the differences in distribution and metabolism of chemicals in experimental animals and man. My personal view (which is not original) is that these gaps can only be filled by intensive efforts to understand the many ways in which chemicals produce toxic effects. Only then will we be able to make confident predictions about safe levels of exposure.

The speakers in our session this morning will outline in more detail the nature and variety of the problems and issues facing those who study toxicology.

© 1980 Elsevier/North-Holland Biomedical Press
The Scientific Basis of Toxicity Assessment
H. Witschi, editor.

PROBLEMS AND ISSUES IN TOXICOLOGY

INTRODUCTION

ROBERT G. TARDIFF

Board on Toxicology and Environmental Health Hazards, National Academy of Sciences, Washington, D.C. 20418

It is a pleasure to introduce this symposium and to provide a framework for this distinguished Panel by addressing issues on the frontier of developmental toxicology.

The concept of establishing toxicity assessment on a sound scientific basis has been a steadfast goal of toxicology marked by considerable controversy over the course of its implementation. Since the turn of the century, and particularly after World War II, our society has witnessed incredible growth in the development of chemicals whose application has enhanced substantially our health, welfare, and general quality of life.

With the continuing growth of chemical technology, concern about chemicals in the environment and their threat to human health have become more intense. Real or suspected chemical threats often arise from the same sources providing some measures of real or perceived benefit to members of our society. Our recognition that medications possess adverse effects on health has been carried over to other classes of chemicals such as pesticides, consumer goods (e.g., flame retardants), food additives (e.g., saccharin), and industrial agents (e.g., vinyl chloride and bis-chloromethyl ether), and to the by-products and wastes of chemical manufacturing processes (e.g., tetrachlorodibenzo-p-dioxin, landfill leachates, combustion products, etc.) that enter the air, water, and food supply.

The diversity of substances is noteworthy: the annual production volume of synthetic organic chemicals includes approximately 10,000 compounds, of which approximately 70% is contributed by nearly 500 large-volume chemical substances. Because there is such a large number of substances and the likelihood that humans will be exposed to them, the requirement for information about anticipated toxic manifestations is great.

The need for predictive toxicology has long been recognized by both industry and government. By using surrogates for humans, the toxicologist attempts to replicate conditions in which humans are exposed, to identify organismic dysfunctions at several amplified dosage levels, and to determine the underlying cause(s) of the malfunctions.

The prediction of chemically induced toxic reactions in humans has undergone increasing complexity as a result of contributions from other areas of scientific development. When animal models are selected on the basis of convenience and/or cost, the pharmacokinetic and metabolic tools of the pharmacologist and biochemist are being used with ever greater intensity to compare empirically the handling of chemicals by different species in order to identify those species that more closely approximate human beings. Such information provides a scientific basis for later extrapolation of results, a greater understanding of the underlying effects, and cogent arguments for proper resource management.

Similar contributions have been made by enzymologists (e.g., understanding of mechanism of action of organophosphate poisoning and the uncovering of mechanisms for the repair of DNA damaged by chemical carcinogens and mutagens), immunologists (e.g., the understanding of the expression or repression of chemical carcinogenesis through the in-situ recognition and control of transformed cells), and endocrinologists (e.g., the study of diethylstilbestrol as a chemical carcinogen).

To illustrate the progress in toxicity assessment, one can compare the two editions of "Principles and Procedures for Evaluating the Toxicity of Household Substances," a report that was developed by the National Academy of Sciences for the Consumer Product Safety Commission. In the 1964 edition, only the study of acutely toxic responses could be adequately described; however, the 1978 report contained a detailed treatise of chronic toxicity (including carcinogenesis), mutagenesis, teratogenesis and reproduction, and behavioral toxicity. In addition, it substantially updated the elements of acute toxicity study. What progress will we observe in the next decade?

Despite substantial methodologic advancements, there still remain many issues to be resolved either by experimentation or by critical deliberation. I trust that it will be of interest to speculate on some emerging directions and foci of toxicology that have a direct impact upon the assessment of hazards to humans from chemicals.

While over the past two decades environmental chemists have described the exposure of humans to a variety of compounds simultaneously as well as sequentially, previous and contemporary toxicity studies have dealt almost exclusively with evaluation of individual compounds. Relatively few combinations of agents have been studied to determine possible interactions, and some of those, such as the interaction between asbestos and cigarette smoke, have effects that are qualitatively or quantitatively different from those related to the individual compounds.

During the past few years, several _in-vitro_ systems have been used to deal with the toxicity of mixtures with varying success. These approaches provide useful tools with which to compare the toxicity of various mixtures, to ascertain the effectiveness of chemical fractionation techniques, and to screen materials for specific responses such as mutagenesis. This usefulness in hazard assessment stems from the ability of the approaches to establish priorities for substances and mixtures to be studied in the future.

The assessment of hazards from complex mixtures is one of the more challenging aspects in toxicology. Continuing development is required to improve the integration of information about diverse mechanisms of action at the level of the whole animal. We need a greater understanding of the variety of ways in which the expression of toxicity may be altered through changes in physiologic states (such as nutrition and microbial diseases) and by stress from other chemical substances. In the premarket testing of chemicals, it may be insufficient in the near future to describe a pathologic lesion in a single compound environment, and such analysis may require the elucidation of the risks from agents under study as modified by a more complex environment, such as several disease states, genetic aberrations, and varying dietary conditions. A variety of approaches is required including diametrically opposite perspectives: (a) studies of test agents versus selected variables and (b) complex mixture studies dissecting the components to identify dominant factors in the toxic manifestations.

Let us now examine briefly the directions of a controversial practice used to predict chemical hazards: namely, "risk assessment." The term is used to denote the application of statistical formulae to project dose-response data far below experimental levels to the anticipated or known human doses. The most readily recognized difficulty is the construction of the dose-response curve at several orders of magnitude below the observation range.

In some fashion, virtually all toxicity studies using laboratory animals require the use of relatively high doses to identify adverse effects and to compensate for differences in size between human and experimental animal populations (statistical sensitivity). Thus, any observations in the animal model studies are a function of at least two parameters: (a) biologic activity within individuals and (b) differential sensitivity of individuals in an exposed population (species sensitivity). While all toxicity studies should strive to identify the boundaries of differential sensitivity within a population of the test species, the lower limits of species sensitivity are often prescribed by the investigators' selection of doses and sample sizes. The "lower limit" of species sensitivity can be defined as that individual in a population who will manifest a minimal adverse reaction to an agent at a dose at which other members of the population are not adversely effected (i.e., most susceptible individual for that compound). The determination of this parameter could be constrained to the dimensions of the exposed population: if only ten humans are to be exposed, then, studies could be used to define the limit of species susceptibility for one order of magnitude greater than the number of subjects—assuming a likely growth in numbers exposed. Information on genetic variability and mechanisms of action could be used to modify the limit.

For the accurate translation of toxic reactions from one species to another the lower limit of species sensitivity should be defined—or at least it could be determined for the test species and assumed to be the same for the target species. For example, several pharmaceuticals and some environmental agents are believed to produce toxic or allergic reactions in humans at a rate of one in 10,000 but presumably no less. Yet animal studies with these agents could detect responses at a rate of only 5 to 10 percent or greater. Thus, in analyzing the results of chronic feeding studies using 25 or 50 animals per dose group, one should address the question of whether the "no observed adverse effect level" is related to sample size or to the boundaries of species sensitivity.

When species sensitivity can be characterized in the observation range, the extrapolation process contains greater certainty of accurate predictions at lower doses. Clearly, verification of the lower limit of species sensitivity must be obtained through the creative development of empirical data beyond conventional studies.

If, on the other hand, species sensitivity to a compound cannot be characterized in the observation range of the conventional toxicity design, two compatible approaches are available.

First, the limit of species susceptibility may be ascertained in animal models through extensive mechanistic investigations to identify primary lesions, rates of injury, defense mechanisms, rates of repair, dose-response structure, and other biologic factors whose integration and variability will serve to characterize the limit of species sensitivity. If comparable data could be obtained directly in humans—without breaching ethical considerations—it would be possible to identify the dose range for human risk, to ascribe risk levels per unit of dose, and to characterize the no-risk level of human exposure. However, much human experimentation is unfeasible and impractical.

Alternatively, the lower limit of species sensitivity could be defined arbitrarily as "infinite" (i.e., equal to population base of target species). If the shape of the dose-response curve were characterized, then risk levels for any type of toxic manifestation could be derived. If, because of practical limitations, the dose-response curve cannot be characterized precisely, one model dose-response (such as the linear model) can be applied, but with consistency to assure the comparability of risk estimates. In the forseeable future, such extrapolation models will be applied with greater frequency to a variety of toxic manifestations. Thus, it can be anticipated that "risk levels" will replace "safety" and "safe levels" until the lower limit of species sensitivity to toxic substances can be defined scientifically.

Our distinguished panel members will address these and other issues in greater detail.

© 1980 Elsevier/North-Holland Biomedical Press
The Scientific Basis of Toxicity Assessment
H. Witschi, editor.

TOXIC SUBSTANCES IN RETROSPECT AND PROSPECT

ROBERT I. KRIEGER*
Department of Environmental Toxicology, University of California,
Davis, CA 95616

INTRODUCTION

In this Symposium participants will address many contemporary problems and issues in toxicology, new outlooks on testing, mechanisms of
toxicity, environmental transport of chemicals, and development of toxicology as a predictive science. My invitation to participate included
the suggestion that review of human disasters and lessons learned from
them would be particularly relevant to the program. Although it is true
that particular incidents often serve as points of departure for much
research and resassessment of chemical hazard evaluation procedures. I
had difficulty applying the term "disaster" to my thinking about health
effects of chemicals. After several false starts, I concluded that the
term disaster was probably better reserved for events such as hurricanes
and tornadoes, earthquakes, floods, fires, and transportation accidents
in which there were major losses of life and property which occurred in
short time intervals.

It is generally recognized that chemical-based technologies have made
profound impacts upon the quality of life in recent times. Insuring
that these technologies will meet both short- and long-term human needs
is increasingly complex and requires continual evaluation by scientists,
technologists, and the general public. Members of the scientific and
technological communities readily accept the notion that detailed knowledge of mechanisms of action is essential for understanding chemical
selectivity and biological adaptation. The benefits of this knowledge
are less clear to the public whom we serve.

Greater public visibility of the regulatory process and an active
news media are associated with increased public awareness of health and
environmental effects of chemicals. All use classes have been subjects

─────────
*Visiting Scientist, Chemical Industry Institute of Toxicology
 P. O. Box 12137, Research Triangle Park, NC 27709

16

of concern - chemical trace substances and nutrients of the food supply;
drugs in medical and social settings; economic poisons deployed against
other living competitors for food and fiber, process chemicals, products, and pollutants of the workplace; and chemical residues in air,
water, biota, and soil. Revelations about exposures to toxic substances
are common features of printed and televised media. Those revelations
arouse concerns, and sometimes actions, by individuals who are usually
ill-prepared to acquire information, analyze, and respond to many uncertainties about biological effects of chemicals.

   The concerns have evoked societal responses to many of these uncertainties but frequently the responses perpetuate concern rather than
promote perspective and understanding. Legislatures offer statutes such
as the Toxic Substances Control Act and the Occupational Safety and
Health Act to protect constituents and their environments. Regulators
within the Environmental Protection Agency, Food and Drug Administration, Occupational Safety and Health Administration, Consumer Product
Safety Commission and related federal, state, and local agencies increasingly act upon issues related to biological effects of chemicals.
The circle is completed by advocates of the public and business who
represent particular points of view in the decision-making process.

   Improvement of the status quo in chemical hazard evaluation and risk
assessment requires continued scientific research and greater attention
to the need to establish foundation for involvement of more sectors of
society in the decision-making process. Public perception of chemical
threats to health and environmental quality have major influence upon
efforts to conduct chemical hazard evaluation and risk assessment.

   The particular subjects selected for this presentation were issues
which have influenced public perception of toxic substances, and the
materials were selected specifically for this audience of scientists. I
hope these examples will remind viewers of some of the common percep-
tions of chemicals, the complexity of the process of risk assessment,
and the need to develope effective communication with the public.

MATERIALS

   The slide-tape presentations utilized 35 mm slides, magnetic cassette
tapes and readily available projection equipment. The slide sequence
was produced and synchronized using a Wollensak 2573 AV "Sync II" Tape
Recorder. Slides were projected using two Kodak Carosel Projectors
equipped with automatic focus. Smooth visual transitions between slides

were made using a Wollensak AV-33 Dissolve Unit and dissolve rates of about 1, 3, and 7 seconds.

OVERVIEW AND COMMENT

The subjects of six slide and taped music presentations included pictures and lyrics which represented complex scientific, technologic, and humanistic factors which are important to decision-making about human and environmental exposures to chemicals.

Presentation 1. Opening. Much of current concern about impacts of chemicals on quality of life is closely associated with population growth and resource utilization. Natural products, food chemicals and adulterants, social and medicinal drugs, pesticides and commercial chemicals (process chemicals, products, and pollutants) are important, easily identified chemical use classes. Representatives of each of these' use classes have been associated during the past 40 years with potential threats to health resulting from excessive exposures. In rapid succession we have experienced nuclear weapons testing and use, prescription of miracle drugs such as penecillin, unexpected side effects (toxicity) of some of these same drugs, application and persistence of DDT and related persistent pesticides, consumption of food currently described in terms of additives and trace contaminants rather than nutritional sufficiency, and life with polluted air, water and soil. Slides accompanied by instrumental jazz by Chuck Mangione ("Echano") depicted some of these experiences.

As scientists we may readily identify knowledge which is essential to obtaining a reply to the question "How much is too much?", but ultimately societal answers to the question will include technological and humanistic factors as well. The corollary, "How little is OK?," represents a significant challenge for the future.

The opening featured many recently newsworthy episodes involving chemicals. The following slide and taped music presentations depict toxic substances in Personal, Occupational, Community and Global Environments. The latter classification is useful in describing qualitative and quantitative characteristics of chemical exposures and reinforces the idea that toxicity is a consequence of pattern of chemical use.

Personal Environment. Alcohol in beverages, aspirin pills, caffeine in stimulating drinks, and nicotine in tobacco smoke are more frequently effective than harmful. Each is listed as a Toxic Substance for regulatory purposes. Scientific risk assessment is a negligible factor in determining their patterns of use by individuals. Consideration of patterns of use of these common chemicals provides an opportunity for discussion of principles of toxicology which are closely related to personal experience.

The short, topical concentrates on aspirin, nicotine, and ethanol included slides which depicted their common origin as natural products and their use and abuse. The reminder that the essences of "pills, tobacco smoke and drinks" are biologically active chemicals may be reinforced by discussion of effective dose, maximum tolerated dose, "side effects," and even death in cases of excessive exposures. These concepts are effectively presented to non-scientists using these familiar chemicals. In developing societal goals for scientific risk assessment of chemicals, we might benefit from careful consideration of the extent that scientific research influences the use of these common toxic substances.

Over 400 years ago Paracelsus urged fellow physicians to recognize that dose was the most important determinant of toxicity. Although this tenet of Paracelsus' teaching is recognized by most toxicologists and is consistent with the common experience, it is too frequently ignored in deliberation and regulation of chemical use practices. Today chemical exposures in the Personal Environment can serve as points of reference in discussions between scientists and an uncertain, wary public and in scientific risk assessment.

Presentation 3. Occupational Environments. Individuals have an opportunity to control most chemical exposures in the Personal Environment. The workforce is comprised of individuals who have less easily controlled, contractual exposures to chemicals. Bernardo Ramazzini wrote Discourse on the Diseases of Workers in 1713 from which comes the following observation:

> "...workers in certain arts and crafts sometimes derive from them grave injuries, so that where they hoped for a subsistence that would prolong their lives and feed their families, they are too often repaid with the most dangerous diseases and finally, uttering curses on the profession to which they had devoted themselves, they desert their post among the living."

In all 54 groups of workers were discussed by Ramazzini and strong emphasis was placed upon the need to apply knowledge to protect health and to promote productivity.

The strategies are straight-forward for minimizing chemical exposures which result in acute toxicities. Less clear are means to avoid possible threats to health posed by agents which produce effects in the work force only after long, continued exposures or only in combination with other chemical, biological or ergonomic factors. Results of scientific research will continue to provide understanding of mechanisms of disease, but the information is seldom directly applicable to protecting health and safety. The scientific study of frequency and distribution of disease among cohorts of workers requires increased attention. The contributions of epidemiologists to chemical risk assessment seems certain to increase in magnitude and importance.

Although considerable knowledge of human health effects of chemicals in occupational environments has been obtained, problems continue to be discovered. To the contemporary, popular song "Take This Job and Shove It" (Johnny Paycheck) were depicted agents, settings, and effects of asbestos and kepone, two substances which have recently been associated with widely-publicized occupational illness.

The first, asbestos, is the subject of the initial criteria document of the National Institute of Occupational Safety and Health. Asbestos is extensively distributed in occupational environments. The case demonstrates effectively how concerns about chemicals in the workplace promote study of other exposures in personal and community environments and uncertainty about health effects. The present campaign to identify persons at risk resulting from World War II occupational exposures has extensively used public media. Although we can only guess at the impact of the program at this time, the public is being presented information about types of exposure, latency, and special risks associated with cigarette smoking.

In contrast to the widespread occurrence of asbestos and its potential impact on very large numbers of workers, a single occupational environment and work force were included in the second segment of the presentation. Kepone manufacture at Life Science Products Corporation in Hopewell, Virginia, promoted extensive morbidity among workers. Revelation of the disease epidemic in 1975, contamination of the community and region with the persistent insecticide, and complex litigation which followed are matters of record. Even today "occupational hazards" may be too frequently assigned to others by persons in power and too easily accepted by others unaware of risks and alternatives.

Presentation 4 is also set in the Occupational Environment and features mining, the most hazardous occupation. The ballad "Give My Love to Marie" (James Talley) describes the plight of a black-lunged, coal miner in East Tennessee. For our Symposium here in Gatlinburg it seemed especially relevant to include this presentation which depicts the human pathos historically associated with coal mining and black lung disease. Scientific studies in England and the United States during this century have resulted in modern work practices which can provide protection by minimizing dust production and accumulation. Alternative energy sources such as nuclear, hydro, and solar also featured in this presentation to emphasize the point that each alternative carries a characteristic set of risks.

Presentations 5 and 6. Community and Global Environments. Whereas exposure and effects of certain chemical exposures in Personal and Community environments may be closely related in time and space, these relationships are less clear on the community and even global scales.

Occurrence of chemicals which are relatively unreactive in abiotic and biotic systems can be established using sensitive analytical technology. Most frequently measured in air, water, soil, and biota are halogenated (-Cl, -Br) organics, crude oil constituents and combustion byproducts, radionuclides, and heavy metals. Human activities have had major influence upon the kinds and amounts of such chemicals in community and global environments and the chemicals are frequently referred to as anthropogenic chemicals. The term "anthropogenic chemicals" is useful to indicate the possibility of human control over their production, use and distribution. Biological effects of accidental environmental release of large amounts of these chemicals (shipping accidents, train derailments, industrial accidents) are amenable to study using precise analytical measurements and assessments of mortality and morbidity are straightforward. Understanding of possible biological effects associated with low-level, long-term persistent chemical exposures is extremely limited or totally lacking.

Much impetus for societal concern about harmful effects of chemicals was created during the past 20 years by controversy about nuclear weapons testing and global radionuclide transport, human mortality and morbidity resulting from discharge of mercury-contaminated process waters in Japan, thalidomide phocomelia in Europe, and global distribution of persistent chlorinated hydrocarbon pesticides. These issues became part of the public domain with the 1962 publication of Silent Spring by Rachel Carson. Although description of environmental consequences considerably exceeded reality, the book effectively communicated the need to more completely evaluate environmental impacts of chemical technologies.

The resulting movement was termed "environmentalism." It is difficult to guage the profound impact of Rachel Carson's Silent Spring (1962) on research, public policy and public opinion during that period. The writer of a master's thesis titled "The Development of the Pronephros During Embryonic and Early Life of the Catfish Ictalurus punctatus" and later the author of Under the Sea-Wind (1941), The Sea Around Us (1951), The Edge of the Sea (1955), Carson sensitized scientists, technologists and the public to possible impacts of chemicals on the environment. The book spawned much intense criticism and acclaim. Although one could now engage in arguments about detail, there would be little challenge of Rachel Carson's eminent status as an effective advocate. Two subjects which became important during the ensuing public debate were featured in the concluding presentations.

Mercury and Minamata Disease were the subjects of presentation 5 which included graphics from the book Minamata (W. Eugene and Aileen M. Smith, 1975) and the song "Sakura, Sakura" (flute, Jean-Pierre Rampal and harp, Lily Laskine). Aspects of mercury production and distribution in biota, water, air and soil were included in a now-familiar materials balance format. Consideration of chemical distribution in these natural compartments is consistent with the recognized importance of obtaining a complete materials balance to begin to adequately assess fate and effects of chemicals. The magnitude of mortality and morbidity associated in the mid-1950s with the waste discharges which contained mercury of the chemical factory of Chisso Corporation contributed to the concern about chemical pollutants which developed in the 1960s. That particular episode could be justly classed as a disaster.

Chlorinated hydrocarbon insecticides became a major focus of the "environmental movement" in the 1960s and their use and distribution were the subjects of the final presentation. The discovery, development, deployment and persistence of DDT were portrayed using reproductions of many original technical bulletins and were accompanied by

22

"Chase the Clouds Away" (Chuck Mangione). Initial successes in disease vector control and agriculture promoted discussion of the extinction of pest species. Later pest resistance and resurgence plus pesticide residues in crops, water, soil and air and non-target organisms (including humans) required reevaluation of use practices. Scientific, technological, and humanistic arguments have been important in determination of the current economic status of these chemicals, prototypes of persistent chemical pollutants.

CONCLUSION

The presentations featured toxic substances in familiar Personal, Occupational, Community and Global Environments. Audio-visual media were used to review a broad spectrum of events of the past 40 years. These events seem important to toxicology and to development of more general understanding of scientific, technological and humanistic contributions to chemical hazard evaluation and risk assessment. The materials should remind participants of the need to communicate results of scientific studies with decision-makers at all levels - individuals, groups, advocates (both public and industrial), legislators, and regulators. Limiting the effectiveness of communication with those outside the scientific community at present is the poor, general understanding of toxicology and its relationship to the science-technology enterprise. Enlightened chemical hazard evaluation and risk assessment require a solid scientific base, critical evaluation of technologies, and improved communication with the public.

ACKNOWLEGEMENTS

Audio-visual materials were prepared by Diane Mihara, Tina van Hoesan, Craig Rourke and Greg Hall. Shirley Gee assisted with production and presentation of the slides and taped music. Some materials from the course, "Introduction to Toxicology" at the University of California, Davis, were prepared with the support of the Department of Environmental Toxicology and two University Undergraudate Instructional Improvement Grants.

© 1980 Elsevier/North-Holland Biomedical Press
The Scientific Basis of Toxicity Assessment
H. Witschi, editor.

ENVIRONMENTAL TOXICOLOGY: ISSUES, PROBLEMS, AND CHALLENGES

STANLEY I. AUERBACH and CARL W. GEHRS
Environmental Sciences Division, Oak Ridge National Laboratory, Oak Ridge,
Tennessee 37830

INTRODUCTION
    Since antiquity man has been aware of his environment and of the materials
within it that could be used as toxins. The *Rig-Veda* of Hindu origin, dating
perhaps to 5000 B.C., talks of the use by priests of the *Soma* plant as an
hallucinogen, while the Hebrew Pentateuch discusses the relationship man has
with his surroundings. In this paper we discuss both segments, environment
and toxins, from an ecologist's point of view. We trace ecology and toxicology
to see when and how they emerged as separate sciences, with the purpose of
understanding their 'sphere of influence' and identifying the contributions
each can make to environmental toxicology. Finally, we discuss the challenges
that exist, from our perception, for environmental toxicology.

Toxicology
    The earliest records reveal that man observed both his environment and the
presence of toxic agents and made use of each (Figure 1) without understanding
why they existed or how they functioned. Near the time of Christ, Dioscorides
attempted to classify poisons based on their origin (plant, animal, or mineral),
a step toward understanding. Long before this time, man made use of poisons
in hunting and as a method of ending life (Socrates 399 B.C.). While the use
of toxins increased during the next 1500 years (one needs only to think of the
Borgia family in Rome), it remained for Paracelsus, in the early 1500s, to
focus attention on the toxin as a chemical entity and on the concept of specificity of action whereby the toxic response is initiated. Structural activity
and dose response concepts were formulated, and toxicology began to consider
the organism to identify specifically where an effect occurred and how the
chemical action took place. Toxicology was becoming scientific. Other
advancements included the systematic correlation of chemical and biological
information on poisons (Orfila, early 1800s), development of analytical methods
for specific toxicants (arsenic in 1836 by Marsh), and initiation of mechanism-
of-action studies (for example, Bernard and carbon monoxide in the mid-1850s).

ORNL—DWG 79-11302

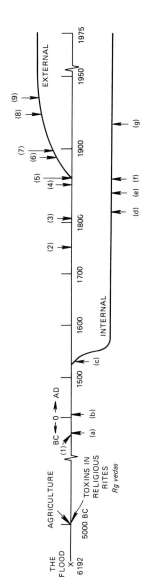

1. ARISTOTLE OBSERVES AIR, FIRE, WATER (400)
2. LINNAEUS PUBLISHES CLASSIFICATION SYSTEMS FOR PLANTS AND ANIMALS (1753 AND 1758, RESPECTIVELY)
3. VON HUMBOLDT NOTES REPLACEMENT OF LATITUDE BY ALTITUDE (1802)
4. DARWIN PUBLISHES *ORIGIN OF SPECIES* (1859)

5. HAECKEL DEFINES OEKOLOGIE (1866)
6. FORBES IDENTIFIED ABIOTIC/BIOTIC INTERACTIONS IN ORGANISMS FUNCTIONING IN LAKE (1877)
7. COWLES INTRODUCES DYNAMIC ECOLOGY (1899)
8. LOTKA INITIATES QUANTITATIVE ECOLOGY (1925)
9. TANSLEY USES TERM ECOSYSTEM (1935)

a. SOCRATES DRINKS POISON (399)
b. DIOSCORIDES CLASSIFIES POISONS (ca 50)
c. PARACELSUS IDENTIFIED TOXIN AS CHEMICAL ENTITY WITH SPECIFICITY OF ACTION (ca 1535) BIRTH OF TOXICOLOGY
d. ORFILA DEFINES TOXICOLOGY (1818). SYSTEMATIC CORRELATION OF CHEMICAL/ BIOLOGICAL INFORMATION ON POISONS

e. MARSH METHODOLOGY FOR ARSENIC ANALYSIS (1836)
f. BERNARD MECHANISM OF CO/HEMOGLOBIN ACTION (1850)
g. CHEN INTRODUCTION OF MODERN ANTIDOTES (1934)

Fig. 1. Time line of recorded history of man showing important dates for science of toxicology (small case letters) and ecology (arabic numbers).

Enactment of the Toxic Substances Act (TOSCA) places emphasis on societal concerns about the short- and long-term hazards of substances potentially toxic to human health and the environment. New methods, that take into account the complexities and unknowns of environmental and ecological interactions must be developed for testing and evaluating these substances. Moreover, these methods not only must be based on the concepts and methods of modern ecology, but also must have a predictive component sufficiently powerful to enable industry and the government to make decisions on the production and potential release of these substances to the environment.

The national concern about the environment is now almost a decade old. The environmental laws and regulations enacted because of that concern in many cases presume a knowledge of environmental/ecological processes that actually does not exist. A major underlying reason for TOSCA is that pollutants and potential toxicants are released into the environment and reach both target and non-target organisms in unknown quantities, via poorly known pathways, after equally poorly known transformations. Because of the interposition of the "environment" between source and target, the effects of environmental contaminants cannot be estimated, and the goals set forth in TOSCA cannot be achieved, unless the concepts and methods of modern ecology are combined with those of toxicology in a new "eco-toxicology."

Ecology

Ecology followed a somewhat similar pattern of evolution as has toxicology, from observation through classification and mechanistic studies, but at a later date and with a somewhat different scope of interest. By definition, ecology is the study of the relationship between an organism and its environment, both biotic and abiotic. Its concerns have evolved to the 'gene pool' level of organization and above. While one can trace the history of ecology to the dawn of agriculture (ca 5000 B.C.) and through the works of Aristotle (400 B.C.), little progress in understanding the ecosystem occurred until Linnaeus and his publications, *Species Plantarum*[1] and *System Naturae*[2], formulated a classification of plants and animals that provided a framework for future ecological studies. No great 'leap forward' in the understanding of how organisms interact with their environments occurred in the next 150 years, however. The thrust was still 'natural historian' in approach. To be sure, observations were made, which in retrospect helped to understand this interaction. For example, Von Humboldt, in his climb to the summit of Mt. Chimborazo (6700 m) in the Ecuadorian Andes in 1802, noted the replacement of latitude by altitude, and

Darwin's *Origin of Species*[3] identified the concept of change in species as a response to their environment.

It was not until 1866, in fact, that Oekologie became a concept, identified by Haeckel as signifying the interrelationship between organisms and their environment. Forbes, in 1887, published a paper entitled *The Lake as a Microcosm*[4]. This work called attention to the way in which the surrounding abiotic environment modifies and controls the ability of organisms to function and survive. Additionally, he identified conceptually a subset (a lake) of the total biosphere with unique characteristics that transcend a summation of the traits of its individual components. Fifty years passed before that idea received a name, ecosystem[5]. The concept of interaction between an organism and its environment was further strengthened by the work of Cowles[6]. He introduced the term 'dynamic ecology' to describe the theory that environment is constantly in a state of change, albeit, a structured predictable change, resulting from organisms modifying their surroundings, which in turn affects the ability of that type of organism to survive.

While the 'sphere of concern' of ecology had become established, the science remained primarily descriptive - an approach it maintained until 1925. In that year A. J. Lotka published *The Elements of Physical Biology*[7]. This signified the birth of quantitative ecology based on application of the principles of thermodynamics. Ecosystem approaches to environmental problems were stimulated by the classical paper of Lindemann in 1942[8]. He brought forth the trophic-dynamic concept of food chain relationships which added an additional element of quantitative rigor and prediction to ecology. Moreover this concept is basic to all studies of biological transport and bioaccumulation. In the past half century, population and ecosystem ecology have continued to flourish and expand, developing new approaches to understanding the numerous interactions that take place in complex systems. We use several examples of these recent efforts to exemplify this development and to identify components of ecology necessary for the development of environmental toxicology.

Earlier it was stated that toxicology is concerned with where and how a particular material causes an effect within an organism. As such, the approach involves investigations through the organ, tissue, cellular, and perhaps to the molecular level, while developing an understanding of how a chemical operates to produce the observed response. Ecology, on the other hand, is concerned with the population, community, and ecosystem levels of response. Individuals are useful in experimentation only to provide data that can be extrapolated to the population (or above) level of organization. Legitimate extrapolation of data gathered (on individuals) to a population necessitates understanding where, within a population, that 'type' of individual fits; what role that type of individual occupies within the population; and how that type of individual operates in the functioning population.

Environmental or eco-toxicology is concerned with determining the effects of xenobiotic chemicals at the supra individual level; that is, at the population, community, and ecosystem levels. At the population level, one may be concerned with effects on such ecological parameters as survival, birth, growth, and productivity rates because these characteristics are measures of population maintenance or survival (in the evolutionary sense).

It is common practice in toxicology to use individual organisms for testing purposes. In the ecological population context this is not satisfactory unless the individuals represent a stage in the life cycle of the population of that organism that is critical to the maintenance of the population. An example of the results of this type of approach is shown in Figure 2, which presents three distinct survivorship curves for a population of the calanoid copepod *Diaptomus clavipes*. These organisms are important in aquatic environments, serving as the major link between primary producers (algae) and fish. The horizontal axis shows the various life history stages, from egg through six naupliar (N) and six copepodid (C) stages, the last being the adult. The vertical axis is survival rate. The three survivorship curves were developed from laboratory data, for the first generation of a field population (g_1) and a full reproductive year of the natural population (total year). Gehrs and Robertson[9] suggested that laboratory data revealed the response of an unstressed population where all the 'types' of individuals were functioning under ideal conditions. The two curves resulting from data developed on a natural population are assumed to reveal response in stressed situations. They identified two stages in the life history of *Diaptomus* where the survivorship curve of the natural population diverged from the laboratory population - the egg to nauplius IV component and the nauplius VI to copepodid I stage. These two stages, where greatest deviation in survivorship from a nonstressed population was seen, were identified as the critical life stages or weakest links, and experimentation into the functioning of the population could be centered primarily on these stages. Hence, they were able to select a manageable subset of parameters for use in future investigations.

Increasingly, ecologists have been involved in the development of methods that provide a firm foundation for the extrapolation of laboratory results to field situations. Since population phenomena are time-related, with time

28

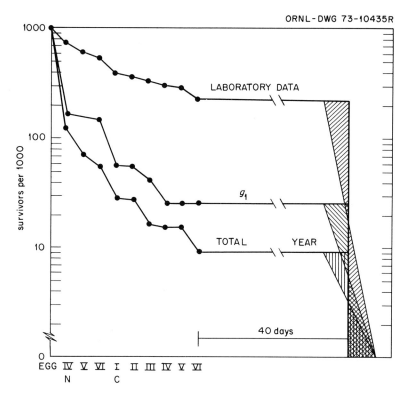

Fig. 2. Survivorship curves for the first generation, complete year study, and laboratory-grown *Diaptomus clavipes* Schacht. (From Ref. 9).

constants ranging up to years for some species and even up to centuries for ecosystems, some means are necessary for projecting, quantitatively, findings not only from laboratory to field but also through time and space. Computer modeling, systems analysis, and simulation techniques--all variants of systems theory and control theory--are increasingly being used by ecologists and other environmental scientists to provide rigor in extrapolation and prediction. For example, Maguire et al.[10] used the data of Gehrs and Robertson to develop simulation models for the *Diaptomus* population. By varying input for key parameters (which would be survivorship from egg to NIV and from NVI to CI, for example), they were able to simulate, in a period of several minutes (or hours), how the population would respond over a full year's time.

Figure 3 shows the response of the population (expressed by clutch size) when three different rates of input to the population were used. While input

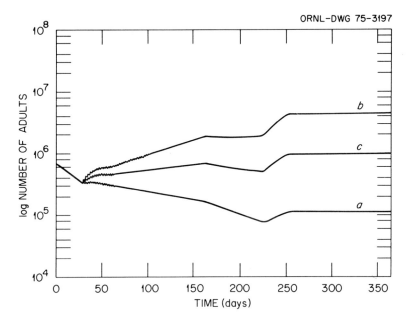

ORNL-DWG 75-3197

Fig. 3. Size of adult female population of *Diaptomus clavipes* Schacht after one year, resulting from model run with three different clutch sizes: (a) 4.73, (b) 14.19, and (c) 9.46. (From Ref. 10).

varied by approximately a factor of 4 between (a) and (b), output or final population size varied by a factor of 15. Incidentally, the input (c) was what was seen in the natural population, and the output of the model represented a population of approximately the same size after a full year. This result was measured in the field population, adding credibility to the model actually mimicking the natural population.

How does this approach relate to environmental toxicology? We believe it enables the use of experimental data on the effects of toxins on individual organisms for estimating population response through time. By utilizing data developed from laboratory toxicity studies of short-term duration at the individual level, one can generate data on population response to that stress through time. Such simulation models enable one to translate changes in key parameters observed with individuals to the population.

In a sense this sounds like the panacea for environmental effects determination -- low-cost, short-term, and accurate predictions. Unfortunately, natural phenomena do not permit such a quick and easy use of most simulation models; modifications are frequently necessary. For example, not all populations behave as predictably as those used in the previous example. Populations can compensate for changes in density. This phenomenon complicates simulation-modeling efforts. As their numbers decrease (for whatever reason), the population may respond with increased birth rate, greater survival, or more rapid maturation. Population ecologists are still developing methods for handling compensation phenomena with their simulation models. Difficulties arise because quantitative measurement of compensation per se has yet to be done.

When one moves from assessing responses at population levels to those at the ecosystem level, the number of potential complications increases exponentially. Nutrients must be transported through the environment to the vegetation in a soil-plant-litter system, for example, with the environment modifying the form and concentration of nutrients the vegetation 'sees.' Different nutrients use different processes to enter plants. Luxmoore et al.[11] have combined five different submodels (Figure 4) on nutrient transport to higher plants. This construct provides a framework for utilizing additional information as it becomes available. A closer examination of the figure reveals that each model communicates with a minimum of two other models (boxes), symbolizing the complexity of interactions taking place within an ecosystem. The construction of models requires an understanding of their components and the interactions among the various components that control the response (whole system or specific components).

We believe that ecosystem models, once developed and validated, are necessary for investigating environmental fate and effects of toxic substances. They are needed for determining those parameters for which empirical data are needed to assess a toxicant. In the figure, these are identified as plant capacity for concentrating contaminants, amount of uptake, etc. These data can then be in put into the model, with a simulation run producing an estimation of the potential response (through time) of the system to a stress (the toxicant).

A forest is one example of an ecosystem in which modeling to assess potential effects is essential. In general, the system is too large and complex to permit experimental manipulation, and in addition, the response time is so long (decades or centuries) that by the time empirical data are developed, major forested ecosystems may be ravaged. Mielke et al.[12] have developed and used mathematical simulation models to investigate the successional dynamics of forest stands through long periods of time.

By imposing differential stresses on individual species in a validated multispecies model of a deciduous forest[13], significant, yet somewhat

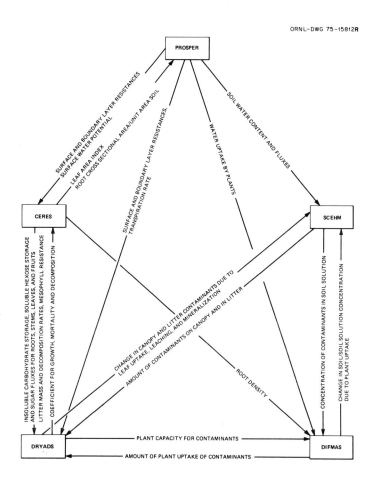

ORNL-DWG 75-15812R

Fig. 4. Coupling of fine process models that describe
hourly carbon, water, and solute dynamics of the soil-
plant-litter system. (From Ref. 11).

unexpected, changes can be seen in forest growth and succession (Figure 5).
Relative sensitivity of individual species to air pollutants was used as a
basis of differential response. In one experiment, growth rate reduction
categories were assigned according to the best available information on
response of individual species to sulphur dioxide. Results of simulations
with this regime suggested that the response of trees to air pollution may be
quite different under competitive conditions in a forest stand from that which
would be expected in experiments conducted with single individuals or single
species. Growth of trees of intermediate sensitivity may actually be stimu-
lated by a relative increase in competitive potential. Thus, these simulation

32

ORNL-DWG 78-6488R

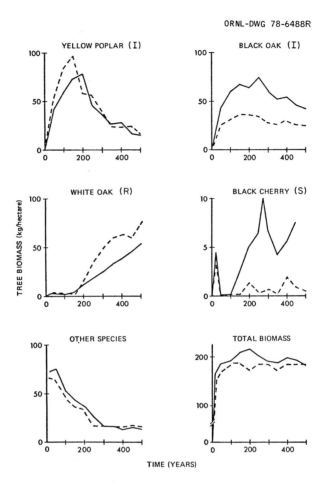

Fig. 5. Species and stand dynamics of a forest with and without continuous exposure to air pollution stress (——— unaffected; -----affected). R is resistant species, S sensitive, and I intermediate. (From Ref. 13).

experiments serve an essential role in extending our understanding of air pollution effects to levels beyond the capability of conventional experimental methodologies.

The first part of this paper briefly traced the origins of both toxicology and ecology to identify what we perceive as the major developments that led each science to evolve to its current position. We have emphasized those attributes of ecology which pertain to the problems associated with toxic substances and included examples of the uses of ecological approaches to

environmental effects because they serve as the bases upon which our perception
of environmental toxicology are grounded.

ENVIRONMENTAL TOXICOLOGY: AN ECOLOGICAL PERSPECTIVE

   The relationship of ecology to toxicology can be illustrated in several
ways. Loomis[14] identified and outlined the contributions of several disciplines to the field of toxicology (illustrated in Figure 6). He also related
toxicological findings to economics, forensics, and environmental science.
Much has happened in the environmental field since this book was written;
ecology no longer functions primarily as a subdivision of biology any more
than does physiology or pathology. We would therefore add an eighth input,
ecology, to the field of toxicology. Ecological knowledge, besides providing
another scientific dimension to toxicology, not only contributes to environmental concerns but also to economics, particularly in the development and use
of pesticides.

   Figure 7 includes only three components, the toxicant, the environment and
the organism (population or ecosystem) of interest. Each component can affect
(and be affected by) the other two. The uniqueness of the relationship (when
ecology is compared to sub-disciplines of toxicology) is that all interactions

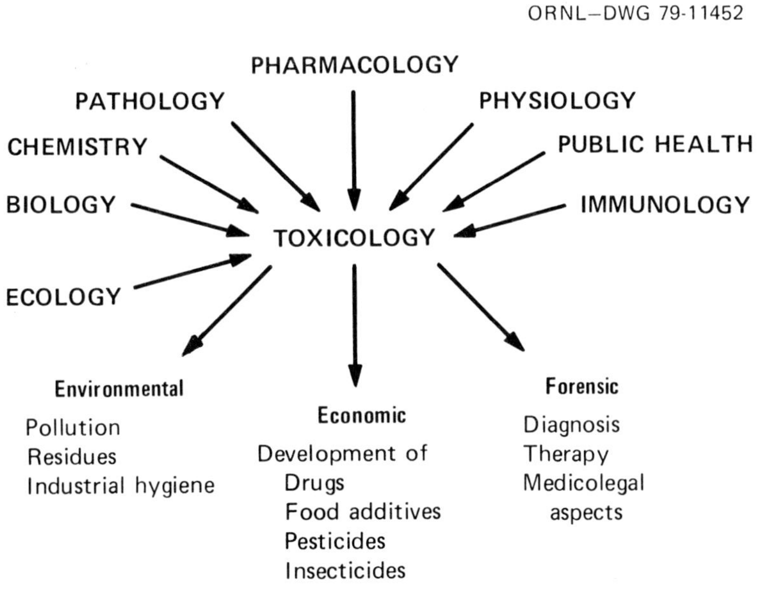

ORNL–DWG 79-11452

Fig. 6. Relationship between toxicology and other biological
disciplines. (Adapted from Ref. 14).

ORNL-DWG 79-11451

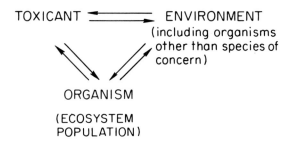

Fig. 7. Relationship of ecology with toxicology.

occur external to the individual organism. It is in these areas, addressing
(a) the way in which the environment modifies the toxicant before it (toxicant)
reaches the target organism, (b) how the environment affects the response of
the organism to the toxicant, and (c) how the toxicant modifies the environment,
that ecology can make its contribution to the science of toxicology.

Direct effects of toxicant on organism

The elucidation of direct effects on organisms caused by exposure to toxic
chemicals is of importance to environmental toxicologists but only (as we mentioned earlier) as it pertains to estimating population response. Some of the
first studies of direct effects of materials on organisms took place in the
early 1800s and were concerned with evaluation of deleterious effects on aquatic
environments from municipal and industrial discharges. Penny and Adams[15]
examined the acute toxicity of chemicals present in dye-works effluents to
organisms from the River Lenen in Scotland. They revealed an awareness of
variation in species sensitivity by selecting two species of fish, the minnow
because of the "fine sensitivity it evinces towards all kinds of disturbing
substances" and the goldfish because its "sluggish nature and tenacity of life"
permit longer evaluation.

Acute toxicity studies comprised the majority of environmental toxicology
investigations until well into the present century. In the early 1900s, the
concept that organisms other than man may be sublethally affected by toxic
substances was borrowed from human toxicology and applied to environmental
toxicology. Steinmann[16], one of the first to incorporate this concept,
investigated the effects of several chemicals on the breathing rate and
heartbeat of trout. Although acute toxicity studies continued to flourish,

sublethal chronic effects studies increased markedly after it was demonstrated
that the responses of fish and other organisms to toxic chemicals were as
complex as human responses.

It is now recognized that toxicity tests should involve all stages in the
life cycle of an organism, because immature stages are often more sensitive to
toxicants than are adult stages. Recently, attention has focused on sublethal
effects such as retardation of growth and development, interference with reproduction, increased susceptibility to stress, and behavioral changes. Such
sublethal effects, which typically occur at toxicant concentrations well below
the lethal level, are potentially as damaging to a population as the death of
individuals. The development of reliable methods for measuring sublethal
effects is one of the most active and challenging areas of research in environmental toxicology today.

Effects of toxicants on environment

A particular substance can also affect a system by modifying its environment,
resulting in both indirect and secondary direct effects on the system. Chemicals may alter habitats physically (e.g., oil spills), chemically (e.g., changes
in water quality resulting from mine drainage), or biologically (e.g., elimination of predators, competitors, or food organisms). Secondary effects may
then result from a weakening of the system with an increased susceptibility of
its components to the toxicant. The concentration of a substance in an aquatic
environment may not be sufficient to affect fish directly, for example, but it
may directly affect the algae and zooplankton, natural food for the fish.
Decreased food supply may weaken fish, making them susceptible to the toxicant.

Effects of organism and environment on toxicant

The form in which a particular material reaches the organism and its concentration are of great interest to ecologists. Both the organism and the
environment (abiotic and biotic components) can modify the toxicant, thereby
altering its potential affects on the organism. While the way in which the
organism handles the toxicant is of some interest to ecologists, this is truly
the domain of classical toxicology. The ecological perspective, however, is
particularly well suited for use in evaluating how the environment modifies
the toxicant before it reaches the target organism. Hence, defining source
terms, chemical forms, and important environmental exposures are components of
environmental toxicology.

The distribution and chemical form of many toxicants are controlled by environmental processes. The potential of chemicals to move through air, water,
and soil can often be inferred from their basic physical/chemical properties,
such as solubility in water, vapor pressure, and sorption coefficients. These
experimentally measurable properties are combined with knowledge of atmospheric
circulation patterns, groundwater flow, surface water hydrology, and local
geology and topography to predict pathways of chemical transport through the
environment. Toxicants that spread widely from their point of release are
naturally of greater concern than are relatively immobile toxicants.

Figure 8 is a simplified schematic of the various pathways whereby a chemical
substance can move through an aquatic environment. It summarizes the role of
the environment in modifying the chemical and defining the concentration that
reaches the target organism, in this case, man. Each of the arrows identifies
important parameters for which transfer coefficients must be determined.

A major component of any pollutant transport model requires the determination
of persistence and fate, including uptake, bioaccumulation, and biomagnifica-
tion through the food chain, of the toxicant. Simply measuring concentrations
in the water is not sufficient. For example, the levels of DDT present in
Lake Michigan were accumulated 10^7 times in the tissue of coho salmon and
lake trout[17].

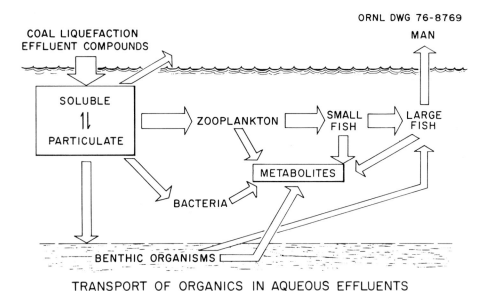

TRANSPORT OF ORGANICS IN AQUEOUS EFFLUENTS

Fig. 8. Generalized schematic of pathways in which chemicals move through the
aquatic environment toward man.

Population and ecosystem responses

Another major area of concern for ecologists in research on toxicant effects is in the response of nontarget organisms. The primary difficulty is extrapolating effects on individuals to populations and ecosystems and from laboratory experimentation to field situations.

To estimate adequately the response of a particular population or ecosystem to a toxicant requires information not only on the direct effects of the material on the organism but also on the indirect effects. How a population of that organism is affected in its competitive capabilities with populations of other species is one example. Development of predictive capabilities for direct effects requires an understanding of the basic ecology of the organism as well as an understanding of the mechanism of action of the toxicant being evaluated.

SUMMARY

Environmental toxicology (from an ecological perspective) can have several applications to the broader field of toxicology. An important role, perhaps, is identifying and quantifying potential pathways of toxicants to man. The recently enacted Toxic Substances Control Act and Resource Conservation and Recovery Act bear witness to the public awareness of and concern with environmental transport and the need for developing predictive capabilities. Any assessment of the potential risks to people must be built on an understanding of the movement and fate of materials in the environment. While the primary concern of environmental toxicologists is related to the impact of toxic substances on man directly or indirectly, one must bear in mind that the potential impact of toxic substances upon the environment per se can be construed as another aspect of ecotoxicology. To the extent that introduced chemicals have a potential for degrading key components of the environment or for damaging gene pools through selective mortality of organisms, these areas become of concern to the ecologist.

The ability to extrapolate from individuals to populations and ecosystems through use of simulation models brings great capabilities to the field of environmental toxicology. It provides a tool for utilizing a minimum set of empirical data to transcend space and time to estimate the effects of a substance.

The science of understanding the ecosystem, of understanding how substances move through the environment, and of developing more cost-effective short-term predictive tests for evaluating long-term sublethal effects must move forward

concurrently with providing data to the regulators. Only then will environmental toxicology achieve its perceived role in today's complex scheme of
science, regulation, and standards-development, all of which are increasing in
importance as components of today's research in the applied biological sciences.

ACKNOWLEDGMENTS

We wish to acknowledge the following individuals of the Environmental
Sciences Division, ORNL, for valuable assistance in the preparation and
review of this manuscript: B. R. Parkhurst, J. W. Giddings, D. C. West,
S. B. McLaughlin, R. E. Millemann, R. J. Luxmoore, D. S. Shriner, and
L. W. Barnthouse. Research sponsored by the Office of Health and Environmental
Research, U.S. Department of Energy, under contract W-7405-eng-26 with Union
Carbide Corporation. Publication No. 1385, Environmental Sciences Division,
ORNL.

REFERENCES

1. Linnaeus, C. 1753. Species Plantarum (two volumes). L. Salvii,
    Stockholm, Sweden.

2. Linnaeus, C. 1758-9. Systema Naturae (two volumes). L. Salvii,
    Stockholm, Sweden.

3. Darwin, C. 1859. Origin of Species by Means of Natural Selection.
    Reprinted by: The Modern Library, Random House, New York.

4. Forbes, S. A. 1887. The lake as a microcosm. Bull. Sci. Assoc. Peoria
    77-87.

5. Tansley, A. G. 1935. The use and abuse of vegetational concepts and
    terms. Ecology 16:284-307.

6. Cowles, H. C. 1899. The ecological relations of vegetation on the sand
    dunes of Lake Michigan. Bot. Gaz. 27:95-117, 167-207, 281-308, 361-391.

7. Lotka, A. J. 1925. The Elements of Physical Biology. Williams and
    Wilkins, Baltimore, Maryland.

8. Lindemann, R. L. 1942. The trophic-dynamic aspect of ecology. Ecology
    23:399-418.

9. Gehrs, C. W., and A. Robertson. 1975. Use of life tables in analyzing
    the dynamics of copepod populations. Ecology 56:665-672.

10. Maguire, L. A., C. W. Gehrs, and W. Van Winkle. 1975. COPEPOD2: A
    Markov-type model for copepod population dynamics. ORNL/TM-4976. Oak
    Ridge National Laboratory, Oak Ridge, Tennessee.

11. Luxmoore, R. J., C. L. Begovich, and K. R. Dixon. 1978. Modeling solute uptake and incorporation into vegetation and litter. Ecol. Model. 5:137-171.

12. Mielke, D. L., H. H. Shugart, and D. C. West. 1978. A stand model for upland forests of southern Arkansas. ORNL/TM-6225. Oak Ridge National Laboratory, Oak Ridge, Tennessee.

13. West, D. C., S. B. McLaughlin, and H. H. Shugart. Simulated forest response to chronic air pollution stress. J. Environ. Qual. (in press).

14. Loomis, T. A. 1970. Essentials of Toxicology. Lea and Febiger, Philadelphia, Pennsylvania. 166 pp.

15. Penny, C., and C. Adams. 1863. Fourth Report, Royal Commission on Pollution of Rivers in Scotland, Vol. 2. Evidence, London.

16. Steinmann, P. 1928. Toxicologie der fische. In Handbuch der binnenfischerei Mitteleuropos. E. Schweizerbart'sche verlagsbuchhandlung (Erwin Nagele), Stuttgart.

17. Harrison, H. L., O. L. Loucks, J. W. Mitchell, D. F. Parkhurst, C. R. Tracy, D. G. Watts, and V. J. Yannacone, Jr. 1970. Systems study of DDT transport. Science 170:503-508.

NEW OUTLOOKS AND APPROACHES TO TESTING
Chairman: V.K. Rowe

© 1980 Elsevier/North-Holland Biomedical Press
The Scientific Basis of Toxicity Assessment
H. Witschi, editor.

NEW OUTLOOKS AND APPROACHES TO TESTING: INTRODUCTION

V. K. ROWE

Toxicological Issues, Health and Environmental Research, Dow Chemical U.S.A.,

Midland, Michigan 48640

The theme of this section of the symposium on "The Scientific Basis of Toxicity Assessment" is entitled "New Outlooks and Approaches to Testing." This title is one which always has been and always will be in tune with the times. Researchers are always searching for new, better and quicker ways to solve their problems. Through the years the techniques and approaches to toxicology testing and safety evaluations have continuously improved and will continue to improve. Many of the test procedures used in the past are viewed as crude and inadequate by today's standards and yet they provided much basic information useful today. It should be emphasized that merely because a test is old does not necessarily mean that it was the source of incorrect data. More likely the problem was not with the data but with the inadequacy of its interpretation, past and present. Many of the newer test procedures and concepts are merely refinements and extensions of proven older procedures made possible by technological advances such as have occurred in analytical chemistry. There is no doubt that the techniques viewed as sophisticated today will be commonplace in two or three years and some will be replaced with better ones in the next few years. The rate at which new and better approaches to testing will be devised and validated will be commensurate with the need and our ability to unravel the mysteries of biological systems.

There is no question that there is a serious need for technology to rapidly test chemicals and mixtures of chemicals for their potential to cause serious adverse effects such as cancer, genetic aberrations and behavioral or neurological changes in human beings. A multitude of investigators are responding to these needs.

Researchers have been studying the response of many ingenious biological systems to various types of chemicals in an effort to find a test or a battery of tests that will yield data in a short time from which reliable predictions can be made as to long term effects of a test material. Others are attempting to refine old techniques, develop new tests and describe the limitations of various animal models for detecting and measuring the capacity of materials to alter behavior and to determine by what mechanism the alterations occur.

Considerable effort is now being expended to elucidate the biochemical mechanisms through which chemical carcinogenesis develops.   There is good reason to believe that differences between species and strains in susceptibility to particular chemicals may be attributable to differences in inherent biochemical capabilities.   Most certainly a better understanding of such basic mechanisms whether in monocellular organisms, tissue cultures or whole animals, will permit a far better interpretation of data from the various models and its extrapolation to the human being.

The following four papers by recognized authorities in their fields present a comprehensive review and evaluation of the state-of-the-art in several categories of testing.   This insight should be very valuable not only to researchers in the particular fields but also to those in related fields of research, to administrators, to product planners and to regulators involved with safety evaluations.

THE APPROPRIATE USE OF GENETIC TOXICOLOGY IN INDUSTRY

J. L. EPLER, W. WINTON, A. A. HARDIGREE, and F. W. LARIMER
Biology Division, Oak Ridge National Laboratory, P. O. Box Y, Oak Ridge, Tennessee 37830

INTRODUCTION

Industrial activity through the last centuries has created a large group of chemical pollutants. Modern technology has added to this group at an accelerated pace. For safety and industrial hygiene practice to parallel these technological advances, potential health hazards for the worker and for the general population must be determined early in the development of the process or, in the case of a newly developed compound, early in the synthetic studies. However, chemical exposures arise not only from industrial processes but also from medical, cosmetic, and food intake and use (Table 1).

TABLE 1

GENERAL CLASSES OF CHEMICALS TO WHICH HUMANS ARE EXPOSED[a]

Drugs	Industrial products and effluents
Medicinal	Energy-related effluents
Veterinary	Energy production
Cosmetics	Energy conversion
Pesticides	Energy use
Stimulants	
Food	Natural products
Additives	
Dyes	
Preservatives	
Sweeteners	

[a] After ref. 1.

Thus, thousands, perhaps tens of thousands, of chemicals can be considered as potential biohazards. Although the health effects of a few of these chemicals have been studied extensively, methods to cut down the research time and money required are mandatory to allow the scientific community and eventually the regulatory agencies to evaluate the relative hazard(s) of exposure to this array of chemical threats. However, the number of specific compounds and complex materials in need of biotesting is very large and would tax the whole-animal test facilities that are currently available. Therefore, several "screening" (i.e., short-term, inexpensive) assays for toxicity, mutagenicity, teratogenicity and carcinogenicity are being developed and tested.

Since the Oak Ridge National Laboratory functions as a key fundamental research arm of the Department of Energy, the efforts of the Biology Division and the Life Sciences Divisions have focused, in general, on the potential biohazards of energy-related technologies — oil shale, coal liquefaction, and coal gasification.

The need for substitute fluid fuels and convenient energy sources has led to renewed efforts in the field of coal conversion. A number of coal liquefaction and coal gasification processes are being developed. For this approach to adequately and safely serve as an aid in solving energy problems, potential health hazards for workers and the general public should be considered. The overall environmental aspects of any energy technology include pollutant releases, physical disturbances, and socioeconomic disturbances along with health and safety impacts. This paper will concentrate on health and safety aspects and illustrate various rapid and inexpensive (short-term) biological assays. The realization that the number of specific compounds and complex effluents and streams in need of biotesting in any technology is overwhelming and would tax the scientific community's whole-animal testing capabilities has led to the development of this array of screening assays for toxicity, mutagenicity, teratogenicity, and carcinogenicity. The working hypothesis has been that the rapid tests can serve as predictors of biohazards early in the development of the technology. Thus, process changes might be initiated and/or definitive whole-animal testing considered. Conceivably, savings in both time and money on the technology and the biological testing would be gained (see Figure 1).

FIGURE 1

MAJOR OBJECTIVES OF RESEARCH IN SHORT-TERM ASSAYS[a]

DESIGN ———————— PILOT PLANTS ———————— PRODUCTION

BIOLOGICAL TESTING INPUTS

1. MINIMIZE LONG-RANGE HUMAN RISK
2. UNDERSTAND BASIC MECHANISMS

---

[a] After L. B. Russell and J. L. Epler, Presentation to President Carter, May 22, 1978, Oak Ridge National Laboratory, Oak Ridge, Tennessee.

Furthermore, current and/or prospective government regulations consider the short-term biological tests and advocate their use (e.g., the Toxic Substance Control Act and the Resource Conservation and Recovery Act). Coal-derived liquids, aqueous wastes, particulates, and solid wastes can be evaluated as complex mixtures with potential biohazards, common, perhaps, to all coal conversion processes.

The possibility of using short-term biological tests to isolate and identify the potential hazard of complex materials has been investigated with various coupled chemical and biological approaches. The work has usually involved chemical analyses and preparation for biological testing, e.g., cytotoxicity, mutagenicity, and carcinogenicity assays. As a prescreen for potential mutagenesis and/or carcinogenesis, the genetic test for Salmonella histidine reversion (Ames test; see review by Ames et al.)[2] has been widely used. Subsequent fractionation procedures are carried out to aid in isolating and identifying the mutagens in the material, with the bioassay being used as a tool to trace the biological activity and guide the separations. The biological tests function as (1) predictors of long-range health effects such as mutagenesis, teratogenesis, and/or carcinogenesis; (2) predictors of toxicity for man and his environment; (3) a mechanism to rapidly isolate and identify a hazardous agent in a complex material; and (4) a key to relative biological activity through the correlation of control data with changes in environmental or process conditions. Since much of the exploratory work in the use of short-term assays has involved fractionated natural and synthetic oils and wastes,[3-5] the health effects research reviewed here will emphasize the assays that have been applied to coal conversion processes.

48

TABLE 2 SHORT-TERM GENETIC TEST SYSTEMS

BACTERIAL SYSTEMS

Salmonella typhimurium

    arabinose resistance (forward mutation)
    8-azaguanine resistance (forward mutation)
    histidine reversion
    DNA repair assay

Escherichia coli

    WP_2 – tryptophan reversion
    343/113 – arginine, nicotinic acid reversion
           galactose utilization (forward mutation)
           gal^+ – lysine requirement (deletions)
    rec^- – DNA repair
    $PolA^-$ – DNA repair

Bacillus subtilis

    rec^- – DNA repair

FUNGAL SYSTEMS

Saccharomyces cerevisiae

    mitotic recombination
    histidine, homoserine reversion
    canavanine resistance

Neurospora crassa

    adenine reversion

PLANT SYSTEMS

    Allium
    Tradescantia
    Barley
    Maize

INSECT SYSTEMS

Drosophila melanogaster

    sex-linked recessive lethals

MAMMALIAN CELLS IN CULTURE

Chinese hamster cells

    HGPRT system – 8-azaguanine resistance
    sister-chromatid exchanges

Human leukocytes

    sister-chromatid exchanges

Human fibroblasts

    unscheduled DNA synthesis

BATTERY OF TESTS

To investigate the potential genetic (and carcinogenic) hazards associated with the developing synthetic fuel technologies, we initiated a coupled chemical and biological analysis of the products, process streams, and effluents of the existing or proposed energy-generating or -conversion systems. One phase of our investigation deals with known compounds expected to occur in the environment through energy production, conversion, or use; another phase deals with actual samples from existing or experimental processes. To approach the problems of coping with and testing large numbers of compounds, we set up a battery of assays for mutagenicity testing. Table 2 illustrates a possible battery in this type of assay.

The research effort described here is specifically concerned with the question of genetic hazard; but, as has been pointed out recently,[6] certain microbial genetic assays (for example, the Ames test with Salmonella) show a high correlation between positive results in mutagenicity testing and the carcinogenicity of the compounds under test. The overall need to subject environmental chemicals to mutagenicity testing has been discussed in the Committee 17 Report on Environmental Mutagenic Hazards.[7] Their key recommendation can be summarized as: "Screening should be initiated as rapidly and as extensively as possible." deSerres has discussed the utility of short-term tests for mutagenicity[8] and the prospect for their use in toxicological evaluation.[9] He stresses that the data base of knowledge on untested environmental chemicals should be expanded, but cautions that "We are not ready, however, to extrapolate directly from data obtained in short-term tests for mutagenicity directly to man."[9] Tests on other organisms must be performed to validate and reinforce results from short-term tests, which simply point out potential mutagenic and carcinogenic chemicals and serve to order priorities for further testing in higher organisms.

Microbial assays

Obviously all of the chemical pollutants in question cannot be subjected to whole-animal testing. The expense in time and money would be overwhelming with genetic testing alone. A scheme has to be developed which will reliably prescreen the genetically hazardous compounds and allow the investigator to select a smaller sample to be thoroughly tested in other systems. (One example of such a list of tests is shown in Table 2.) A "tiered" system of testing [suggested by Bridges[10,11]] would save the scientific world considerable time and expense while bringing the pertinent information to the industrial community and the general population in an organized and rapid manner.

Perhaps most important in a tiered system of screening is the initial level of testing. False negatives here presumably would terminate the testing of any particular compounds, while false positives would be clarified by further comparative testing. Thus, the initial test should be a high-resolution, sensitive assay, yet rapid and inexpensive. The Salmonella histidine reversion system probably fits these criteria best of the currently available short-term assays. However, the possibility of false negatives makes the use of a further battery of assays pertinent.

The Salmonella tester series (obtained through the courtesy of Dr. Bruce N. Ames) is composed of histidine mutants that revert after treatment with mutagens to the wild-type state (growth independent of histidine). Both missense mutants and frame-shift mutants comprise the set, and their reversion characteristics with a potential chemical mutagen imply the mechanism of action. In addition, the detection scheme yields the highest resolution possible by the inclusion of other mutations such as: (1) the deep rough mutation, rfa, which affects the lipopolysaccharide coat, making the bacteria more permeable; and (2) the deletion of the uvrB region, which eliminates the excision-repair system.[12] The procedures with the strains and their use in mutagenicity testing are discussed in detail by Ames et al.[2]

Generalized testing of compounds is accomplished by use of the three standard tester strains, TA1535, TA1537, and TA1538, in combination with the R-factor strains, TA100 and TA98 (plasmid-carrying strains with increased sensitivity). Briefly, the compound to be tested is dissolved in dimethyl sulfoxide or buffer. Concentration is varied over a range of 1–500 μg added per plate except with highly toxic compounds. The various Salmonella strains are usually treated by use of the plate-incorporation assay of Ames,[2] but other modified assays or assays for forward mutation can be used.

One other feature of the Salmonella system is the ease with which metabolic activation can be incorporated into the assay. Spot tests or quantitative plate tests can be performed in the presence of rat or other mammalian liver homogenates so that the mutagen can be metabolized to its ultimate, active form in the in vitro short-term test. In assays requiring activation, standard rat liver microsome preparations[2] from rats induced with Aroclor 1254 (Monsanto Corp.), sodium phenobarbital, or other inducers are used.

As an initial step in establishing testing procedures, we have investigated the use of the Ames Salmonella system with a large number of environmentally important chemicals and effluents, principally those known or predicted to occur in energy use, production, and/or conversion. However, other microbial tests should be used in comparison with the Salmonella results. Among these are bacterial systems such as the Escherichia coli WP2 tryptophan reversion assay,[13] the sensitive fluctuation test described by Green,[14] and the multiple-end-point system developed by Mohn.[15]

For example, the Mohn system, which employs a well-characterized mutant of E. coli, K-12 (343/113), has been utilized in our laboratory to test various compounds that are either identified or suspected to occur in various products and effluents of the synthetic fuel technologies. The mutation screening involves (1) reversion of an auxotrophic marker for arginine requirement to prototrophy (Arg^+), (2) induction of a forward mutation leading to 5-methyl tryptophan resistance (5 MTR), (3) ability to utilize galactose as sole carbon source (gal^+), and (4) a deletion in gal R region resulting in a new auxotrophic mutation for lysine requirement (gal^+, lys^-). Results can be compared and correlated with the "Ames test" results.

A number of bacterial assays which detect effects on strains either proficient or deficient in DNA repair are also widely used in this initial battery of tests. Among these are the "rec assay" of Kada[16] in Bacillus subtilis, the assay using E. coli mutants deficient in DNA polymerase ($polA^-$),[17] and, again, the Salmonella system[2] using strains with DNA deficiencies in comparison with normal. The common hypothesis is that bacterial strains that are repair-deficient are much more sensitive to agents that alter cellular DNA than are the parent strain, the wild-type, or strains normal for DNA repair functions. Presumably, these same agents that preferentially alter DNA are potential mutagens and carcinogens.

Neurospora[18] and yeast[19] are also useful tools in mutagenicity screening. Many laboratories utilize the yeast strains developed by Zimmermann for detecting mitotic recombination and mitotic gene conversion along with assays for forward mutation and reverse mutation. We have chosen to develop a comprehensive gene mutation system[20] in Saccharomyces cerevisiae somewhat analogous to the bacterial systems described.

A haploid yeast of genotype a; rad2-1; CAN1, his1-7, hom3-10; lys1-1; trp5-48; ade2-1 is the basis of the reversion test system. This strain is defective in DNA excision-repair. General forward mutation can also be detected by selecting canavanine-resistant clones (CAN1 → can1).

Base-pair substitution is monitored by observing the reversion of missense (his1-7) and nonsense (lys1-1, trp5-48, ade2-1) markers and by the generation of nonsense suppressors (various tRNA loci). Additions or deletions of base pairs are indicated by the reversion of a frame-shift (?) marker (hom3-10). Nonsense suppressors can also arise by addition/deletion. Metabolic activation of promutagens is provided by rat liver microsome preparations.

Thus, a battery of short-term microbial tests comprised of a selection of the above or other similar assays yields preliminary information on the question of whether or not the substance under test inflicts genetic damage at the highest level of resolution possible.

Tests with higher organisms

At a second level of testing or perhaps of validation with selected compounds from the microbial screens (including some negatives) or with compounds of high importance or interest to man, the question becomes one of the mutagenicity of the compound in higher organisms. Because of the expense of these assays in both time and money, the probability of exposure and the actual intake by man may become deciding factors. The key objective of the approach is to gain sufficient information to enable the investigator to compare and eventually extrapolate from one system to another.

The Drosophila (insect) system can be utilized as a key assay at this level. The standard Basc, or Muller-5,[21,22] test for sex-linked recessive lethals can be used. Males are exposed to the test compound by ingestion, injection, or inhalation of an aerosol, then mated to females, and finally recovered after a mating period. Females are allowed to lay eggs for a period of days, and F_1 heterozygous females are scored for sex-linked lethals.

The insect assay is a sensitive system, since loci throughout the length of the sex (X) chromosome can mutate to recessive lethals. Furthermore, the organism is diploid and possesses its own metabolizing system for mutagens/carcinogens. Additional genetic and cytogenetic end points can easily be observed and quantitated (e.g., chromosome loss, nondisjunction, translocations, and inversions). Additionally, when the treated male is mated to a sequence of females, cells from various stages of spermatogenesis at the time of treatment can be assayed.

Mammalian somatic cell mutagenesis has progressed remarkably during recent years, although considerable development and validation is still necessary. The CHO/HGPRT system[23] appears to be the most reliable and promising. This system can be coupled to rat liver microsomal preparations prepared as for the microbial systems and used to detect the conversion of promutagens (and procarcinogens) to their active forms. DNA repair assays in mammalian cells[24,25] are also highly sensitive and accurate predictors.

Mammalian cytogenetic assays such as the induction of aberrations in chromosomes of leukocytes from human peripheral blood or of mammalian cells in vitro are useful screens, as shown by Ishidate.[26] The relatively new assay of sister-chromatid exchange[27,28] may be a most effective tool with chemical agents. Again, however, exogenous sources of metabolizing enzymes must be added for detection of promutagens.

At a second level or tier of testing, preliminary assays with whole animals (the mouse) should be initiated in order to address the question of mutagenic potential for higher organisms. Although the work of the Comparative Mutagenesis unit at Oak Ridge applies specifically to submammalian systems and cultured mammalian cells, the mouse assay will be briefly outlined here.

The dominant lethal assay[29] can be included as a potential screen. In this relatively rapid test for chromosomal damage, different germ cell stages can be compared with respect to their sensitivity to the sample. This is done by studying uterine contents of females mated to exposed males at various intervals after the exposure. Another potentially useful assay for the whole animal involves the detection of somatic mutations in vivo, the so-called "spot test" designed by L. Russell.[30] Embryos heterozygous for the same markers that are used in the specific-locus test[31] are exposed to the putative mutagen. Genetic changes that uncover the recessive at these loci are detected as spots of altered color in the fur. Since each animal scored represents several hundred cells in which the genetic changes could have occurred, the method combines the advantages of cell culture with an in vivo system. It can probably be used as a prescreen to select materials for use in the specific-locus test described below.

Mammalian testing — Risk assessment (?)

Although only selected compounds would be tested in depth in the mammalian assays, these systems are the closest available bridge to actual risk assessment in human populations.[7] Based on data accumulated in submammalian systems, gene mutation, and cytogenetic data, reasonable decisions to carry out more complex and expensive mammalian testing can be made. Data from, e.g., heritable translocations and the specific locus test in the mouse might prove most useful. The search for heritable genetic changes in mammalian germ cells may be the most critical and definitive one for the assessment of genetic risk to human beings. The heritable translocation method[29] measures the frequency of chromosome breakage and rearrangement that is transmitted to the next generation. The test is a sensitive and reliable procedure for measuring breakage and exchange of parts between chromosomes induced in male germ cells. The heritable translocation procedure generates meaningful information for evaluating chromosome aberration hazards of test agents to the human population because it measures transmissible genetic damage.

In the specific-locus method, induced mutations can be objectively detected in the first generation by mating exposed mice to a stock carrying seven recessive markers in homozygous condition.[31] This is a practical method to detect gene mutations in the germ cells of mammals and to determine their rate of induction by a given agent.

The use of a battery of tests on a series of selected compounds under standard conditions should allow a meaningful comparison between the less expensive and more rapid tests on microorganisms and the more definitive tests for effects in the mammal. Such a comparison will allow greater confidence to be placed in the tests on lower organisms, thus reducing the future effort required. Only such a comparative approach will allow rational decisions to be made between different testing and screening schemes.

The assays used here are discussed in detail in the series edited by Dr. Alexander Hollaender, Chemical Mutagens: Principals and Methods for Their Detection. Note that both gene mutation and chromosomal assays are included and that testing involves a move from the simple microbial tests (Salmonella, E. coli, and yeast), to tests with higher organisms (Drosophila, mammalian cells, human leukocytes), to tests with the whole mammal, presumably the mouse. Thus, if the testing priorities are established on the basis of use by or impact on man, complete testing may be reduced to groups of environmentally important compounds, e.g., selected polycyclic hydrocarbons or nitrosamines.

DISCUSSION

The theory that tumor production involves a somatic mutation has led to the extensive use of short-term genetic assays as a prescreen for the detection of environmental carcinogens as mutagens. Several research workers around the world have reported a fair qualitative correlation between the ability of a chemical agent to produce tumors in experimental animals and mutations in genetic testing systems.

A proper evaluation of genotoxicity does require examination of the chemical agents in a battery of test systems. Such comparative mutagenesis studies will involve mutagenic potency determinations in a number of systems for a broad spectrum of genetic damage and evaluation of genetic risk to human populations. Such studies should include not only point mutations but also other genetic damages such as DNA damage, addition or deletion in DNA, and gross chromosomal modifications. We have illustrated a number of such genetic systems. Similarly, a battery of environmental or ecological tests could be applied. The utility and use of the majority of these assays is taken up in the Level I Environmental Assessment treatment[32] and the accompanying recommendations for sampling[33,34] by the Environmental Protection Agency. Furthermore, we have emphasized bioassays for mutagenesis. A comparable battery of short-term tests for carcinogenesis is discussed by Weisburger.[35]

A multiple component program

The principal focus of an Industrial Toxicology Program (including genetic toxicology) is the testing of primary effluents, products, and fugitive emissions for potential effects on man. The evaluation should be concerned with questions of (1) relative toxicities of process materials, products, aqueous wastes, and solid wastes; (2) toxicity variation as a function of process conditions; and (3) fugitive emissions which present the greatest potential for toxicity in the workplace.

The approach to answering these questions in an expeditious and cost-effective manner should involve a parallel, two-component program. Component one should be cellular bioassays as described here. These assays will accumulate base-line data on typical effluents, products, and emissions and ascertain how the relative toxicities of major test materials and fractions thereof vary as a function of changes in process conditions. In addition, biological-effects studies using cellular assays will provide an essential data base for eventual determination of correlation with whole-animal, acute and chronic, somatic effects.

Component two should consist of the mammalian toxicity bioassays. These assays will involve characterization of the acute, subacute, and chronic toxicity of primary process by-products and effluents. As data become available through the chemistry, monitoring, and cellular bioassay programs, this information can be used to guide decisions concerning whether other materials or tests are indicated for additional evaluation of the process or product.

Consequently, both cellular and mammalian bioassays should be time-sequenced within the constraints of the program and of the complexity and cost of the tests. In this way the use of proper testing protocols and selection of critical compounds and materials can be ensured in a cost-effective manner.

Cautions on the use of short-term assays

When impure samples or actual process materials are being tested and fractionation procedures have to be utilized, the detection or perhaps the generation of mutagenic activity may well be a function of the chemical fractionation scheme utilized. The inability to recover specific chemical classes or the formation of artifacts by the treatment could well distort the results obtained, as could an inability to detect the specific biological end point chosen. Along with the obvious bias that could accompany the choice of samples and their solubility or the time and method of storage, a number of biological discrepancies could also enter into the determinations. For example, concomitant bacterial toxicity could nullify any genetic damage assay that might be carried out; the choice of inducer for the liver enzymes involved could be wrong for selected compounds; or the choice of strain could be inappropriate for selected compounds. In addition, the applicability of the microbial test results to other genetic assays and the apparent correlation between mutagenicity and carcinogenicity still needs validation through sufficient fundamental research. Furthermore, the short-term assays chronically show negative results with, e.g., heavy metals. Similarly, compounds involved in or requiring co-carcinogenic phenomena would presumably go undetected.

Confirmation with a battery of tests

Because of the intrinsic limitation of each mutation assay, testing with only one microbial system has often led to faulty conclusions with pure compounds. To overcome this shortcoming, we suggest employing short-term mutagenic and/or DNA-repair assays on any test materials to screen comprehensively both the mutagenic and carcinogenic hazards. However, some segments of the battery of assays would be used only on selected active compounds determined by the coupled effort of chemical and initial biological screens on complex mixtures. The actual components could then be characterized as either highly purified fractions or actual pure chemicals, and feedback to chemical screening would become a feasible monitoring method.

The minimal battery of tests might be composed of the following: (1) bacterial gene mutation; (2) yeast gene mutation (and recombination/conversion assays); (3) microbial DNA repair; (4) mammalian cell genetic toxicity assay using, e.g., cultured Chinese hamster ovary (CHO) cells to determine toxicity, mutagenicity, chromosomal aberrations, and sister-chromatid exchange; (5) when feasible, an epithelial-cell malignant transformation system. Only selected samples would be tested in the full battery of assays, the selection being dependent largely upon the preliminary results of the microbial screening. For risk assessment, further exhaustive validative tests in higher organisms will be necessary. However, as a prescreen to aid investigators in ordering their priorities, the short-term tests appear to be a valid approach to testing the large number of hazardous compounds and complex mixtures that man encounters in his environment.

SUMMARY

The predictive value of short-term mutagenicity tests for potential genetic hazards and carcinogenic hazards in man remains in question. Microbial, insect, mammalian cell, and whole-animal assays each have advantages and disadvantages depending on the test material. Metabolic activation of the compound(s) under test poses additional experimental questions. Extrapolation from one system to another in a comparative sense needs clarification. Further considerations of resolution, metabolism, synergism, and additivity arise when complex mixtures are evaluated in an industrial situation. The relationship of relative hazard in a short-term assay to relative hazard in man has to be approached with caution. A series of representative "genetic toxicological" procedures is described, and precautions inherent to their use and interpretation are presented.

ACKNOWLEDGEMENTS

The authors thank the staff of the Analytical Chemistry Division, coordinated by M. R. Guerin, for their efforts in providing materials; the Environmental Mutagen Information Center for their aid; and their colleagues Drs. T. K. Rao, C. E. Nix, and Ti Ho for their aid and comments. This research was jointly sponsored by the Environmental Protection Agency (IAG-D5-E681; Interagency Agreement 40-516-75) and the Office of Health and Environmental Research, U.S. Department of Energy, under contract W-7405-eng-26 with the Union Carbide Corporation.

REFERENCES

1. Epler, J. L., Larimer, F. W., Rao, T. K., Nix, C. E. and Ho, T. (1978) Environ. Health Perspect., 27, 11–20.

2. Ames, B. N., McCann, J. and Yamasaki, E. (1975) Mutat. Res., 31, 347–364.

3. Epler, J. L., (1979). The use of short-term tests in the isolation and identification of chemical mutagens in complex mixtures. In: Chemical Mutagens: Principles and Methods for Their Detection, Vol. 6 (F. J. deSerres, ed.), Plenum Press, New York and London, in press.

4. Guerin, M. R., Epler, J. L., Griest, W. H., Clark, B. R. and Rao, T. K. (1978) In Carcinogenesis, Vol. 3: Polynuclear Aromatic Hydrocarbons, Raven Press, New York, pp. 21–33.

5. Epler, J. L., Clark, B. R., Ho, C.-h, Guerin, M. R. and Rao, T. K. (1978). Short-Term Bioassay of Complex Organic Mixtures. Part II: Mutagenicity Testing, ORNL-TM-6390, Oak Ridge National Laboratory, Oak Ridge, Tennessee; Presented at the Symposium on Application of Short-Term Bioassays in the Fractionation and Analysis of Complex Environmental Mixtures, Williamsburg, Virginia, February 21–23, 1978.

6. McCann, J., Choi, E., Yamasaki, E. and Ames, B. N. (1975) Proc. Natl. Acad. Sci. USA, 72, 5135–5139.

7. Drake, J. W., et al. (1975) Science, 187, 503–514.

8. deSerres, F. J. (1976) Mutat. Res., 38, 1–2.

9. deSerres, F. J. (1976) Mutat. Res., 38, 165–176.

10. Bridges, B. A., (1973) Environ. Health Perspect., 6, 221–227.

11. Bridges, B. A. (1974) Mutat. Res., 26, 335–340.

12. Ames, B. N., Lee, F. D. and Durston, W. E. (1973) Proc. Natl. Acad. Sci. USA, 70, 782–786.

13. Witkin, E. M. (1969) Annu. Rev. Genet., 3, 525–552.

14. Green, M. H. L. and Muriel, W. J. (1976) Mutat. Res., 38, 3–32.

15. Mohn, G. R. and Ellenberger, J. (1979) The use of Escherichia coli K12/343/113 (λ) as a multipurpose indicator strain in various mutagenicity testing procedures. In: Handbook of Mutagenicity Test Procedures (B. J. Kilbey et al., eds.), Elsevier-North-Holland Biomedical Press, Amsterdam, pp. 95–118.

16. Kada, T., Tutikawa, K. and Sadaie, Y. (1972) Mutat. Res., 16, 165–174.

17. Slater, E. E., Anderson, M. D. and Rosenkranz, H. S. (1971) Cancer Res., 31, 970–973.

18. deSerres, F. J. and Malling, H. V. (1977) In: Chemical Mutagens: Principles and Methods for their Detection, Vol. 2 (A. Hollaender, ed.), Plenum Press, New New York, pp. 311–342.

19. Zimmermann, F. K. (1975) Mutat. Res., 31, 71–86.

20. Larimer, F. W., Ramey, D. W., Lijinsky, W. and Epler, J. L. (1978) Mutat. Res., 57, 155–161.

21. Abrahamson, S. and Lewis, E. B. (1971) In Chemical Mutagens: Principles and Methods for Their Detection, Vol. 2 (A. Hollaender, ed.), Plenum Press, New York, pp. 461–487.

22. Nix, C. E. and Brewen, B. S. (1978) The role of Drosophila in chemical mutagenesis testing, Symposium on Application of Short-Term Bioassays in the Fractionation and Analysis of Complex Environmental Mixtures, Williamsburg, Virginia, February 21–23, 1978, EPA-600/9-78-027, EPA Office of Research and Development, Washington, D.C.

23. Hsie, A. W., O'Neill, J. P., San Sebastian, J. R., Couch, D. B., Brimer, P. A., Sun, W. N. C., Fuscoe, J. C., Forbes, N. L., Machanoff, R., Riddle, J. C. and Hsie, M. H. (1978) Mutagenicity of carcinogens: Study of 101 individual agents and 3 subfractions of a crude synthetic oil in a quantitative mammalian cell gene mutation system, Presented at the Symposium on Application of Short-Term Bioassays in the Fractionation and Analysis of Complex Environmental Mixtures, Williamsburg, Virginia, February 21–23, 1978, EPA-600/9-78-027, EPA Office of Research and Development, Washington, D.C.

24. Stich, H. F., Lam, P., Lo, L. W., Koropatnick, D. J. and San, R. H. C. (1975) Can. J. Genet. Cytol., 17, 471–492.

25. Regan, J. D. and Setlow, R. B. (1974) Cancer Res., 34, 3318–3325.

26. Ishidate, M. and Odashima, S. (1977) Mutat. Res., 48, 337–354.

27. Stetka, D. G. and Wolff, S. (1976) Mutat. Res., 41, 333–342.

28. Wolff, S. (1977) Annu. Rev. Genet., 11, 183–201.

29. Generoso, W. M. (1973) Environ. Health Perspect., 6, 13–22.

30. Russell, L. B. (1977) Arch. Toxicol., 38, 75–85.

31. Cattanach, B. M. (1971) In Chemical Mutagens: Principles and Methods for their Detection, Vol 2 (A. Hollaender, ed.), Plenum Press, New York, 535–539.

32. Duke, K. M., Davis, M. E. and Dennis, A. J. (1977) IERL-RTP Procedures Manual: Level I Environmental Assessment. Biological Tests for Pilot Studies, EPA 600/7-77-043, EPA Office of Research and Development, Washington, D.C.

33. Hamersma, J. W., Reynolds, F. L. and Maddalone, R. F. (1976) IERL-RTP Procedures Manual: Level I Environmental Assessment. EPA Technology Series, EPA-600/2-76-160, EPA Office of Research and Development, Washington, D.C.

34. Waters, M. D. and Epler, J. L. (1978) Status of Bioscreening of Emissions and Effluents from Energy Technologies. EPA-600/9-78-022, EPA Office of Research and Development, Washington, D.C.

35. Weisburger, J. H. (1976) In Chemical Carcinogens, ACS Monograph 173 (C. E. Searle, ed.), American Chemical Society, Washington, D.C.

© 1980 Elsevier/North-Holland Biomedical Press
The Scientific Basis of Toxicity Assessment
H. Witschi, editor.

ASSAYS FOR IN VITRO CARCINOGENESIS, INITIATION, AND PROMOTION

CHARLES HEIDELBERGER

University of Southern California Comprehensive Cancer Center, Los Angeles, CA, 90033, USA.

It appears that in this entire Symposium on the Scientific Basis of Toxicity Assessment, mine is the only presentation that deals with the highly important field of short-term tests for carcinogenesis and genetic toxicology. I respond to this challenge with enthusiasm, and because of the enormous development in this field in recent years I will be forced to restrict myself to jovian generalities rather than experimental details. Hence, I will attempt a brief and critical review of the field with sufficient literature references to enable an interested reader to search it in more detail. Suffice it to say at the outset that short-term assays for carcinogenesis provide dual opportunities to learn much about cellular and molecular mechanisms, as well as to develop and validate assay systems.

The prototype of the short-term assay for carcinogenic activity is the Ames test[1]. In this test, chemicals are mixed with a suitable rat liver activating system and exposed to several tester strains of Salmonella typhimurim that have been constructed especially to sensitively detect various types of chemical mutagens, and back-mutations to histidine auxotrophy are measured. In this test there is an excellent correlation beteen mutagenicity and carcinogenic activities of more than 300 chemicals, with about 10% false positives and 10% false negatives[2]. Thus, the Ames test is quick and inexpensive, and is being very widely used throughout the world in academic and industrial research laboratories and by regulatory agencies. Unfortunately, Salmonella do not get cancer, and there is as yet no unequivocal proof that chemical carcinogenesis is invariably the result of a somatic mutation. Hence, there is a very real need for short-term tests in which carcinogenesis can be measured in cell cultures. Fortunately, there are some systems in which this can be done, and I will describe the more important of these, while recognizing at the outset that these systems are more difficult, expensive and time-consuming than the Ames test, and that they are in earlier stages of evaluation. I have written several reviews of this field [3-7].

I shall begin by defining some termed. The process that I will be describing has been termed "transformation", and represents an alteration in the social behavior of the cells following carcinogen treatment. "Oncogenic transformation" means that the transformed cells have also acquired the property to grow as tumors in syngeneic hosts. Thus, "carcinogenesis in vitro" is an imprecise term that is better defined as "oncogenic transformation in cell cultures". Depending on the system, morphological transformation often precedes oncogenic transformation to a greater or lesser extent.

In general there are two types of cell culture systems that are useful in this field. The first involves primary or secondary cultures of normal Syrian hamster embryo cells, and the second involves the use of permanent cell lines, such as the mouse embryo fibroblasts, C3H/10T1/2 and BALB/3T3. These systems and their advantages and disadvantages will be described and discussed.

The first report in the literature on the transformation of cultured cells by chemical carcinogens was that of Berwald and Sachs[8], who described the morphological transformation by polycyclic aromatic hydrocarbons (PAH) of primary cultures of Syrian hamster embryo cells. In this system, primary cultures are set up from eviscerated Syrian hamster embryos, and then transferred into secondary cultures in which 5000 cells are treated with the solvent as controls or with various concentrations of PAH. After 8-10 days, the dishes are fixed and stained and the total number of colonies are counted to determine the plating efficiency and cytotoxicity of the test compound. The colonies are also examined under the microscope: normal colonies are flat and somewhat epithelioid in character, whereas transformed colonies appear more fibroblastic and form piled-up, criss-crossed multilayers. There is a wide variety in the morphology of these transformed colonies, and considerable experience is required to score them accurately. The untreated cells are normal in that they have a diploid karyotype, have a limited lifespan in culture, do not give rise to tumors on inoculation into syngeneic hamsters, and have a very low rate of spontaneous transformation[9].

In the orignal work[8,9], there was an agreement in several PAH between their carcinogenic activities in mice and the transformation frequency in this system. Further investigation revealed one-hit kinetics for the transformation of these cells by benzo(a)pyrene[10], and that they are also transformed by x-rays[11]. This system has been extensively studied by DiPaolo and his colleagues[12-14], who first showed that transformed colonies produced sarcomas on inoculation into Syrian hamsters[15].

More recently, Ts'o and his colleagues have found in the same system that transformation results from a direct perturbation of DNA[16], that transformation is a stepwise process[17], and that both the transformation frequency and mutation frequency to 8-azaguanine resistance can be measured in these cells[18]. The latter observation has also been made by Huberman et al.[19].

One of the problems associated with this system is that it has been difficult for some people to obtain reproducible results. This problem has been overcome by Pienta et al.[20] by using large pools of cryopreserved secondary hamster embryo cells. They have then studied the relation between transformation frequency and in vivo carcinogenic activities of 83 compounds[20]. They have found no false positives and 9% false negatives, so their correlations are as good as those obtained in the Ames test.

The advantage of this system are that the cells are normal and that the test takes only 10 days. The disadvantages are that the cloning efficiency is very low, that because of the limited lifespan of the normal cells they cannot be grown up into large populations of cells that can be compared with transformed cells, and that they are a heterogeneous cell population.

The other type of system that is employed for studies of chemical oncogenesis involves the use of permanent cloned cell lines. Those in which extensive studies have been carried out include mouse prostate fibroblasts that were first developed in my laboratory[12] and subsequently used by Marquardt[22], mouse embryo cells infected with a nontransforming AKR leukemia virus[23], high passage rat embryo cells that express a nontransforming rat leukemia virus[24], BALB/3T3 cells[25,26], and BHK21 baby hamster kidney cells[27,28]. Perhaps the most widely used of such systems is the C3H/10T1/2 mouse embryo fibroblast system, which was also developed in my laboratory[29,30]. Since this cloned cell line is typical of these systems, and since I have most direct experience with it, I will concentrate in the remainder of this article on examples of its use.

These permanent cell lines have the disadvantage that the cells are usually tetra ploid, and hence are not normal. Another disadvantage is that it usually takes about six weeks to carry out a transformation assay. On the other hand, some advantages of these systems are that scoring is less subjective and more quantitative than in the hamster embryo cell system, the cells are cloned and represent a homogeneous population, and they clone at a high efficiency, so that populations of nontrans-formed cells and independently transformed cells clonally derived from them can be grown in large quantities and used for comparative studies of almost any property.

The C3H/10T1/2 cloned cell line was obtained by passaging C3H mouse embryo cells until they became a permanent line. These cells are exquisitely sensitive to post confluence inhibition of cell division and form a very flat monolayer, they do not transform spontaneously if they are properly cared for, and they do not produce tumors on inoculation into immunosuppressed syngeneic mice[29]. When 2000 of these cells are plated and one day later are treated with a PAH for one day, and then the cultures are carried for six weeks with twice weekly medium changes, very distinct piled-up foci are found that overgrow the monolayer and can be easily counted;

these foci produce fibrosarcomas on inoculation into immunosuppressed C3H mice[30]. We initially determined that in a series of PAH there was an excellent correlation between the number of transformed foci produced and the in vivo carcinogenic activities of the compounds[30]. C3H/10T1/2 cells have also been transformed with alkylating agents[31], ultraviolet light[32], x-rays[33], cancer chemotherapeutic drugs[34], tobacco smoke condensate[35], and neutrons[36].

Since PAH require metabolic activation and tranform C3H/10T1/2 cells, it is obvious that these cells have the capability to activate PAH by the cytochrome P448 mixed-function oxidase system, and we have analyzed this metabolism and shown it to be obligatory for transformation[37]. However, chemical carcinogens that are activated by the cytochrome P450 system, such as aromatic amines, nitrosamines, and aflatoxin B_1, do not produce cytoxicity or transformation of C3H/10T1/2 cells. In order for these cells to be useful for the screening of environmental carcinogens it will be necessary to supply them with an exogenous activating system derived from liver. Three such systems are currently under investigation with C3H/10T1/2 cells: the fortified rat liver homogenate system that we successfully employed for activation of chemical carcinogens to produce mutations in Chinese hamster V79 cells[38]; primary rat liver hepatocytes[39]; and a permanent line of hepatocytes derived from regenerating mouse liver[40], which when used as a lethally irradiated "feeder layer" activated aflatoxin B_1 to transform C3H/10T1/2 cells.

It was first discovered by Berenblum[41] that carcinogenesis on mouse skin can be subdivided into two phases, initiation and promotion. This field has also been extensively studied by Boutwell[42]. An important contribution was made by Hecker[43], who fractionated croton oil, the crude mixture that had been used as the classical promoter, isolated the active fraction, and determined its structure to be 12-0-tetradecanoyl phorbol 13-acetate (TPA). In the C3H/10T1/2 cell system we have succeeded in reproducing the two-stages of transformation[44]. In this system, ultraviolet light[45] and x-ray initiation[46] were promoted by TPA; saccharin does not transform the cells by itself, but acts as a weak promoter[47]. Thus this versatile cell system can be used to study transformation, initiation, or promotion from the points of view of determining mechanisms and providing screening systems.

Because most human cancers are carcinomas and not sarcomas, it has been highly desirable to develop epithelial cell systems that can be transformed with chemical carcinogens and that would produce carcinomas or inoculation into appropriate hosts. Although it is beyond the scope of this review, several epithelial cell systems have been studied, but none has been successfully or reproducibly quantitated. Moreover, in many cases carcinomas were not obtained. These systems involve the use of rat liver cells[48,49,50], mouse skin cells[51,52], fetal rat brain cells[53], and mouse embryo epithelial cells[54].

For reasons that are not at present clear, it has been exceedingly difficult to transform human cells by chemical carcinogens. However, Kakunaga has succeeded in transforming normal human diploid fibroblasts with an alkylating agent and 4-nitroquinoline-N-oxide[55], and Milo and DiPaolo have confirmed this work[56].

These cell culture systems have been extremely useful in studying the cellular and molecular mechanisms of carcinogenesis, free from the complicated nutritional, metabolic, and immunological milieu of intact animals. The scope of this review does not permit listing such studies in any detail. Suffice it to say that in our own laboratory we have found that this transformation is direct and is not a selection of preexisting transformed cells[57], and that individual transformed foci have individual and not cross-reacting tumor specific transplantation antigens[58,59], while at the same time exhibiting common embryonic antigens[60]. We have found that in C3H/10T1/2 cells there is no induction of an endogenous retrovirus or its core during the process of transformation by methylcholanthrene[61], and Getz et al., have reported that there is no enhanced transcription of the murine leukemia-sarcoma viral RNA in transformed C3H/10T1/2 cells[62]. We have also studied the cell cycle dependence for transformation of these cells by alkylating agents[31], and Jones et al. by ara-C[63]. We have studied the effects of DNA damage and repair produced by alkylating agents on transformation[64,65].

In attempts to determine the role of somatic mutations in carcinogenesis it has been necessary to correlate mutagenic activities of chemicals in Salmonella[1,2] or in mammalian cells[38] with in vivo carcinogenic activities. As mentioned above, in the Syrian hamster embryo cell system it has been possible to measure both transformation and mutagenesis[18,19]. It has now been possible to quantitate mutagenesis to ouabain resistance in C3H/10T1/2 cells which has been done independently by Chan and Little[66] for ultraviolet light, and ourselves[67] for several chemical carcinogens. This opens up a Pandora's box of possibilities for critically studying in the same cells at the same time the similarities and differences between these two processes, as well as factors that modify them.

I believe it is clear from this necessarily superficial review, that cell culture systems have already achieved considerable utility in studies of cellular mechanisms of chemical carcinogenesis, and are potentially also highly useful as prescreens for environmental carcinogens. In spite of the immense societal and regulatory pressures, it is necessary to proceed to validate these systems in an impartial and scientific fashion before they become prematurely adopted and prematurely discarded.

REFERENCES

1. Ames, B.N. et al. (1973) Proc. Natl. Acad. Sci. U.S. 70, 2281-2285.

2. McCann, J. and Ames, B. N. (1976) Proc. Natl. Acad. Sci. U.S. 73, 950-954.

3. Heidelberger, C. (1973) Advan. Cancer Res. 18, 317-366.

4. Heidelberger, C. (1975) Ann. Rev. Biochem. 44, 79-121.

5. Heidelberger, C. (1977) in Origins of Human Cancer, H. H. Hiatt, J. D. Watson, J. A. Winsten, eds., Cold Spring Harbor Press, pp. 1513-1520.

6. Heidelberger C. (1978) in Polycyclic Hydrocarbons and Cancer, H. V. Gelboin and P. O. P. Ts'o, eds. Academic Press, N. Y. Vol. 2, pp. 269-277.

7. Heidelberger, C. (1979) Advances in Experimental Toxicology Vol. 1, in press.

8. Berwald, Y. and Sachs, L. (1963) Nature 200, 1182-1184.

9. Berwald, Y. and Sachs, L. (1965) J. Natl. Cancer Inst. 35, 641-661.

10. Huberman, E. and Sachs, L. (1966) Proc. Natl. Acad. Sci. U. S. 56, 1123-1129.

11. Borek, C. and Sachs, L. (1966) Nature 210, 276-278.

12. DiPaolo, J. A. et al. (1969) J. Natl. Cancer Inst. 42, 867-874.

13. DiPaolo, J. A. et al. (1971) Cancer Res. 31, 1118-1127.

14. DiPaolo, J. A. et al. (1973) Cancer Res. 33, 3250-3258.

15. DiPaolo, J. A. et al. (1969) Science 165, 917-918.

16. Barrett, J. C. et al. (1978) Nature 274, 229-232.

17. Barrett, J. C. and Ts'o, P. O. P. (1978) Proc. Natl. Acad. Sci. U. S. 75, 3761-3765.

18. Barrett, J. C. and Ts'o, P. O. P. (1978) Proc. Natl. Acad. Sci. U. S. 75, 3297-3301.

19. Huberman, E., Mager, R. and Sachs, L. (1976) Nature 264, 360-361.

20. Pienta, R. J. et al. (1977) Int. J. Cancer 19, 642-655.

21. Chen, T. T. and Heidelberger, C. (1969) Int. J. Cancer 4, 166-178.

22. Marquardt, H. et al. (1974) Int. J. Cancer 13, 304-309.

23. Rhim, J. S. et al. (1974) J. Natl. Cancer Inst. 52, 1167-1173.

24. Freeman, A. E. et al. (1973) J. Natl. Cancer Inst. 51, 799-803.

25. DiPaolo, J. A. et al. (1972) Cancer Res. 32, 2686-2695.

26. Kakunaga, T. (1973) Int. J. Cancer 12, 463-473.

27. Mishra, N. K. and diMayorca, G. (1974) Biochim. Biophys. Acta 355, 205-219.

28. Styles, J. A. (1977) Brit. J. Cancer 36, 558-563.

29. Reznikoff, C. A. et al. (1973) Cancer Res. 33, 3231-3238.

30. Reznikoff, C. A. et al. (1973) Cancer Res. 33, 3239-3249.

31. Bertram, J. S. and Heidelberger, C. (1974) Cancer Res. 34, 526-537.

32. Chan, G. C. and Little, J. B. (1976) Nature 264, 442-444.

33. Terzaghi, M. and Little, J. B. (1976) Cancer Res. 36, 1367-1374.

34. Jones, P. A. et al. (1976) Cancer Res. 36, 101-107.

35. Benedict, W. F. et al. (1975) Cancer Res. 35, 857-860.

36. Han, A. and Elkind, M. M. (1979) Cancer Res. 39, 123-130.

37. Nesnow, S. and Heidelberger, C. (1976) Cancer Res. 36, 1801-1808.

38. Krahn, D. F. and Heidelberger, C. (1977) Mutation Res. 46, 27-44.

39. Langenbach, R. J. et al. (1978) Proc. Natl. Acad. Sci. U. S. 75, 2864-2867.

40. Mondal, S. et al. (1979) Proc. Am. Assoc. Cancer Res. 20, 62.

41. Berenblum, I. (1941) Cancer Res. 1, 44-48.

42. Boutwell, R. K. (1964) Prog. Exptl. Tumor Res. 4, 207-250.

43. Hecker, E. (1971) in Methods in Cancer Res., H. Busch, ed., 6, 439-484.

44. Mondal, S. et al. (1976) Cancer Res. 36, 2254-2260.

45. Mondal, S. and Heidelberger, C. (1976) Nature, 260, 710-711

46. Kennedy, A. R. et al. (1978) Cancer Res. 38, 439-443.

47. Mondal, S. et al. (1978) Science 201, 1141-1142.

48. Montesano, R. et al. (1975) Int. J. Cancer 16, 550-558.

49. Williams, G. M. et al. (1973) Cancer Res. 33, 606-612.

50. Yamaguchi, N. and Weinstein, I. B. (1975) Proc. Natl. Acad. Sci. U. S. 72, 214-218.

51. Elias, P. M. et al. (1974) J. Invest. Derm. 62, 569-581.

52. Fusenig, N. E. and Worst, P. K. M. (1975) Exptl. Cell Res. 93, 443-457.

53. Laerum, O. D. and Rajewsky, M. F. (1975) J. Natl. Cancer Inst. 55, 1177-1187.

54. Mondal, S. and Sala, M. (1978) Nature 274, 370-372.

55. Kakunaga, T. (1978) Proc. Natl. Acad. Sci. U. S. 75, 1334-1338.

56. Milo, G. E. and DiPaolo, J. A. (1978) Nature 275, 130-132.

57. Mondal, S. and Heidelberger, C. (1970) Proc. Natl. Acad. Sci. U. S. 65, 219-225.

58. Mondal, S. et al. (1970) Cancer Res. 30, 1953-1957.

59. Embleton, M. J. and Heidelberger, C. (1972) Int. J. Cancer 8, 8-18.

60. Embleton, M. J. and Heidelberger, C. (1975) Cancer Res. 35, 2049-2055.

61. Rapp, U. R. et al. (1975) Virology 65, 392-409.

62. Getz, M. J. et al. (1978) Cancer Res 38, 566-569.

63. Jones, P. A. et al. (1977) Cancer Res. 37, 2214-2217.

64. Peterson, A. R. et al. (1974) Cancer Res. 34, 1592-1599.

65. Peterson, A. R. et al. (1974) Cancer Res. 34, 1600-1607.

66. Chan, G. C. and Little, J. B. (1978) Proc. Natl. Acad. Sci. U. S. 75, 3363-3366.

67. Landolph, J. R. and Heidelberger, C. (1979) Proc. Natl. Acad. Sci. 76, 750-754.

© 1980 Elsevier/North-Holland Biomedical Press
The Scientific Basis of Toxicity Assessment
H. Witschi, editor.

IMPLICATIONS OF THE MECHANISMS OF TUMORIGENICITY FOR RISK ASSESSMENT

P. G. Watanabe, R. H. Reitz, A. M. Schumann, M. J. McKenna, J. F. Quast and
P. J. Gehring
Dow Chemical U.S.A., Toxicology Research Laboratory, Health and Environmental
Sciences, USA, 1803 Building, Midland, MI 48640

INTRODUCTION

Studies of the pharmacokinetics and resulting chemical interaction with intracellular macromolecules are important aspects to consider in the interpretation of results from animal toxicity studies. The objective of any toxicologic study is to elucidate the toxic effects of a chemical both qualitatively
and quantitatively. Since toxicity is elicited through reactions of a chemical
with molecular targets in sensitive tissue, it is necessary to correlate toxicity with the pharmacokinetics of the chemical which describes as a function of
time the absorption, distribution, metabolism and excretion of the chemical.
However, experience has shown that the pharmacokinetic characteristics alone are
not always sufficient to explain the differential susceptibility to carcinogenicity between species and sometimes strains within a given species. Thus, in
order to generate data which can be used ultimately to assess the risk of exposure in man from animal toxicity data it is also necessary to understand how
chemical interactions with intracellular macromolecules can be related to induction of toxicity, including carcinogenicity. Therefore, assessment of risk
requires integrating the results from studies of acute and chronic toxicity,
pharmacokinetics and chemical-macromolecular interactions.

Carcinogenicity is only one aspect of the toxicology of the chlorinated
hydrocarbons. However, due to the sensitivity of this issue in society today
our studies have concentrated on this aspect. The examples of how pharmacokinetics and chemical macromolecular interaction studies can be used in assessing toxicity with particular emphasis on carcinogenicity will be the central
theme of this paper.

Mice appear to be more sensitive than rats to the tumorigenic effects of the
chlorinated hydrocarbons; thus our objective was to assess the importance of
pharmacokinetics and resultant macromolecular interactions in explaining,
mechanistically, why this species difference exists. These studies were conducted on vinylidene chloride (1,1-dichloroethylene) and perchloroethylene

(1,1,2,2-tetrachloroethylene). Prior to giving details on these studies it may be useful to review the available animal carcinogenicity data for vinylidene chloride and perchloroethylene.

Background animal carcinogenicity data

Vinylidene chloride (VDC) has not been observed to be carcinogenic in several long term, lifetime, studies with rats when administered by inhalation exposure (25, 75, 100 ppm) or in the drinking water (up to 220 ppm) (Viola and Caputo,[1] 1977; Rampy et al.[2], 1977 Maltoni et al.[3], 1977). In contrast, two investigators have reported the induction of tumors in mice following long term inhalation exposure to 25 or 55 ppm (Maltoni et al.[3], 1977; Lee et al.[4], 1978). Maltoni et al. reported that male mice were far more sensitive to VDC than females, that the target organ in male mice was the kidney, and that the tumorigenicity of VDC was associated with significant nontumor related injury to kidney tissue in male mice (Maltoni et al., 1977). Of particular significance was that at a lower exposure level (10 ppm) there was an absence of both nontumor related tissue injury to the kidney and kidney tumors.

Similar to vinylidene chloride, a carcinogen bioassay study of perchloroethylene (Perc) indicated that daily administration of high oral doses (500, 1000 mg/kg/day) produced an increase in the incidence of hepatocellular carcinomas in mice (NCI,[5] 1977), but perchloroethylene did not produce tumors in rats in the same study nor was it tumorigenic in rats following long-term inhalation exposure (up to 600 ppm, Rampy et al.[6], 1977). Thus for vinylidene chloride and perchloroethylene the data indicate that mice are much more susceptible to the tumorigenic effects than rats. This enhanced sensitivity of mice to the toxic effects of halogenated hydrocarbons holds true for other chlorinated hydrocarbons as well, including trichloroethylene, trichloroethane (1,1,2 isomer) carbon tetrachloride and chloroform (National Cancer Institute Bioassay Results).

METHODS

Since details of the methods used in these studies have been previously reported (McKenna et al.[7], 1979; Reitz et al.[8], 1979; Schumann et al.[9], 1979), only the salient features of the methodologic approach will be presented.

Animals

When possible, the pharmacokinetic studies were conducted in the same strain of animal for which prior carcinogenicity information was available. For the vinylidene chloride studies male Sprague Dawley rats, Ha(ICR) mice (Spartan Research Laboratories, Haslett, MI) and CD-1 mice (Charles River Laboratories, Wilmington, MA) were used. The perchloroethylene studies used male Sprague Dawley rats (same supplier as above) and B6C3F1 mice (Charles River Laboratories, Wilmington, MA).

Material

Carbon 14 labeled vinylidene chloride (^{14}C-VDC) and perchloroethylene (^{14}C-Perc) were purchased from New England Nuclear (Boston, MA). The radiochemical purity for the ^{14}C-VDC and ^{14}C-Perc was greater than 98% as checked by gas chromatographic and liquid chromatographic analysis, respectively.

Exposure

Animals were exposed by inhalation (6 hour exposures) or oral gavage to the ^{14}C-labeled test chemicals. The inhalation exposures were conducted in a 30 liter glass inhalation chamber under either recirculating or dynamic air flow conditions. The test atmosphere was monitored at regular intervals by gas chromatography. Subsequent procedures involving quantitating radioactivity in excreta, expired air, tissues or macromolecular fractions were done by liquid scintillation spectrometry (LSC).

Specific Procedures

Covalent binding to macromolecules. Covalent binding of ^{14}C-activity to tissue constituents was determined in liver and kidney tissues obtained at autopsy by a modification of the method of Jollow et al.[10], (1973) as described previously (McKenna et al.[11], 1978).

Covalent binding to purified DNA. Covalent binding of ^{14}C-activity to purified DNA was determined by LSC after purification of DNA by a modification of the method of Marmur[12] (1961) as described by Reitz et al.[8], (1979).

DNA repair synthesis. DNA repair was measured according to the following procedure: animals from one population were divided into treated (T) or control (C) groups. Each group was further divided into two subgroups (3-6 animals/subgroup). One subgroup received ^{3}H-thymidine (0.01 ml/gram body wt, 50-100 μCi/ml, 20 Ci/mM, ip) and the other subgroup received an identical injection of ^{3}H-thymidine dissolved in 40 mg/ml hydroxyurea. Four hours later, the animals were sacrificed by cervical dislocation, and the DNA was isolated.

Repair was calculated from these groups as suggested by Arfellini et al.[13], (1978):

1. The specific activities of the DNA isolated from each tissue were calculated (dpm/mg DNA).
2. Next a correction factor (CF) for the effect of the test chemical on normal replicative DNA synthesis was calculated. This was approximated as the ratio of the mean specific activities of DNA in the subgroups receiving ^{3}H-thymidine (treated group/control group).
3. Finally the repair ratio (RR) was calculated as:

$$RR = \frac{(T)_{HU}}{(C)_{HU} \times CF}$$

where $(T)_{HU}$ = the mean specific activity of the DNA isolated from the treated subgroup injected with ^{3}H-thymidine plus hydroxyurea, $(C)_{HU}$ = the mean specific activity of the DNA isolated from the control subgroup injected with ^{3}H-thymidine plus hydroxyurea, and CF is the correction factor calculated in (2).

Repair synthesis of DNA is maximal within a few hours after treatment, when absorption, distribtuion, and (in the case of procarcinogens) metabolic activation have taken place. Consequently, repair measurements were carried out 4 hours after ip injection of dimethylnitrosamine (DMN) or immediately following a 6 hour inhalation exposure to VDC.

DNA synthesis (regeneration following tissue injury). DNA synthesis was measured 18-48 hours after exposure. In this procedure, a population of animals was divided into a control and treated group. Each group received an ip injection of ^{3}H-thymidine (50-100 µCi/ml, 20 Ci/mM) at the rate of 0.01 ml/gram of body weight. Four hours after the ^{3}H-thymidine injection, the animals were sacrificed and DNA was isolated from kidney and/or liver.

The DNA synthesis value was calculated by dividing the mean specific activity of DNA preparations from treated groups by the mean specific activity of the DNA preparations from the control group. In each experiment, a matched control group was used for this calculation. A DNA synthesis value of 1.0 or less indicates that the treatment did not stimulate DNA synthesis, while numbers larger than 1.0 show stimulation of DNA synthesis, indicating regeneration following cellular injury.

Histopathology. Samples of kidney and liver were removed at autopsy and fixed in buffered 10% formalin. The tissues were processed by routine histologic procedures. Sections, 5-6 microns thick were stained with hematoxylin and eosin and examined by light microscopy.

RESULTS/DISCUSSION

Pharmacokinetics/Metabolism

VDC. Preliminary experiments compared the fate of inhaled ^{14}C-VDC in male Sprague Dawley rats and male Ha(ICR) mice (Table 1). Exposure to 10 ppm ^{14}C-VDC for 6 hours resulted in no significant qualitative differences in the fate of ^{14}C-VDC in rats and mice. However, the acquired body burden of ^{14}C-activity in mice was 5.3 mg equivalents ^{14}C-VDC per kg, nearly twice that obtained in the rat under identical exposure conditions. Inhaled ^{14}C-VDC was also more extensively metabolized by mice than by rats; the former eliminated less than 1% of the body burden as unchanged VDC is expired air. In both species ^{14}C-VDC per se was found only in expired air. ^{14}C-activity in the excreta and remaining in the body at the end of the experiment was assumed to represent biotransformation products of ^{14}C-VDC (McKenna et al.[11], 1978).

TABLE 1

RECOVERY OF ^{14}C-ACTIVITY IN RATS AND MICE FOLLOWING A 6 HOUR INHALATION EXPOSURE TO 10 PPM ^{14}C-VINYLIDENE CHLORIDE (^{14}C-VDC)

	% Body Burden ($\overline{X}$±S.E., n=4)	
	Mice	Rats
Expired VDC	0.65±0.07	1.63±0.14
[14]CO_2	4.64±0.17	8.74±3.72
Urine	80.83±1.68	74.72±2.30
Feces	6.58±0.81	9.73±0.10
Carcass	5.46±0.41	4.75±0.78
Cage Wash	1.83±0.84	0.44±0.28
	(mg Eq ^{14}C-VDC/Kg)	
Body Burden	5.30±0.75	2.89±0.24
Total Metabolized VDC	5.27±0.74	2.84±0.26

The higher body burden and more rapid metabolism of VDC by mice suggested that the production of reactive VDC metabolites in mice may be much greater than observed in rats thus rendering them more susceptible to the adverse effects of VDC exposure (McKenna et al.[14], 1977). A comparison of values obtained for ^{14}C-VDC metabolites bound to liver and kidney tissues of the two species is shown in Table 2. Following the 10 ppm ^{14}C-VDC exposure a marked increase was

74

observed in covalently bound ^{14}C-VDC metabolites in mouse liver and kidney when compared to rats. This enhanced production of reactive VDC metabolites in mouse tissues could not be attributed solely to the increased metabolism of VDC over that of the rat as indicated by the normalization of the binding data for differences in metabolism (B/A ratio). Thus, not only was the metabolism of VDC greater in the mouse than in the rat, but the production of reactive metabolites in target tissues for VDC-induced toxicity was markedly greater.

TABLE 2

VDC METABOLISM AND COVALENTLY BOUND ^{14}C-ACTIVITY IN MALE RATS AND MICE AFTER A 10 PPM ^{14}C-VDC INHALATION EXPOSURE

Species	A Metabolized ^{14}C-VDC mg Eq/kg	Tissue	B Covalent Binding µg Eq ^{14}C-VDC/g Protein	(B/A)[a]
Rat	2.84±0.26	Liver	5.28± 0.14	1.86
		Kidney	13.14± 1.25	4.63
Mouse	5.27±0.74	Liver	22.29± 3.77	4.23
		Kidney	79.55±19.11	15.09

All values are $\bar{X}$±S.E., n=4.

[a] Covalent binding data normalized to account for differences in metabolized VDC.

Perc. Studies were also conducted to compare the routes of excretion and extent of metabolism of perchloroethylene in rats and mice. Groups of 3, rats or mice, were exposed to a 10 ppm atmosphere of ^{14}C-labeled perchloroethylene for 6 hours and the percentage of recovered radioactivity excreted by the various routes was determined. In mice, only 12.0% of the radioactivity was excreted by the lungs as perchloroethylene. This is in contrast to 68.1% perchloroethylene excreted by the lungs in rats. Consistent with this pattern suggesting that the mouse metabolizes much more perchloroethylene than the rat is the excretion of urinary metabolites, 62.5% in mice versus only 18.7% in rats (Table 3).

TABLE 3

RECOVERY OF RADIOACTIVITY AFTER A 6-HOUR INHALATION OF 10 PPM
^{14}C-PERCHLOROETHYLENE

	% Body Burden ($\overline{X}$±S.E., n=3)	
	Mice	Rats
Expired Air		
Perchloroethylene	12.0±1.3	68.1±2.7
$^{14}CO_2$	7.9±0.4	3.6±0.7
Urine	62.5±1.0	18.7±1.2
Feces	6.8±1.5	5.2±0.4
Carcass	3.1±0.2	4.3±0.9
Cage Wash	7.7±2.1	—

When expressed on a weight basis, it can be seen that the mouse metabolizes
8.5x more perchloroethylene than the rat (Table 4). If the metabolism of perchloroethylene is associated with the formation of a reactive metabolite, then
it would be expected that those reactive metabolites should bind to intracellular macromolecules. The macromolecular binding of perchloroethylene metabolites
to liver tissue is shown (Table 4) and these data support the contention that
increased metabolism results in a proportionate increase in the macromolecular
binding (mice/rat = 7).

TABLE 4

AMOUNT OF PERCHLOROETHYLENE METABOLIZED AND BOUND TO MACROMOLECULES
(10 PPM INHALATION EXPOSURE)

	Mice	Rats	Mice/Rat
μMole Equiv Perc Metabolized	2.15±0.24	2.82±0.28	
$\frac{\text{μMole Equiv Perc Metabolized}}{\text{Kg Body Wt}}$	89.53±5.8	10.52±0.92	8.5
$\frac{\text{μMole Equiv Perc Bound}}{\text{G Liver Protein}}$	0.147±0.00	0.021±0.001	7.0

Conclusion. Consistent with data on other halogenated hydrocarbons Perc and VDC are hypothesized to be metabolized to their respective epoxides. Epoxides by virtue of their structure are reactive intermediates which have the capability of attacking and binding to sites on tissue macromolecules such as protein, RNA, DNA, and lipid. Such macromolecular interactions can lead ultimately to toxicity and/or carcinogenicity. Since the initial metabolic step in the metabolism of Perc and VDC appears to be an activation process, the extent of formation of the epoxide will presumably influence the toxicity of Perc and VDC. Therefore, the species with the greatest extent of metabolism of Perc and VDC should be most sensitive.

These results indicate that the species sensitivity to the tumorigenicity of Perc and VDC is correlated with the greater extent of metabolism of these two chemicals by the mouse. In addition, the tumorigenicity of Perc and VDC with respect to their target organs is correlated with greater macromolecular binding in mice than rats.

It has long been known that the smaller the animal the more rapid is its rate of oxidative metabolism. Since the metabolism of Perc and VDC appear to be an activation process, these results support the predicted greater sensitivity of the mouse compared to the rat.

Macromolecular interactions (tumorigenic mechanisms)

Generally, animals are administered a test chemical and tumors are observed at some later date with little consideration for the mechanism of tumorigenicity. Understanding the mechanism of tumor formation is critical in assessing the risk of exposure because different protective measures are indicated depending on whether the predominant mechanism is genetic or epigenetic. Tumors may arise in animals by either genetic or epigenetic mechanisms or a combination of both. The genetic mechanism is most simply described by the somatic cell mutation theory of chemical carcinogenesis. The chemical interacts with DNA and causes somatic cell mutations. Following replication these mutagenic effects may result in transformed cells which ultimately lead to a tumor. DNA repair mechanisms are normal defense mechanisms which inhibit the progression toward transformation.

Evidence indicates strongly that DNA repair is a primary defense against somatic cell mutations which may lead to cancer. The work of Cleaver[15,16] (1968; 1969) and Maher et al.[17], (1976) have clearly demonstrated that it is the deficient DNA repair mechanisms of skin fibroblast cells that cause individuals with Xeroderma pigmentosum to be ultrasensitive to ultraviolet light (sunlight) induced skin cancers. Even more importantly their studies have indicated that competent DNA repair in normal cells prevents mutagenic events caused by UV-light or various chemical carcinogens.

Similarly, tumorigenicity absent at low doses following exposure to a geno-toxic chemical may become evident only at high doses after the enzymatic DNA repair mechanisms have been saturated. Thus even for genetically active chemicals these concepts illustrate why the risk may decrease disproportionately with decreasing dose when tumors are associated only at high doses where the normal defense and repair mechanisms of the body have been overwhelmed.

In addition to genotoxic effects, chemicals can also produce tumors through epigenetic mechanisms such as cytotoxicity. In this case, tissue damage occurs to such an extent as to cause cell death and subsequent cell regeneration.

During chronic administration of cytotoxic agents, DNA replication is stimu-lated greatly in the affected tissues. Since there is a tiny, but still finite chance for error in each replication cycle, the net effect is to increase the spontaneous mutation rate and ultimately enhance the tumorigenic response.

Another consequence of increasing cell division is that the relative rates of DNA repair and DNA replication are altered. This may be very important be-cause there is evidence that the existing DNA repair systems may fail to recognize DNA alterations after replication. Consequently, repair becomes less effective in protecting cells from the consequences of genetic damage after cellular replication. This is shown by the work of Berman et al.[18], (1978) and Weymouth and Loeb[19] (1978) who found that increased division of normal cells in-creases their susceptibility to mutagenic events. This is also demonstrated by the studies of McCormick[20] (1979) who found that momentarily arresting cell division to give added time for DNA repair greatly diminished the mutational action of UV light.

These data stress the importance of DNA synthesis and subsequent cellular replication in fixing lesions present in DNA leading to mutagenic events. An in vivo correlate emphasizing the importance of DNA synthesis and cellular replication in enhancing a carcinogenic process is illustrated by the inhibition of dimethylbenzanthracene (DMBA) induced skin carcinogenesis by anti-inflam-matory steroids. Synthetic anti-inflammatory steroids were shown to decrease inflammation, cellular proliferation and hyperplasia induced by the tumor promotor 12-0-tetradecanoylphorbol-13-acetate (TPA) and effectively prevent DMBA induced skin cancer in mice (Slaga et al.[21], 1978).

Further indication that increased cell division can be significant comes from the observations of Laroye[22] (1974) who found that many cancers develop in chronically inflamed or scarred tissue (colonic cancer in patients with ulcerative colitis or squamous cell carcinomas in ulcers of burn scars). Berenblum[23] (1929) observed that repeated freezing of the skin with dry-ice induced tumors, and Peraino et al.[24], (1973) reported the enhancement of "spontaneous" tumors in mice by dietary phenobarbital, a treatment also known to stimulate DNA synthesis. Similarly, the tumor yield from a known genetic carcinogen is enhanced greatly after partial hepatectomy (Date et al.[25], 1976) or by physical trauma at the site of initiation (Berenblum[26] 1944).

Several procedures have been under investigation in our laboratory in order to determine their utility in indicating the mechanism of tumorigenesis in mice administered VDC or Perc. Primary attention has been focused on _in vivo_ procedures since these appear to have the greatest potential for understanding the tumorigenic process in intact animals. Four such indicators will be described. The results from the VDC and Perc studies were compared to the known genotoxic, hepatocarcinogenic chemical dimethylnitrosamine (DMN).

For studies of the genetic mechanism, animals were exposed to the radio-labeled chemical. The DNA from the target tissue was extracted and purified and the amount of radioactivity associated with the purified DNA reflected the degree of direct DNA interaction. An alternative procedure that indirectly measures genetic damage was also used. In this procedure, DNA repair was measured and used as an indicator of previous DNA damage. DNA repair systems recognize damaged DNA, and cause the damaged area to be excised and replaced with normal DNA. Although this DNA repair procedure is not currently as sensitive as measuring a direct DNA-chemical interaction, one important advantage is that this procedure does not require a radioactive form of every chemical to be tested.

Chronic tissue damage causes individual cells to continually die and be replaced by new cells. Consequently, for detecting the contribution of this epigenetic (cytotoxic) mechanism, DNA synthesis in the affected tissues was measured. The increase in DNA synthesis was quantitated by using the DNA precursor ^{3}H-thymidine.

Another consequence of tissue damage is the induction of histopathologic alterations in the cells of the affected tissue. When increased DNA synthesis and nontumor related histopathology can both be observed in a tissue, the contribution of an epigenetic mechanism of tumor formation may be inferred.

VDC genetic effect. The levels of radioactivity which were incorporated into DNA purified from the tissues of animals exposed to ^{14}C-VDC for single 6 hour inhalation exposures are summarized in Table 5. VDC alkylation of DNA was very low in kidney and liver of both rats and mice. The highest level of alkylation was observed in the kidneys of mice exposed to 50 ppm VDC but this was much less than the DNA alkylation observed by Pegg and Hui[27] (1978) in rats given 3 mg/kg DMN intraperitoneally.

After exposure to either 50 or 10 ppm ^{14}C-VDC, the DNA from the livers of mice contained 5 to 10 fold less radioactivity than the DNA from the kidneys (Table 5). In rats exposed to 10 ppm ^{14}C-VDC, the DNA of kidney contained about 2 fold greater activity than the DNA of liver. Compared to mice exposed to 10 ppm ^{14}C-VDC, about 6 fold less radioactivity was found in the DNA of rat kidneys, while similar amounts were found in the DNA from the livers of both species (Table 5).

TABLE 5

DNA DAMAGE PRODUCED BY ^{14}C-VDC AND ^{14}C-DMN IN RATS AND MICE

Treatment/Tissue	DPM/MG DNA	Alkylations/Nucleotide x10^6
50 PPM VDC (Mouse)		
Kidney	88	30
Liver	18	6.1
10 PPM VDC (Mouse)		
Kidney	34	11
Liver	2.8	0.94
10 PPM VDC (Rat)		
Kidney	5.9	2.0
Liver	2.6	0.87
3 Mg/Kg DMN (Rat)[a]		
Liver	-	1000[a]

[a] Calculated from data of Pegg and Hui[27] (1978), assuming that the alkylation of guanine is typical of other bases.

TABLE 6

DNA REPAIR IN TISSUES OF ANIMALS EXPOSED TO DMN OR VDC: RATIO OF TREATED ANIMALS TO CONTROLS

Dose/Tissue	(A) ^{3}H-TdR Only Mean Spec. Act±SEM (Treated/control)	(B) Correction Factor (95% Confidence Limit)	(C) ^{3}H-TdR + HU Mean Spec. Act±SEM (Treated/control)	(D) Repair Ratio (C) Divided by (B) (Observed/expect) 95% Conf. Lim.
VDC-50 ppm				
Kidney	5.30±1.15 (n=4) / 9.45±2.28 (n=3)	0.561±0.285*	1.74±0.0488 (n=4) / 2.25±0.0917 (n=4)	1.38±0.090*
Liver	9.69±1.50 (n=4) / 12.9±1.63 (n=4)	0.751±0.275	16.0±2.13 (n=4) / 18.4±0.434 (n=4)	1.16±0.363
VDC-10 ppm				
Kidney	14.7±1.20 (n=6) / 14.6±1.86 (n=6)	1.01±0.164	2.67±0.197 (n=3) / 2.27±0.640 (n=4)	1.16±0.255
Liver	17.2±2.36 (n=6) / 15.6±1.28 (n=6)	1.10±0.305	2.16±0.195 (n=3) / 2.57±0.378 (n=4)	0.764±0.222

*Ratio is significantly different than 1.0, t-test with p <0.05.

TABLE 6 (Continued)

DNA REPAIR IN TISSUES OF ANIMALS EXPOSED TO DMN OR VDC: RATIO OF TREATED ANIMALS TO CONTROLS

Dose/Tissue	(A) ^{3}H-TdR Only Mean Spec. Act±SEM	(B) Correction Factor (95% Confidence Limit)	(C) ^{3}H-TdR + HU Mean Spec. Act±SEM	(D) Repair Ratio (C) Divided by (B)
DMN-20 mg/kg				
Liver	$\dfrac{34.4\pm1.03}{80.5\pm1.92}\ \begin{array}{l}(n=3)\\(n=3)\end{array}$	0.427±0.038*	$\dfrac{44.7\pm4.51}{14.2\pm2.64}\ \begin{array}{l}(n=3)\\(n=3)\end{array}$	7.37±2.16*
DMN-10 mg/kg				
Liver	$\dfrac{27.0\pm2.94}{41.6\pm14.5}\ \begin{array}{l}(n=4)\\(n=4)\end{array}$	0.649±0.166*	$\dfrac{15.5\pm1.95}{7.85\pm1.28}\ \begin{array}{l}(n=4)\\(n=3)\end{array}$	3.04±0.896*
DMN-3 mg/kg				
Liver	$\dfrac{19.0\pm1.41}{25.0\pm4.93}\ \begin{array}{l}(n=6)\\(n=6)\end{array}$	0.760±0.114*	$\dfrac{9.57\pm2.32}{7.85\pm1.28}\ \begin{array}{l}(n=3)\\(n=3)\end{array}$	1.60±1.14

*Ratio is significantly different than 1.0, t-test with $p < 0.05$.

Using ^{3}H-thymidine (^{3}H-TdR), DNA repair was measured directly in animals exposed to VDC (50 and 10 ppm) or injected with DMN (20, 10, and 3 mg/kg, ip).
DMN treatment caused a dramatic increase in the level of hydroxyurea-resistant
^{3}H-thymidine incorporation; this is due primarily to "repair" replication,
since hydroxyurea inhibits normal replication in vivo. The relative increase
in repair synthesis caused by DMN, after correction for the effects of DMN on
nonrepair synthesis as outlined in the "Methods" section of this paper, was more
than 7 fold, and this increase was dose-related (Table 6). In contrast, a much
smaller increase in the repair ratio occurred after exposure of mice to VDC.
The only statistically significant increase caused by VDC was that occurring in
the kidneys of the mice exposed to 50 ppm. DNA repair was not significantly
altered in the livers of the mice exposed to 50 ppm VDC, or in the kidneys or
livers of mice exposed to 10 ppm VDC.

VDC epigenetic effects. A second procedure which measures increased DNA
synthesis was used to evaluate nongenetic effects of VDC exposure. The results
of these experiments are summarized in Table 7. In each case, the rate of DNA
synthesis in the treated group is compared to the rate of DNA synthesis in an
untreated control group. Exposure for 6 hours to 50 ppm VDC caused about a 25
fold increase in DNA synthesis in the mouse kidney, while DNA in the kidneys of
mice exposed to 10 ppm of VDC was increased about 8 times above control.
Effects on DNA synthesis in the mouse liver were much smaller: 2.4 and 1.2
times control at 50 and 10 ppm VDC, respectively. Neither of the VDC effects on
DNA synthesis in mouse liver was statistically significant. DMN also failed to
significantly increase DNA synthesis in mouse liver (Table 7).

Rats exposed to 10 ppm VDC exhibited much smaller effects on DNA synthesis
than mice exposed to the same concentration. In the rat kidney, DNA synthesis
was 2.2 times the control value, while DNA synthesis in the liver of VDC-exposed
rats was less than that observed in controls (Table 7). DNA synthesis changes
in the kidney of the rats were statistically significant, but the changes in the
DNA synthesis of rat liver were not.

Histopathologic examination of kidneys from mice showed that degenerative and
regenerative changes were induced following exposure to 50 ppm VDC (Table 8).
Some pathologic effects of VDC and DMN were also seen in mouse liver (Table 8)
but these were rated as mild or minimal.

TABLE 7

DNA SYNTHESIS IN TISSUES OF VDC AND DMN EXPOSED RATS AND MICE
(TREATED/CONTROL)

Dose/Tissue	Mean Spec. Act±SEM	Ratio
VDC-50 PPM (Mice)		
Kidney	$\dfrac{272\pm15.2\ (n=4)}{11.0\pm2.63\ (n=2)}$	24.7**
Liver	$\dfrac{26.9\pm5.40\ (n=4)}{11.0\pm3.08\ (n=2)}$	2.45
VDC-10 PPM (Mice)		
Kidney	$\dfrac{95.0\pm15.2\ (n=5)}{12.3\pm2.41\ (n=5)}$	7.72**
Liver	$\dfrac{17.6\pm2.96\ (n=6)}{14.7\pm1.95\ (n=5)}$	1.20
VDC-10 PPM (Rats)		
Kidney	$\dfrac{23.8\pm3.7\ (n=3)}{10.8\pm3.8\ (n=3)}$	2.20**
Liver	$\dfrac{16.3\pm0.87\ (n=3)}{18.6\pm2.3\ (n=3)}$	0.88
DMN-20 mg/kg (Mice)		
Liver	(Died before 48 hours)	
DMN-10 mg/kg (Mice)		
Liver	$\dfrac{94.0\pm30.1\ (n=3)}{47.8\pm17.6\ (n=4)}$	1.97
DMN-3 mg/kg (Mice)		
Liver	$\dfrac{54.5\pm11.0\ (n=3)}{47.8\pm17.6\ (n=4)}$	1.14

**Ratio significantly greater than 1.0 ($p < 0.05$, t-test).

DNA synthesis was estimated by determining the specific radio-activity of DNA following ^{3}H-thymidine (^{3}H-TdR) injection. ^{3}H-TdR was injected 48 hours after the treatment suspected of causing cyto-toxicity. A positive response is indicated by an increased rate of incorporation of ^{3}H-TdR into DNA relative to a control group, resulting in a ratio greater than 1.0.

TABLE 8

SUMMARY OF HISTOPATHOLOGY FINDINGS IN TISSUES FROM MICE
TREATED WITH VDC AND DMN[a]

Exposure	Hours Post-Exposure	Histologic Findings	
		Kidneys	Liver
VDC, 50 PPM, 6 hr	0	Toxic nephrosis	Slight centrilobular swelling
	24	Progressing nephrosis	
	48	Increased mitotic figures with early regeneration occurring	No effect
	96	Regeneration apparent	
VDC, 10 PPM, 6 hr	0	Slight dilation, swelling	
	96	Nephrosis-variable 0-20% tubules affected	
DMN, 10 mg/kg, ip	4		Centrilobular swelling Hyaline degeneration
	52		Accentuated lobular pattern, necrosis minimal or absent
DMN, 3 mg/kg, ip	4		Centrilobular swelling
	48		No effect

[a] 3-6 animals were given the indicated treatment and then sacrificed at the
   appropriate time.
Tissue slices were prepared by standard histochemical procedures.

Perc genetic effects. Following a single oral dose of ^{14}C-Perc (500 mg/kg)
or a 6 hour inhalation exposure (600 ppm) no detectable radioactivity was observed to be associated with purified hepatic DNA. The detection limit was
10.0 and 14.5 alkylated nucleotides/10^6 nucleotides respectively. DNA repair
was not measured with Perc because DNA repair is a less sensitive parameter
than measuring direct DNA alkylation, and Perc did not show any evidence for
DNA alkylation.

Perc epigenetic effects. Rats and mice received 12 oral administrations of
0 or 500 mg/kg of perchloroethylene in a 16 day period. This dose of perchloroethylene was approximately equivalent to the low dose level used in the NCI
carcinogen bioassay for perchloroethylene. Microscopic treatment related
changes were observed in the livers of mice and included an accentuated lobular
pattern, hepatocellular swelling, altered cytoplasmic staining, microvesicula-

tion and microvacuolation of the cytoplasm in the centrilobular region. Approximately 1/2 of the lobule was affected. In contrast, 4 of 5 rats showed no evidence of hepatocellular degeneration following histopathologic examination. The liver weight/body weight ratio was significantly increased in perchloroethylene treated mice but not in rats when compared to their respective controls (Table 9). To assess the effect of perchloroethylene on hepatic DNA synthesis, ^{3}H-thymidine was injected i.p. 18 hours after the last dose of perchloroethylene, 6 hours prior to sacrifice. Hepatic DNA synthesis, expressed as dpm of ^{3}H-thymidine/µg of DNA, was significantly increased approximately 2-fold in the perchloroethylene-treated mice compared to control values, whereas no difference in hepatic DNA synthesis was observed between treated and control rats. The significant increase in hepatic DNA synthesis in mice coupled with the histopathology observed in this species indicates increased cell division in the liver.

TABLE 9

EFFECTS OF PERCHLOROETHYLENE ON LIVER WEIGHTS AND HEPATIC DNA SYNTHESIS IN MICE AND RATS FOLLOWING 12 ORAL DOSES*

Dose, 12 in 16 days	Liver Weight/ Body Weight	DNA Synthesis DPM/µg DNA
Mouse		
0	0.040±0.002	65±34
500 mg/kg/day	0.050±0.002**	118±22**
Rat		
0	0.038±0.003	63±11
500 mg/kg/day	0.040±0.003	65±17

*Mean ±SD (n=3-5): ^{3}H-thymidine 1000 µCi/kg, 20 Ci/mmole, i.p. 6 hours prior to sacrifice.
**p $\leq$0.05; Student's t-test

Conclusion. The most striking observation in these studies was the low degree of DNA alkylation in target tissues detected following VDC or Perc (nondetectable) in comparison to DMN. Similarly, DNA repair was markedly increased in the liver following DMN treatment and only slightly increased in the kidneys of mice following VDC exposure.

In contrast, both VDC and Perc showed significant cytotoxic activity by increased DNA synthesis in the organs which developed tumors. The significance of this observation is increased by the finding that similar increases in DNA synthesis were not seen in organs of the mouse where tumors did not develop. Furthermore, the rat does not develop tumors from exposure to VDC or Perc by the routes of administration employed in these studies, and this animal does not exhibit similar quantitative effects on DNA synthesis seen with the mouse.

Histopathologic evaluation revealed that severe tissue damage was produced in the kidneys of mice exposed to VDC, while slight to moderate damage was seen in the liver of animals exposed to Perc. Of particular importance was the observation of Maltoni et al.[3], (1977) that in his studies with VDC "there was a clear-cut direct relationship between the degree of toxic (tissue damage) and carcinogenic effects in the different animal species and sexes considered." Kidney tumors were only observed at 25 ppm and not at 10 ppm where toxic kidney effects were absent or greatly diminished. Unfortunately, the studies conducted by the National Cancer Institute (USA) for Perc were not conducted at lower doses which did not produce indications of toxic liver injury. Thus from the available data it is not possible to ascertain whether tumors would have occurred at subhepatotoxic doses.

A summary of the four parameters used to differentiate between genotoxic and epigenetic (cytotoxic) mechanisms of tumorigenesis for VDC and Perc is shown in Table 10.

TABLE 10

SUMMARY FOR GENETIC VERSUS EPIGENETIC MECHANISMS OF TUMORIGENICITY
OF VDC AND PERC

		VDC-50 ppm	Perc-500 mg/kg
DNA damage (alkylated nucleotides/10^6 nucleotides)	Genotoxic Indications	30	Not detected. <10
DNA repair (% increase) (Due to DNA damage)		38	-[a]
DNA synthesis (Due to tissue injury)	Epigenetic (Cytotoxic) Indications	25X	2X
Histopathology		Severe	Slight-moderate

[a] Not determined.

The absence of significant genetic effects, coupled with the presence of significant increases in DNA synthesis and tissue damage, indicates that a cytotoxic, epigenetic mechanism plays a major role in the induction of tumors in mice exposed to Perc. For VDC, cytotoxicity also appears to be a primary contributing factor to the induction of kidney tumors in mice. This is supported by the present study which demonstrated marked cytotoxic responses (increased DNA synthesis and histopathology) taken in conjunction with the studies of Maltoni et al. (1977) where tumors were only observed in the kidney at doses which produced tissue injury.

SUMMARY

The results of these studies further support the concept that VDC and Perc are activated in the body to reactive intermediate metabolites which are responsible for toxicity, including carcinogenicity. The pharmacokinetic studies have revealed that the mouse metabolizes and therefore produces more reactive metabolite(s) than the rat. This results in an enhanced binding to intracellular macromolecules in the organs susceptible to tumor formation in the mouse. These pharmacokinetic results are consistent with the sensitivity of the mouse and resistance of the rat to the tumorigenic effects of VDC and Perc.

Investigations into the mechanism of tumor formation in the mouse has revealed that all materials being identified as animal carcinogens are not equally dangerous. This is because there are at least two distinct mechanisms capable of inducing tumors, and these mechanisms vary in their relative contribution with each chemical. The objective procedures for estimating the contribution from each mechanism indicate that recurrent tissue injury plays a major role in tumors induced in mice by VDC and Perc. Thus it appears that these tumors arise by epigenetic mechanisms.

The implications of this mechanism are: first, that tumors produced by VDC or Perc should be preceded by visible signs of tissue injury, and second, that exposures to these chemicals at levels which do not result in recurrent tissue damage should not produce cancer. Consequently, safety factors such as are currently employed to protect against organ toxicity should also be effective in protecting against any carcinogenic activity of VDC or Perc.

These concepts are important when using animal data obtained at high dose levels to assess the potential harmful effects at much lower levels encountered in the occupational environment and by the public at large. As more work is conducted to test this hypothesis it is likely that chemical carcinogens will illustrate an entire spectrum of activity relative to the roles of genetic and

88

epigenetic mechanisms. Chemicals such as DDT, chloroform, CCl_4 and saccharin, to name a few, are likely to be epigenetic carcinogens. Other animal carcinogens may show both genetic and epigenetic components of their tumorigenic mechanism. In that case it will be important to assess the relative contributions of each mechanism to determine appropriate levels to prevent adverse health effects.

REFERENCES

1. Viola, P. L. and Caputo, A. (1977) Carcinogenicity Studies on Vinylidene Chloride, Environ. Hlth. Perspectives, 21, 45-47.

2. Rampy, L. W., Quast, J. F., Humiston, C. G., Balmer, M. F., and Schwetz, B. A. (1977) "Interim Results of Two Year Toxicological Studies in Rats of Vinylidene Chloride Incorporated in the Drinking Water or Administered by Repeated Inhalation, Environ. Hlth. Perspectives, 21, 33-43.

3. Maltoni, C., Cotti, G., Morisi, L., and Chieco, P. (1977) "Carcinogenicity Bioassays of Vinylidene Chloride: Research Plan and Early Results." La Medicina del Lavoro, 68(#4), 241-262.

4. Lee, C. C., Bhandari, J. C., Winston, J. M., Dixon, R. L., and Woods, J. S. (1978) Carcinogenicity of Vinyl Chloride and Vinylidene Chloride, J. Toxicol. and Environ. Health, 4, 15-30.

5. NCI (1977) Bioassay of Tetrachloroethylene for Possible Carcinogenicity, DHEW Publication No. 77-813.

6. Rampy, L. W., Quast, J. F., Leong, B.J.K. and Gehring, P. J. Results of Long Term Inhalation Studies On Rats of 1,1,1-trichloroethane and perchloroethylene formulations. Presented at the 1st. International Congress on Toxicology, Toronto, Canada, April, 1977.

7. McKenna, M. J., Zempel, J. A. and Gehring, P. J. (1979) A Comparison of the Pharmacokinetics of Inhaled Vinylidene Chloride in Rats and Mice. Toxicology Laboratory, Dow Chemical Company, Midland, MI (in manuscript).

8. Reitz, R. H., Watanabe, P. G., McKenna, M. J., Quast, J. F. and Gehring, P. J. (1979) Effects of Vinylidene Chloride on DNA Synthesis and DNA Repair in the Rat and Mouse: A Comparative Study with Dimethylnitrosamine. Toxicology Laboratory, Dow Chemical Company, Midland, MI (in manuscript).

9. Schumann, A. M., Watanabe, P. G. and Quast, J. F. (1979) The Pharmacokinetics and Macromolecular Interactions of Perchloroethylene in Mice and Rats as Related to Oncogenicity. Toxicology Laboratory, Dow Chemical Company, Midland, MI (in manuscript).

10. Jollow, D. J., Mitchell, J. R., Potter, W. Z., Davis, D. C., Gillette, J. R. and Brodie, B. B. (1973) Acetaminophen Hepatic Necrosis. II. J. Pharmacol. Exp. Therap., 187, 195-202.

11. McKenna, M. J., Zempel, J. A. Madrid, E. O. and Gehring, P. J. (1978) The Pharmacokinetics of ^{14}C-Vinylidene Chloride in Rats Following Inhalation Exposure. Toxicol. Appl. Pharmacol., 45, 599-610.

12. Marmur, J. (1961) "A Procedure for the Isolation of Deoxyribonucleic Acid from Micro-organisms", J. Mol. Biol., 3, 208-218.

13. Arfellini, G., Grilli, G., (1978) In Vivo DNA Repair after N-Methyl-N-Nitrosourea Administration to Rats of Different Ages, Zeitschrift fur Krebsforschung and Klinische Onkologie, 91, 157-164.

14. McKenna, M. J., Watanabe, P. G., and Gehring, P. J. (1977) Pharmacokinetics of Vinylidene Chloride in the Rat, Environ. Health Perspec., 21, 99-105.

15. Cleaver, J. E. (1968) Defective Repair Replication of DNA in Xeroderma Pigmentosum, Nature, 28, 652-656.

16. Cleaver, J. E. (1969) Xeroderma Pigmentosum: A Human Disease in Which an Initial Stage of DNA Repair is Defective, Proc. Nat. Acad. Sci. USA, 63, 428-435.

17. Maher, V. M., Curren, R. D., Quellette, L. M., and McCormick, J. J. (1976) Effect of DNA Repair on the Frequency of Mutations in Human Cells by Ultraviolet Irradiation and by Chemical Carcinogens, In Fundamentals of Cancer Prevention, Plenum Press, New York.

18. Berman, J. J., Tong, C., and Williams, G. M. (1978) Enhancement of Mutagenesis During Cell Replication of Cultured Liver Epithelial Cells, Cancer Letters, 4, 277-283.

19. Weymouth, L. A. and Loeb, L. A. (1978) Mutagenesis During In Vitro DNA Synthesis, Proc. Nat. Acad. Sci., 75, 1924-1928.

20. McCormick, J. J. (1979) Evidence that DNA Excision Repair Processes in Human Fibroblasts Can Eliminate Potentially Cytotoxic and Mutagenic Lesions, Reported at the 10th Annual Meeting of Environmental Mutagen Society, New Orleans, LA, USA, March 8-12, 1979.

21. Slaga, T. J., Fischer, S. M., Viaje, A., Berry, D. L., Bracken, W. M., LeClerc, S., and Miller, D. R. (1978) Inhibition of Tumor Promotion by Anti-Inflammatory Agents: An Approach to the Biochemical Mechanism of Promotion, In Carcinogenesis, Vol. 2, Mechanisms of Tumor Promotion and Carcinogenesis, pp. 173-195, eds, T. J. Slaga, A. Sivak, R. K. Boutwell, Raven Press, New York.

22. Laroye, G. J. (1974) How Efficient is Immunologic Surveillance Against Cancer and Why Does it Fail, The Lancet, 1097-1100.

23. Berenblum, I. (1929) Tumor-Formation Following Freezing with Carbon Dioxide Snow, Brit. J. Exper. Path., 10, 179-184.

24. Peraino, C., Fry, R.J.M., and Staffeld, E. (1973) Enhancement of Spontaneous Hepatic Tumorigenesis in C3H Mice by Dietary Phenobarbital, J. Nat. Cancer Inst., 51, 1349-1350.

25. Date, P. A., Gotoskar, S. V., and Bhide, S. V. (1976) Effect of Partial Hepatectomy on Tumor Incidence and Metabolism of Mice Fed Thioacetamide. J. Nat. Cancer Inst., 56, 493-495.

26. Berenblum, I. (1944) Irritation and Carcinogenesis, Arch. Pathol., 38, 233-244.

27. Pegg, A. E., and Hui, G. (1978) Formation and Subsequent Removal of O^6-Methylguanine from Deoxyribonucleic Acid in Rat Liver and Kidney after Small Doses of Dimethylnitrosamine, Biochem. J., 173, 739-748.

© 1980 Elsevier/North-Holland Biomedical Press
The Scientific Basis of Toxicity Assessment
H. Witschi, editor.

BEHAVIORAL TOXICOLOGY: A CRITICAL APPRAISAL

STATA NORTON
Department of Pharmacology, University of Kansas Medical Center, College of
Health Sciences and Hospital, Kansas City, Kansas 66103 (U.S.A.)

INTRODUCTION

The major problem confronting behavioral toxicologists today is the lack
of an organized body of knowledge about sensitive, reliable methods which
relate predictably to knowledge from other disciplines, e.g. neurophysiology,
biochemistry and morphology. Of the functional impairments which may
result from exposure to chemicals, behavioral changes are considered of
great importance. Why behavior is receiving attention is uncertain. It may
be because behavior is considered to be a sensitive measure of CNS damage,
because behavioral change is a matter of great concern or because alteration
in behavior is a common toxic effect. Any of these reasons may be invoked.

The problem is acute. Various regulatory agencies may promulgate regulations requiring behavioral tests for which there is no adequate scientific
basis. Unlike other areas of biological science, there does not seem to be
general agreement that behavior is the function of the central nervous system,
or at least represents a major portion of CNS function. The concept of organ
and function as a joined area for study seems fundamental to all scientific
investigation of complex, multicellular organisms. For the purposes of this
presentation behavior will be defined as the output of the central nervous
system resulting in coordinated movement of the organism via the musculoskele-
tal system. This definition is intended to include all learned and unlearned
behaviors from "conscious, emotionally-directed behaviors", whatever they may
be, to centrally-mediated reflexes.

Historically, methods used for the study of behavior have been divided into
methods for conditioned and observed behavior. Each of these can be subdivided
(Table 1). Operant conditioning espoused by B. F. Skinner has been the dominant force in experimental psychology in this country for some time. Pavlovian
conditioning, in its classical form, has been established in an equal way in
Russian psychology but here is almost restricted to active and passive avoidance conditioning. Ethological methods, first popularized by Konrad Lorenz
in Europe, have had a limited success but in this country the methods of
ethology often cannot be distinguished from the older observational methods

long practiced by field zoologists in both Europe and the United States. The
classic studies of Karl Von Frisch on communication in bees are a good example
of the latter. With the advent of the tranquilizer age in 1954 there was a
wide-spread academic and industrial effort to unravel the mechanisms of actions
of the new CNS drugs and to find new and better psychoactive drugs using behavioral tests. The result of this was the development of tests which were
capable of detecting single exposures to pharmacologic agents which disappeared
in a few hours, leaving the CNS without a permanent scar or time to adapt.
Furthermore the prototype drug, chlorpromazine, was already available. It was
not necessary to know the mechanism of action of chlorpromazine as long as a
new compound possessed the same "pharmacologic profile".

TABLE 1

HISTORICAL CATEGORIES OF BEHAVIORAL TESTS

1. Conditioned Behavior
a) Operant (Skinner)
b) Pavlovian (Pavlov)
2. Observed Behavior
a) Ethological (Lorenz)
b) Zoological (Von Frisch)

Now there is a new problem. Behavioral toxicology is in the limelight and
is being considered as a sensitive method for predicting hazard from environmental chemicals. There is some inituitive feeling that behavior must be a
subtle or sensitive way to monitor early damage from many chemicals. Scientific data supporting this view are not only scanty but the available evidence
often flatly contradicts this assumption. Psychoactive drugs may enter and
leave the CNS readily and may interact by design with the synaptic areas of
neurons, resulting in specific behavioral effects. No such biochemistry can
be assumed for many toxic chemicals which inadvertently cause CNS effects.
Neither the assumption of reversibility nor of synaptic site of action may be
valid for a toxic agent. The possibility of irreversible neuronal damage,
presumed to be absent in the short-term response to most psychoactive drugs
must be considered in exposures to toxic substances. The concept of short-
term, reversible activity predominates in pharmacology, but behavioral toxicology must be concerned with behavior which returns to normal in the presence of

a toxic agent or the permanent damage caused by the agent. Thus behavioral
methods with recognized validity for psychopharmacological testing cannot be
assumed to be equally valid for toxicology.

A second difference of behavioral toxicology from behavioral pharmacology
is that behavioral toxicology has, in its short lifetime, become strongly
associated with teratology so that a new area of study, behavioral teratology,
has been defined. The unexpected and unplanned nature of many toxic exposures
in man makes the risk to the developing organism or neonate of special
interest. Therefore no discussion of behavioral toxicology is complete
without consideration of preweaning behavior of neonatally or prenatally
exposed animals as well as the more usual tests in adult animals.

TABLE 2

PREWEANING BEHAVIORAL AND DEVELOPMENTAL TESTS IN THE RAT

Postnatal Day for Onset of Response	Condition Tested	
	Behavioral	Developmental
2-5	Surface righting; pivoting; time nursing; time awake	ear flap opening
6-10	Crawling; homing; cliff avoidance; reflex suspension; forelimb placing	
11-15	Auditory startle; swimming; walking; emergence from nest box	eye opening incisor eruption
16-21	Traversing narrow path; mid-air righting	
22+	Rotorod; open field	weaning

METHODOLOGICAL CONSIDERATIONS

Preweaning behavior

Normal development of reflex and complex motor behaviors in mice and rats
is covered in several excellent articles[1,2,3,4]. Information is also available on early development in the dog[5]. Some of the behaviors of the preweanling rat which have been used in toxicological studies are listed in Table 2.
Exposure to hydroxyurea during gestation[6], neonatal carbon monoxide[7], and

maternal restraint stress[8] had little effect on any of these early behaviors
in the rat. Body weight was not reduced in rats exposed to hydroxyurea in
utero or carbon monoxide at 5 days of postnatal age but was reduced in offspring of mothers subjected to restraint stress. Of the parameters measured
in these studies, only amount of ambulation and time awake in the nest were
significantly altered by carbon monoxide. The other behaviors examined in the
3 studies were not significantly changed. The failure to find more effects in
tests of developing behaviors agrees with other generalizations that perinatal
damage to the CNS becomes more obvious when the animals are mature than when
they are young[9,10]. However, some investigators have found retarded development in preweanling rats after prenatal exposure to mercury[11] or lead[12].

No specific period in the gestational or preweaning phase is uniquely
appropriate for exposure of developing animals to toxic agents. However,
there are some guidelines which can be considered based on the extensive
knowledge of embryogenesis and postnatal development of the CNS in the rat and
mouse. The CNS is laid down in a rostral direction from the spinal cord,
beginning at about the ninth day of the 21-day gestational period of these two
species. Once the brain stem is laid down by around the thirteenth day,
viable embryos can be produced with varying degrees of malformed structures in
the diencephalon and telencephalon. Even after day 13 the structural consequences to the CNS from exposure to toxic agents is understandably complex.
The time span of origin of the different groups of neurons, the selectivity,
or lack of it, and the duration of the toxic agent are major factors contributing to the result. An extensive literature is available from which only a few
papers are listed[13,14,15,16,17,18,19,20,21].

Development of adult behavior

The transition time between the preweanling rat and the mature adult rat
may be called the juvenile period. The central nervous system of rats is
functionally, morphologically and biochemically mature at about 4 months of
postnatal age[10]. From the viewpoint of the behavioral toxicologist it is
important to know the ontogeny of adult behaviors. A list of some behavioral
tests employed in toxicology is given in Table 3. If animals are tested over
a period of time during which a behavior is maturing rapidly, the testing is
being carried out on a shifting baseline, whereas adult behavior may be more
stable over the same length of time. Some studies have been carried out
specifically to determine the ontogeny of selected behaviors.

TABLE 3

POSTWEANING BEHAVIORAL TESTS

---

1. Conditioned behavior
    a. Learning and memory

        Operant conditioning; mazes (Lashley III, T or Y);

        active and passive avoidance (shuttle box)

    b. Motor responding

        Operant conditioning; mazes (Lashley III, T or Y);

        active and passive avoidance (shuttle box)

    c. Sensory discrimination

        Operant conditioning (auditory, visual or proprioceptive

        systems)

---

2. Observed behavior
    a. Emotion-associated behavior

        Open field; aggression; social behavior

    b. Locomotor activity (exploratory or circadian)

        Open field; activity wheel; stabilimeter; photocell maze;

        photographic record

    c. Reflex systems and gait measurement

        Auditory startle; walking patterns; inclined or vertical

        plane; rotorod; swimming behavior

Active avoidance and passive avoidance in shuttle boxes are among the most common tests used in evaluation of postnatal behavior following prenatal exposure[22]. Simple active avoidance tasks which involve escape in response to a light or buzzer to avoid foot shock require learning. This type of learning can occur early in postnatal development. Acquisition of simple escape responding is considered easier than passive avoidance which requires learning to withhold a response. Active avoidance responding (both 1-way and 2-way) and passive avoidance responding improves with age. Many studies of avoidance responding include measures of both trials for learning the response and retention of the learned response over time from 24 hours to 30 days (sometimes called memory). Testing in these experiments cannot begin until locomotion has developed to carry out the required response. Marked improvement occurs in correct responding rates from 15-17 days to 32-37 days of postnatal age[23,24]. Retention improves with age up to 100 days[25]. When older animals

are tested (480 days of age) some decrement may develop[26]. Although the
generalization is valid that there is an increase in performance with early
development, the results with varying methodology are not uniform. Mysliveček
and Hassmanová[27] have recently proposed that responding in tests of active 1-
way avoidance is optimum at 4 to 6 weeks of age in the rat with poorer performance in 3 month old rats. This decrement occurs before the brain is fully
mature.

The open field test is widely used in studies of animal behavior. In a
recent survey it was the most frequently reported test[22]. Animals are placed
in an open area marked into squares or concentric rings. The number of lines
crossed per unit time is a measure of activity. The open field is considered
to cause an emotional response in the animals when they are in the apparatus,
possibly "fear" in rats and mice, resulting in deposition of fecal boluses in
some proportion to the intensity of the emotion. From 18 to 70 days of postnatal age, an increase in activity of mice has been reported and an earlier
levelling off of the number of boluses at about 50 days of age[28]. The same
investigation showed that activity and number of boluses in the rat increased
approximately 10-fold up to about 50 days, with a stable number from then
to 200 days of age. The increase from 17 to 50 days was roughly linear,
indicating a rapid, progressive change during early postnatal development. A
comparable increase in activity of rats in a residential maze has been reported,
with progressive increase in nocturnal to diurnal ratio of activity until the
adult ratio was reached at about 8 weeks of age[29].

Adult behavior

The variety of tests which have been used in pharmacology in evaluation of
psychoactive drugs is extensive. Behavioral tests used in adult animals in
toxicology have, for the most part, been drawn from pharmacology. The categories and tests listed in Table 3 are not meant to be an inclusive catalog of
behavioral methods for either pharmacology or toxicology. The main component
in many of the tests appears to be motor behavior or visual-motor performance
in both conditioned behavior (Table 3, 1b) and unconditioned behavior (Table 3,
2b and c). A recent proposal for behavioral toxicity tests suggested that
broad-scale detection of toxicity might be accomplished by the use of three
such tests: motor responding to fixed ratio and fixed interval schedules;
circadian activity in a residential maze, and performance on a rotating rod[30].

Because of the large number of tests which have been employed, only a few
examples in each category will be given, intended to represent the type of

data obtained by the test with an emphasis on studies where results on more than one type of test were obtained.

1a. Learning and memory. Gestational exposure to a toxic agent may result in learning deficits in adult animals. Mice which were injected with 5-azacytidine on day 16 or 18 of gestation showed differing effects. Day 16-injected mice learned active avoidance as adults more slowly than control mice or day 18-injected mice while day 18-injected mice learned more rapidly than controls. In a passive avoidance test, 24-hr retention was significantly better in day 16-injected mice and poorer in day 18-injected mice[21]. Brain size was significantly reduced by gestational 5-azacytidine.

Methyl mercury chloride was injected into rats on 15, 21 or 60 days of age. The treatment of the younger rats did not affect T-maze learning or open field behavior while 60 day old rats differed significantly from controls with both measures[31].

1b. Conditioned motor responding. Both Pavlovian-type conditioning and operant conditioning are commonly employed. In rats exposed to mercury vapor for 12-42 weeks conditioned active avoidance responding before shock showed more reproducible depression by mercury than conditioned escape after shock. Body weight loss was delayed 1-2 weeks longer than the onset of behavioral change[32].

Pigeons receiving repeated doses of methyl mercury showed gradual lengthening in interresponse times on a fixed-ratio schedule. Motor responses continued in a disorderly pattern until, in advanced stages, gross motor impairment in locomotion was observed and conditioned responding ceased[33]. In conditioned tests involving motor systems it is difficult to separate motor damage from specific effects on the conditioned behavior.

1c. Sensory discrimination. Operant conditioning has been used to detect subtle toxic changes in sensory systems with methods of sensory discrimination. These methods and auditory startle (see below) are the only methods which can be said to develop data on sensory systems which can be distinguished from other sites of action. Some of the most careful work has been carried out on the auditory system by Stebbins and co-workers[34,35]. Visual intensity discriminations in cats[36] and wave-length discrimination in pigeons[37] are examples of methods which can be used for monitoring toxic changes in the visual system.

2a. Emotion-associated behavior. Open field behavior is used both as a method for activity measurement for short periods of time, usually less than 30 min, and as a method for evaluating "emotional reactivity" of animals,

usually rats. Several critical evaluations have been written of the open
field as a test for emotion-associated behavior. Novelty has been considered
a primary condition producing a "stress-reaction" in rats placed in the open
field but Candland and Nagy[28] did not find a correlated habituation of cardiac
rate and defecation on repeated tests in an open field, although both parameters might be expected to measure "stress" to the rat. There also has been
no consistent relationship demonstrated between plasma corticosterone and
open field behavior[38]. Bättig[39] devised a dual maze-open field apparatus and
showed that the activity of rats in the maze portion gradually decreased with
habituation while open field activity gradually increased. Additional details
of determinants of open field behavior have been evaluated statistically[40].
Furchtgott and Echols[41] have proposed that X-irradiation in utero on gestational days 14 to 18 increased "emotionality" as measured in the open field
and by home cage emergence and the latter measure was more reliable in their
experiments than the open field.

Other forms of emotion-associated behaviors such as social behaviors including aggression, dominance or territoriality have had limited use in methods
for testing toxic agents. Mating and reproductive behavior have been evaluated
usually as a portion of reproduction and teratogenicity tests. Detailed
studies of mating behavior also have been made in certain endocrinological
studies.

TABLE 4

WALKING PATTERNS OF ADULT FEMALE RATS

Treatment	No. of Rats	Length of Stride	Width of Stride	Sine of Angle of Progression
Control	10	144.8 ± 3.9	38.3 ± 1.7	0.475 ± 0.023
X-irradiated	6	100.3* ± 3.8	42.3 ± 3.2	0.974* ± 0.021
Control	8	138 ± 3.9	35.3 ± 1.3	0.467 ± 0.023
Pallidal lesioned	8	132 ± 6.0	41.4* ± 2.0	0.532 ± 0.027

2b. Locomotor activity (exploratory or circadian). In one form or another,
tests of activity are widely used in toxicology. One reason is that hyperactivity is a common consequence of brain damage to various structures in the
CNS[42]. The converse, hypoactivity, results from some types of brain damage
and sometimes animals exposed to toxic agents may reliably show both effects,

depending on the method of measurement[43]. Some of the critical variables determining activity are the measuring device[44], previous environment[46], lighting conditions[38], presence of an observer[47], sex[48], age of the animal[10] and amount of habituation[49]. Of these, the most critical appear to be the design of the cage used for measurement, the degree of habituation and the time in the animals' circadian cycle when measurement is made.

Although changes in activity would seem to be easy to interpret, at least some forms of brain damage appear to affect many other behaviors which are not involved in locomotion[42]. There is little doubt that simplistic interpretations of measurements of locomotor activity in animals should not be made. Locomotor activity in a specific test of animal behavior is not equivalent to an imprecise concept of "hyperactivity" in man.

2c. Reflex systems and gait measurement. Tests of visual-motor coordination have been considered by some investigators to be sensitive ways for detection of brain damage in humans[50]. Various reflex systems are involved and there is no clear delineation in some of these tests, such as the rotating rod, of the reflex components and more complex supraspinal systems involved in gait.

The best-designed system is measurement of auditory startle. The magnitude of the motor startle following a sudden noise can be measured, as well as the threshold to elicit it in the presence of different background levels of sound[51]. Stimuli to a different sensory system just prior to the stimulus eliciting a reflex can alter the reflex[52]. Learning is not involved. The potential use of these systems for selectively monitoring damage needs to be exploited in toxicology.

Several designs of rotating rod have been proposed[53] but the principle of all of them is to determine the degree of visual-motor coordination. Measurement of balance with these devices does not give any information regarding the site of damage.

Neuromuscular deficits are often of interest in toxicology, ranging from effects on the brain as in cerebellar damage from the exposure to mercury, to distal axonopathies from acrylamide and n-hexane. Measurement of gait from footprints gives reliable data on the functional state of reflex systems directly involved in locomotion. Table 4 gives an example of the data taken from studies on rats irradiated in utero on gestational day 14[54] and adult rats with bilateral lesions of the globus pallidus[55]. The two types of brain damage affect gait in different ways.

100

Reproducibility

Three facets of any test which need to be considered are: reproducibility, sensitivity and validity.

Reproducibility is determined by the sources of variability in the experiments and variability can be divided into those existing within and between animals and between tests (Table 5). Evaluation of within-animal variability requires repeated measures on the same animals. In some tests, such as some schedules of operant behavior, well-trained controls may achieve a high degree of stability. Some unconditioned behaviors are also stable on repeated measures. A major effect of toxicants can be an increase in variability. The effect of methyl mercury on fixed-ratio responding in pigeons[23] and 5-azacytidine on avoidance conditioning[21] are examples.

TABLE 5

REPRODUCIBILITY

Sources of variability:
  Within animals (Habituation, tolerance and learning
    are factors in repeated testing)
  Between animals (Often increased in experimental
    group over control group)
  Between tests (Subject to large differences in some
    tests)

Between-animal variability is reflected in the apocryphal "First Law of Behavior" which states that, when all experimental variables are controlled, the animal will do as he pleases. An example of this individuality is given in Table 6. In this test the variability among control rats is about the same as variability among rats irradiated on gestational day 15 with 125 R. Repeated measures on the same animals (not shown) are less variable than between animals, indicating that the responses in this test are to some extent characteristic of the individual.

Between-tests variability may be very large where repeated measures are used. Much of the "first-day uniqueness" in behavioral tests results from within-animal habituation or learning on repeated measures, but some residual variability is due to variation associated with repeated tests. Even subtle differences in environmental conditions may affect repeated tests on the same or different groups of animals. Table 7 shows habituation occurring after the first day in rats placed in mazes for 2 hours on 4 successive days. One group of rats was exposed to carbon monoxide on the fifth postnatal day and the other group was exposed to air only (data taken from Culver and Norton[7]). Table 7 also shows the increased variability associated with neonatal carbon monoxide exposure.

TABLE 6

REPRODUCIBILITY BETWEEN ANIMALS

Time lapse photography of 6 week-old rats at 1 frame/second

| Rat No. | Seconds of Walking in 15 Minutes | |
	Control Rats	Irradiated Rats
1	22	27
2	53	92
3	115	35
4	27	44
5	21	12
6	39	14
Av.	46	37

TABLE 7

8-WEEK-OLD CO-EXPOSED AND CONTROL RATS IN

2-HR EXPLORATORY PERIOD IN A MAZE

| Repeated Tests | Photocell Counts Per Hour ± S.E. | |
	CO-exposed	Control
Day 1	1905 ± 660	1690 ± 310
2	655 ± 175	410 ± 75
3	505 ± 90	350 ± 35
4	610 ± 180	345 ± 40

Sensitivity

Several examples have been given of tests showing a significant difference between animals exposed to a toxic agent and the control animals. When the behavior of very young animals has been tested, often differences have not been observed in animals which show significant changes at later ages when other tests can be used. The behavior of rats exposed to carbon monoxide as neonates is an example of this[7]. The lower sensitivity of preweaning behavioral tests does not appear to be due to increased variability in performance of young animals[6,7].

Sensitivity of a test to modification by a toxic agent is not an end in itself. Selectivity may often be a more important consideration, so that a test which measures a significant effect of one type of damage may be unaltered by another type. However, a test must be sensitive to some experimental variable or it is of no value. Often an investigator would like to increase the sensitivity of a test. It can be detrimental to the conduct of a study to wait for months for a rat to mature in order to detect prenatal brain damage, for example. One possibility is to challenge the young animal, using a stimulus which may increase the sensitivity of the test. Table 8 (data from Schneider and Norton[56]) gives an example of increased sensitivity in time-lapse photographic analysis of rat behavior by injection of morphine sulfate (2 mg/kg) one-half hour before photographing the rats. Adult rats (5 months old) irradiated in utero are hyperactive in this test relative to controls[42] but when young, these rats are not hyperactive unless morphine is injected[56].

TABLE 8

AVERAGE OCCURRENCE (SECONDS ± S.E.) OF BEHAVIORAL ACTS IN 900
SECONDS IN 6 WEEK OLD FEMALE RATS

| Behavioral Act | Control | | Irradiated | |
	Saline (n = 6)	Morphine (n = 6)	Saline (n = 6)	Morphine (n = 6)
Sitting	213 ± 84	219 ± 45	80 ± 33	155 ± 50
Washing face	77 ± 29	101 ± 17	30 ± 7	77 ± 23
Walking	52 ± 15	77 ± 23	37 ± 12	90 ± 12*
Turning	65 ± 15	38 ± 8	38 ± 8	66 ± 9*

* $p < 0.01$

Validity

The most important consideration in selection of tests is the validity of the information which is obtained from the test. The measure of validity must relate to the aim of the study. For example, valid tests can be used to

detect potential consequences to man of exposure to toxic agents. Valid tests
are also needed to unravel mechanisms of action of toxic agents. Perhaps,
most important of all, valid tests can be applied to help understand the
central nervous system.

We have some measure of the reliability and sensitivity of a few behavioral
tests. Much more data on these aspects should be routinely collected and
analyzed. The problem is technical and surmountable, requiring the application
of a sufficient amount of time and expertise in an orderly fashion. Determination of validity is another matter. Validity of behavioral tests for any of
the 3 purposes mentioned above is unknown for most of the tests. The primary
deficiency is in the basic information which should allow behavioral tests to
be correlated with the chemical and physical structure of CNS. Many attempts
have been made to do this in connection with therapeutic drugs with little
success. The attempts are usually based on clinical categories, such as
analgesia, anesthesia, or antidepressant action. Inadequately defined or
scientifically indefinable categories like these are not adequate to build a
rigorous science. The science of behavior cannot go beyond careful data
collection until the construction of the central nervous system is understood.

This is why tests (behavioral, morphological, physiological or biochemical)
of sensory systems are the most valid: the role of the structural components
in function of these systems is the best understood. Examples of behavioral
tests of sensory systems have been given. The major structural components of
the motor system are almost as well delineated and, to the extent that they
can be examined by behavioral or other tests, these tests have validity. With
the bulk of the remaining systems in the CNS, which include the "integrative"
capacity of the brain, the structural components and their roles are not well
understood. It is in this area that the adaptability of the CNS is likely to
preclude total reliance on behavior and to require tests of structure as well
as function for evaluation of the state of the CNS (see Table 9).

There is a particular hazard in attempting to use behavioral tests as
predictors of CNS toxicity. As noted above, the characteristic drug has a
short duration of action and is completely reversible in its action. Toxic
substances, on the other hand, are much more likely to cause irreversible
damage to the structure of the CNS. In such cases the validity of behavioral
tests is inherently limited by the adaptability of the CNS. Of all of the
organs, the CNS is most characterized by its ability to restore function in
the continued presence of a toxic agent or to recover function after cell
loss. This phenomenon is well-known in experiments in which overt brain

lesions are made. Serial lesions are much less damaging to function than a single lesion destroying the same amount of brain substance. The effects of serial lesions are often short-lived compared with single lesions[36]. The arguments that morphological changes can exist in brain damage without behavioral changes have been detailed[57]. There are, of course, limitations to the ability of the CNS to tolerate structural damage without functional damage. Four of the factors involved in determining CNS adaptability are listed in Table 9.

TABLE 9

METHODOLOGICAL CONSIDERATIONS

Adaptability of CNS (Morphological and biochemical plasticity) is affected by:

1. Age of animal at time of exposure
2. Nature of toxic effect
3. Time since exposure
4. Age of animal at time of testing

The age of the animal at time of exposure and at time of testing are at least as critical as the nature of the toxic effect. Exposure of the developing brain during embryogenesis may produce an effect unlike the effect in adults because the construction of a developing organ can be severely compromised by loss of a single set of dividing cells. The effect of aging on expression of prenatal damage has already been mentioned. When exposure to damage occurs in the adult brain the time elapsed between the time of damage and the time of testing is critical since longer periods allow more time for recovery. While it can hardly be argued that prolonged behavioral changes can occur without changes in the chemical and physical structure of the CNS, it is quite possible that behavioral changes can be detected without finding structural changes, since difficulties exist in selecting a valid structural test as well as in selecting a behavioral one. It is first necessary to know what to look for and where to look.

CONCLUSIONS

    1. A large number of simple behaviors can be tested in preweanling rats. More needs to be known about the usefulness of these tests in a variety of prenatal and neonatal exposures to toxic agents.

    2. Many tests of behavior of adult animals have been adapted from psychopharmacology to toxicology. The therapeutic categories which have guided psychopharmacology are lacking in toxicology which deals with a large set of chemical categories. This presents a problem in demonstrating validity of behavioral tests.

    3. The failure, to date, to tie morphology and biochemistry to behavior through appropriate scientific generalizations is a major hindrance to establishing the validity of available behavioral tests.

    4. Behavioral tests in toxicology have the inherent limitation that the central nervous system is the most adaptable system in the body and, as such, can compensate for damage through a series of mechanisms. Therefore tests of structure as well as function are essential for delineating damage from toxic agents.

REFERENCES

1. Eayrs, J.T. and Lishman, W.A. (1955) Brit. J. Anim. Behav., 3, 17-24.

2. Bolles, R.C. and Woods, P.G. (1964) Anim. Behav., 12, 427-44.

3. Fox, M.W. (1965) Anim. Behav., 13, 234-241.

4. Altman, J. and Sudarshan, K. (1975) Anim. Behav., 23, 896-920.

5. Fox, M.W. (1964) Anim. Behav., 12, 301-310.

6. Brunner, R.L., McLean, M., Vorhees, C.V. and Butcher, R.E. (1978) Teratol., 18, 379-384.

7. Culver, B. and Norton, S. (1976) Exp. Neurol., 50, 80-98.

8. Barlow, S.M., Knight, A.F. and Sullivan, F.M. (1978) Teratol., 18, 211-218.

9. Spyker, J.M. (1975) Fed. Proc., 34, 1835-1844.

10. Norton, S. (1977) Animal Models in Psychiatry and Neurology, Pergamon Press, New York.

11. Olson, K. and Boush, G.M. (1975) Bull. Environ. Contam. Toxicol., 13, 73-79.

12. Reiter, L.W., Anderson, G.E., Laskey, J.W. and Cahill, D.F. (1975) Environ. Hlth. Perspect., 12, 119-123.

13. Hicks, S.P., D'Amato, C.J. and Lowe, M.J. (1959) J. Comp. Neurol., 113, 345-469.

14. Miale, T.L. and Sidman, R.L. (1961) Exp. Neurol., 4, 277-296.

15. Angevine, J.B. and Sidman, R.L. (1961) Nature, 192, 766-768.

16. Angevine, J.B. (1965) Exp. Neurol. Suppl., 2, 1-70.

17. Brent, R.L. (1969) Methods for Teratological Studies in Experimental Animals and Man, Medical Examination Publishing Co., Flushing, N.Y.

18. Angevine, J.B. (1970) J. Comp. Neurol., 139, 129-152.

19. Bekoff, M. and Fox, M.W. (1972) Develop. Psychobiol., 5, 323-341.

20. Clos, J., Favre, C., Selme-Matrat, M. and Legrand, J. (1977) Brain Res., 123, 13-26.

21. Rodier, P.M. (1977) Teratol., 16, 235-246.

22. Bulke-Sam, J. and Kimmel, C.A. (1978) Personal communication.

23. Riccio, D.C., Rohrbaugh, M. and Hodges, L.A. (1968) Develop. Psychobiol., 1, 108-111.

24. Bauer, R.H. (1978) Develop. Psychobiol., 11, 103-116.

25. Egger, G.J. and Livesey, P.J. (1972) Develop. Psychobiol., 5, 343-351.

26. McLaughlin, L.J., Eller, H.D. and Korol, B. (1975) Develop. Psychobiol., 8, 233-239.

27. Mysliveček, J. and Hassmanová, J. (1979) Develop. Psychobiol., 12, 169-186.

28. Candland, D.K. and Nagy, Z.M. (1969) Ann. N.Y. Acad. Sci., 159, 831-351.

29. Norton, S., Mullenix, P. and Culver, B. (1975) Behav. Biol., 15, 317-331.

30. Committee for the Revision of NAS Publication 1138 (1977) National Academy of Sciences, Washington.

31. Post, E.M., Yang, M.G., King, J.A. and Sanger, V.L. (1973) Proc. Soc. Exp. Biol. Med., 143, 1113-1116.

32. Kishi, R., Hashimoto, K., Shimizu, S. and Kobayashi, M. (1978) Toxicol. Appl. Pharmacol., 46, 555-566.

33. Evans, H.L., Laties, V.G and Weiss, B. (1975) Fed. Proc., 34, 1858-1867.

34. Stebbins, W.C., Green, S. and Miller, F.L. (1966) Science, 153, 1646-1647.

35. Stebbins, W.C. and Rudy, M.C. (1978) Environ. Hlth. Perspect., 26, 43-51.

36. Fischman, M.W. and Meikle, Jr., T.H. (1965) J. Comp. Physiol. Psychol., 59, 193-201.

37. Hanson, H.M. (1975) Fed. Proc., 34, 1852-1857.

38. Walsh, R.N. and Cummins, R.A. (1976), Psychol. Bull., 83, 482-509.

39. Bättig, K. (1969) Ann. N.Y. Acad. Sci., 159, 880-897.

40. Denenberg, V.H. (1969) Ann. N.Y. Acad. Sci., 159, 852-859.

41. Furchtgott, E. and Echols, M. (1958) J. Physiol. Comp. Psychol., 51, 541-545.

42. Norton, S., Mullenix, P. and Culver, B. (1976) Brain Res., 116, 49-67.

43. Reiter, L., Kidd, K., Ledbetter, G., Gray, Jr., L.E. and Chernoff, N. (1977) Toxicol. Appl. Pharmacol., 41, 143.

44. Weasner, M.H., Finger, F.W. and Reid, L.S. (1960) J. Comp. Physiol. Psych., 53, 470-474.

45. Jarrard, L.E. (1968) Physiol. Behav., 3, 65-70.

46. Inglis, T.R. (1975) Anim. Behav., 23, 932-940.

47. Hughes, C.W. (1978) Physiol. Behav., 20, 481-485.

48. Schneider, B.F. and Norton, S. (1979) Physiol. Behav., 22, 47-51.

49. Norton, S. (1973) Physiol. Behav., 11, 181-186.

50. Norton, S. (1975) Toxicology, The Basic Science of Poisons, Macmillan Co., New York.

51. Hoffman, H.S. and Searle, J.L. (1965) J. Comp. Physiol. Psych., 60, 53-58.

52. Ison, J.R. and Leonard, D.W. (1971) J. Comp. Physiol. Psych., 75, 157-164.

53. Watzman, N. and Barry III, H. (1968). Psychopharmacologia, 12, 414-423.

54. Mullenix, P., Norton, S. and Culver, B. (1975) Exp. Neurol., 48, 310-324.

55. Norton, S. (1976) Brain Res. Bull., 1, 193-202.

56. Schneider, B.F. and Norton, S. (1979) Paper presented at annual meeting, Society of Toxicology.

57. Norton, S. (1978) Environ. Hlth. Persp., 26, 21-27.

WHAT MAKES A CHEMICAL A THREAT TO HEALTH
Chairman: James E. Gibson

© 1980 Elsevier/North-Holland Biomedical Press
The Scientific Basis of Toxicity Assessment
H. Witschi, editor.

"WHAT MAKES A CHEMICAL A THREAT TO HEALTH?"

Dr. James E. Gibson, Chemical Industry Institute of Toxicology,
                    Research Triangle Park, North Carolina 27709

INTRODUCTION:

The papers which follow bring to our attention the variety of specific chemical interactions with biological molecules leading to chemical injury. These studies of mechanisms provide insight into the specificity of these responses and the firm scientific bases upon which the science of toxicology can build to achieve the ultimate objective of being a predictive science.

In the rush to use the tools of toxicology in the prediction of risk and/or hazard, we sometimes lose sight of a concept put forward by Paracelsus more than 500 years ago, that "all things have poisonous qualities; it is only the dose that makes a thing a poison." In our consideration of "what makes a chemical a threat to health?", we must keep in mind the dose-dependent character of responses and the variety of biological control systems which usually explain this dose-dependence.

In this session these issues are addressed by considering critical pathways of chemical distribution in the environment, the role of metabolic activation in chemical carcinogenesis, the action of agents affecting toxicity other than carcinogenicity and a consideration of the interactions between toxic chemicals and genetic material.

The approach to toxicology provided by an understanding of toxic mechanisms can assist in explaining phenomena which are characteristic in toxicology. Loomis has stated these well and are summarized as follow:

1. Toxic reactions may be rare events.

2. Toxic reactions may occur only after prolonged exposure.

3. Different species may respond differently to a toxic substance.

Explanations for these phenomena can be provided by an understanding of the mechanism of toxic response. This session addresses these fundamental issues which are the forefront of toxicology today.

© 1980 Elsevier/North-Holland Biomedical Press
The Scientific Basis of Toxicity Assessment
H. Witschi, editor.   113

CRITICAL PATHWAYS OF POLYCYCLIC AROMATIC HYDROCARBONS
IN AQUATIC ENVIRONMENTS

S. E. HERBES, G. R. SOUTHWORTH, D. L. SHAEFFER
Environmental Sciences Division, Oak Ridge National Laboratory, Oak Ridge,
Tennessee 37830

W. H. GRIEST, M. P. MASKARINEC
Analytical Chemistry Division, Oak Ridge National Laboratory, Oak Ridge,
Tennessee 37830

INTRODUCTION

   During the past decade several environmental contaminants have proved to be
real or potential hazards to humans or other organisms: mercury, DDT, and
PCB's are examples which immediately come to mind. In each case hazards were
due not to the toxicity of the material initially released, but to alterations
in form or concentration in the environment. Thus, to assess adequately the
potential hazard from contaminants, effects of the physical, biological, and
chemical processes which act between release and uptake by humans must be
understood. This paper addresses various environmental processes which act on
one class of waterborne contaminants--polycyclic aromatic hydrocarbons--and
attempts to demonstrate the effect of different aquatic environments upon contaminant transport behavior.
   Polycyclic aromatic hydrocarbons, or PAH (Figure 1), are a series of fused-
ring aromatic compounds which are discharged in wastewater from such high-
temperature industrial processes as petroleum refining and coal coking[1].
Some PAH, particularly the four- and five-ring compounds, are highly carcinogenic to skin and lung tissue[2]. More importantly from the standpoint of
waterborne PAH, several compounds have been demonstrated to be carcinogenic to
the gastrointestinal tract[3] (although less strongly than to skin or lung).
   Although PAH seem to be widespread in surface waters receiving industrial
discharges[1], the pathways which the compounds follow and the transformations
which they undergo are only poorly understood, although those pathways and
transformations may largely determine the potential hazard. The objectives of
this paper, therefore, are threefold: (1) to elucidate the various transport
processes which act on PAH in surface waters, (2) to examine the relationship

ORNL–DWG 76–15350R

NAPHTHALENE   ANTHRACENE   BENZ(A)ANTHRACENE   BENZ(A)PYRENE

Fig. 1. Representative PAH compounds.

between transport behavior and molecular parameters within the PAH class, and
(3) to investigate the effect of major environmental variables on PAH transport
behavior. Questions which will be addressed include the following:

- How persistent are PAH in surface waters, and how is persistence affected
  by different environmental conditions?
- In what form do PAH exist in water, and how does the form affect transport?
- To what extent do PAH accumulate in sediments and biota?
- Will PAH transformation products accumulate in the water?
- How will relative concentrations of different PAH compounds change with
  distance from a source?

GENERAL ASPECTS OF TRANSPORT PROCESSES

A number of processes act in concert to alter waterborne concentrations of
PAH; the major pathways are shown in Figure 2. Immediately upon discharge
into surface waters, PAH partition between dissolved and particle-bound forms.
The dissolved form may dissipate to the atmosphere by volatilization. Both
forms may be incorporated into the sediments: the particle-bound form by
sedimentation (settling), and the dissolved form by direct sorption to bedded
sediments. The dissolved form may break down by the action of sunlight
(photolysis) or by abiotic oxidation. Both PAH forms may be taken up by
aquatic organisms (bioaccumulation), which may be consumed by other large
organisms (thus resulting in passage of PAH through aquatic food webs). At
each trophic stage PAH may be metabolized by the organisms. Metabolism may
also occur by microorganisms in the water or sediment. While these processes
are occurring, turbulent mixing and bulk movement of the water are acting constantly to disperse PAH throughout the receiving water system.
The processes which affect PAH in the aquatic environment may be considered
as two general types--those which result in transport, and those which result
in transformation. Transport processes are those in which only the

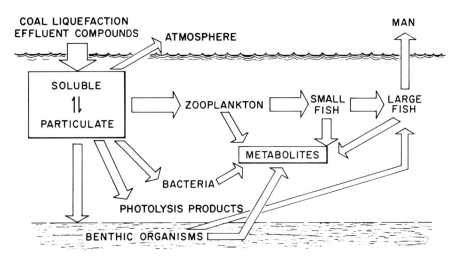

Fig. 2. Major transport and transformation processes acting on PAH in natural waters.

physicochemical form is altered, while transformational processes result in alteration to a different chemical species. As such, transport processes are driven by chemical equilibrium considerations, while transformational processes are essentially nonequilibrium. A second general distinction among transport and transformation processes is whether or not they are mediated by living organisms (biotic vs abiotic). Major transport processes in the aquatic environment are summarized in Table 1.

Three basic mathematical concepts are useful in discussions of contaminant transport behavior: the equilibrium constant, the rate constant, and the half-life. The first constant defines thermodynamic equilibrium relationship between concentrations of a compound in two compartments. Mathematically, the equilibrium constant (dimensionless) in PAH studies is nearly always described:

$$K = \frac{[PAH]_a}{[PAH]_{H_2O}} \quad , \tag{1}$$

where the numerator is the concentration of a PAH in compartment $\underline{a}$ (sediment, biota, suspended particles, or air) relative to the concentration dissolved in water.

116

TABLE 1

MAJOR PROCESSES INFLUENCING PAH BEHAVIOR IN NATURAL WATERS

	Transport	Transformation
Abiotic	Dispersion Sorption Volatilization	Oxidation Photolysis
Biotic	Bioaccumulation	Metabolism Microbial degradation

   While the equilibrium constant describes how a PAH compound will distribute
in the environment at equilibrium, the rate constant describes how rapidly a
process proceeds toward equilibrium (although equilibrium conditions are not
always·attained under environmental conditions). Nearly always environmental
processes are presumed to be first order. The rate constant k_a for process _a_
resulting in PAH removal from water is defined as the ratio of the rate of
change of dissolved PAH with time to the dissolved PAH concentration:

$$k_a = \frac{\frac{d[PAH]_{H_2O}}{dt}}{[PAH]_{H_2O}} \quad . \tag{2}$$

   The half-life, or the time required for PAH in a compartment (usually water)
to decrease to one-half its initial level due to a removal process, is related
reciprocally to the rate constant:

$$t_{\frac{1}{2}} = \frac{0.693}{k_a} \quad . \tag{3}$$

Although rate constants are used for purposes of mathematical modeling,
half-lives are more easily visualized and thus will often be used in this
discussion.

To investigate the effects of the various transport and transformational processes on PAH in surface waters, we (and others) have measured individual process effects on selected representative compounds in laboratory studies. For this approach to be useful in predicting the behavior of the PAH class, three assumptions must be made. First, we assume that the overall transport and transformation behavior of a contaminant is equivalent to the sum of effects of the individual processes acting on the contaminant compound. This assumption permits the study of transport and transformation behavior by measurement of the rate of each individual process as a function of important environmental variables, which is followed by combination of the various process rates into a description of the overall behavior of the contaminant. Second, we assume that the fate of a complex assemblage of contaminants (i.e., PAH) can be described by careful determination of the behavior of selected representative compounds, which span the range of molecular characteristics of the assemblage as a whole. Prediction of the behavior of other compounds should then be possible by interpolation from those for which transport characteristics have been well defined. Third, the behavior of each compound is assumed to be unaffected by the presence of other PAH in the water.

INDIVIDUAL PROCESS STUDIES

Sorption

The extent to which hydrophobic solutes in water tend to sorb at solid-water interfaces is inversely related to their water solubilities. Because PAH solubilities are low (generally in the low μg/liter range) their tendency to sorb is high. Results from our laboratory of measurements of sorbed/dissolved distributions of ^{14}C-labeled PAH added to different surface water and wastewater samples are shown in Table 2. In general, the fraction of PAH present in the sorbed form increases with increasing molecular size, ranging from less than one percent for naphthalene to roughly 40 percent for the four- and five-ring compounds. Although different types of suspended particles have different affinities for PAH, in general water samples which are turbid (containing high suspended particle concentrations) contain higher fractions of sorbed PAH than do less turbid waters.

Sedimentation

As suspended particles settle to the sediment, they carry with them sorbed contaminants; sedimentation can therefore function to decrease waterborne PAH concentrations. In most river systems, however, settling and resuspension

TABLE 2

SORPTION OF PAH IN WATER AND WASTEWATER SAMPLES (22°C)

Compound	% Sorbed (range)	log K (mean)[a]
Naphthalene	0.1 - 0.8	2.38
Anthracene	2.8 - 19	3.74
9-Methylanthracene	6.0 - 27	3.96
Benz(a)anthracene	19 - 60	4.52
7,12-Dimethylbenz(a)anthracene	20 - 43	4.51
Benz(a)pyrene	24 - 44	4.48

[a] $K = \dfrac{[\text{PAH}]_{\text{sorbed}}}{[\text{PAH}]_{H_2O}}$.

processes counterbalance each other, and no net sedimentation occurs. Sedimentation is important in situations where the concentration of suspended solids in water is relatively high and water movement is slow (e.g., lakes and reservoirs).

Volatilization

Table 3 summarizes the expected half-lives of four representative PAH compounds in a river under typical environmental conditions. Half-lives were calculated as described elsewhere[4] from gas-water partition coefficients (Henry's Law coefficients) and river reaeration rate expressions. Expected half-lives vary from less than a day (naphthalene) to two months [benz(a)pyrene]. The effect of PAH molecular size is marked; volatilization rates decrease by factors of 3 to 10 per each additional benzene ring addition.

Photolysis

Rates of breakdown of PAH by sunlight depend on two factors: the fraction of incident sunlight absorbed by PAH molecules, and the efficiency of the absorbed light in producing a chemical reaction. The fraction of incident sunlight absorbed by PAH molecules in water depends on the absorption spectrum of the PAH and the degree of light absorption by other substances in the water. Efficiency of the reaction (quantum yield) varies relatively little among PAH;[5] thus, differences in photolysis rates are due primarily to differences in PAH

TABLE 3

VOLATILIZATION AND PHOTOLYSIS OF PAH FROM SURFACE WATERS

Compound	No. of rings	Half-life (hr) due to:	
		Volatilization[a]	Photolysis[b]
Naphthalene	2	16	71
Anthracene	3	62	0.75
Phenanthrene	3	-[c]	8.4
Benz(a)anthracene	4	500	0.59
Chrysene	4	-	4.4
Benz(a)pyrene	5	1500	0.54

[a] Calculated for a river 1 m deep, water velocity 0.5 m/sec, wind velocity 1 m/sec (Ref. 4).

[b] Calculated for surface waters in midsummer at 40°N latitude (Ref. 5).

[c] Not determined.

absorption spectra. While there is a general tendency for absorption spectra of larger PAH to include the longer, more intense wavelengths of sunlight, thus allowing more light to be absorbed, considerable variation is noted (Table 3). Thus, we find order-of-magnitude difference between benz(a)anthracene/chrysene and anthracene/phenanthrene pairs. With the exception of naphthalene, the rates of photolysis of the representative PAH are considerably more rapid than are the rates of volatilization (Table 3).

Microbial transformation

Rates of microbial transformation of PAH have been measured in this laboratory by addition of ^{14}C-labeled PAH compounds to water and sediment samples, and quantitation of transformation products after incubation periods of 24 to 96 hr[6]. Representative results are shown in Table 4. Several trends are apparent. First, for both water and sediment, the rate of microbial degradation is highest for smaller compounds (e.g., naphthalene) and decreases with increasing molecular weight. Second, the comparison of degradation rates in water with those in sediments collected at the same site (columns 1 and 2) demonstrates that degradation in sediment is 8- to 20-fold more rapid than in the water. Third, the degradation half-life of PAH in sediments is inversely related to the amount of PAH contamination of the sediment. Half-lives were greatest in an uncontaminated forest stream where PAH levels were below detection limits; half-lives were lower at a stream containing moderate PAH contamination (from petroleum storage tank runoff); half-lives were lowest in the most contaminated sediments (downstream from a coking effluent discharge). Thus, the environmental importance of microbial degradation of PAH appears to be directly related to the level of PAH contamination present. However, even the most rapid rates of degradation recorded in water samples were considerably lower than rates of photolysis of the same compounds (Table 3).

TABLE 4

RATES OF MICROBIAL TRANSFORMATION OF ^{14}C-LABELED PAH IN WATER AND SEDIMENT SAMPLES (20°C)

	Half-life (hr) in sample containing:			
	High PAH level[a]		Moderate PAH level[b]	Low PAH level[c]
Compound	Water	Sediment	Sediment	Sediment
Naphthalene	70	3	5	> 2,000
Anthracene	150	20	280	2,800
Benz(a)anthracene	1400	100	7000	> 20,000
Benz(a)pyrene	> 1400	1300	> 20,000	> 20,000

[a] Collected 0.5 km below coke effluent discharge (July 1978).
[b] Collected 0.2 km below petroleum storage depot (November 1976).
[c] Collected from uncontaminated forest stream (December 1976).

Movement into bedded sediments

We have assumed that movement into bedded sediments is a nonequilibrium process driven by microbial degradation in a surface layer of sediment. Instead of the surface sediment rapidly becoming equilibrated with overlying waterborne PAH, therefore, a net movement of PAH from the water into the sediment occurs as the sediment-bound PAH is broken down by microorganisms[4]. The main parameters which affect the process are the rate of microbial degradation in sediment, the sorption coefficient (K) of individual PAH compounds onto sediment, the depth of water, and the depth of sediment which participates in the water-sediment exchange. The implicit assumptions involved in this treatment are probably most valid for relatively shallow, well-mixed

rivers under constant flow and temperature conditions, and receiving constant
PAH inputs (as from an effluent discharge).

From the microbial transformation rate measurements described above, half-
lives of representative PAH in a typical river were calculated if sorption to
bottom sediments were the only removal process (Table 5). Although transformation rates in the sediment decrease as PAH increase in size, the increasing
tendency of PAH to sorb largely counterbalances this trend, and predicted
half-lives for naphthalene, anthacene, and benz(a)anthracene are quite similar.

TABLE 5

PREDICTED RATES OF DIRECT SORPTION OF PAH TO BEDDED SEDIMENTS

Compound	Microbial degradation rate constant (hr^{-1})[a]	Sediment sorption K value[b]	Half-life due to sediment sorption (hr)[c]
Naphthalene	0.23	40	65
Anthracene	0.035	800	25
Benz(a)anthracene	0.005	5000	40
Benz(a)pyrene	< 0.0005	3000	> 600

[a] Sample collected 0.5 km below coke effluent discharge (July 1978).
[b] From Ref. 7 and Herbes, S. E., unpublished data.
[c] River depth 1 m, velocity 0.5 m/sec. Sediment depth participating in
exchange assumed to be 0.1 cm.

Bioaccumulation

The process of concentration of contaminants in tissues, or bioaccumulation,
is unimportant in determining the overall fate of organic compounds in most
systems, because only an extremely small fraction of the total contaminant
load of a river or lake is associated with living organisms (other than microorganisms). However, bioaccumulation may be important in predicting hazards
of chemicals to humans because ingestion of fish and shellfish is often a major
pathway of human exposure to contaminants.

Previous workers[8] have demonstrated that bioaccumulation of contaminants
is often related to the octanol-water partition coefficient, which is a
laboratory-determined measurement of the hydrophobic character of a compound.
Such a relationship has been shown for PAH in our studies with Daphnia[9]

122

(Figure 3; we have observed similar relationships in unpublished studies with snails (<u>Goniobasis</u> sp.) and minnows (<u>Pimephales</u> <u>promeles</u>). Thus bioaccumulation may result in concentrations of four- and five-ring PAH compounds in edible crustaceans and fish several thousand-fold higher than waterborne PAH concentrations.

Overall effect of transport processes

Because in this analysis each transport or transformation process is assumed to act independently from the others, the overall rate constant of removal of a PAH compound from water is equal to the sum of rate constants for all processes acting on it. Thus,

$$
\begin{aligned}
k_{overall} &= k_{volatilization} + k_{photolysis} \\
&+ k_{microbial\ degradation} + k_{sediment\ sorption}
\end{aligned}
\qquad (4)
$$

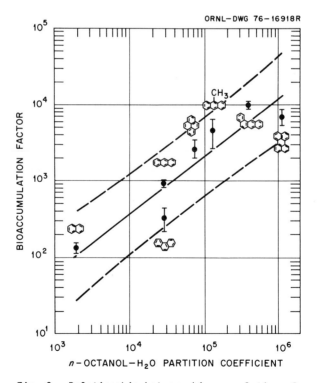

Fig. 3. Relationship between bioaccumulation of PAH by <u>Daphnia magna</u> and calculated octanol-water partition coefficient (Ref. 9).

The relative importance of process $\underline{a}$ is thus equal to the ratio of its rate
constant (k_a) to $k_{overall}$. In Figure 4 the predicted relative importance of
each process in a rapidly flowing stream has been shown graphically for four
representative PAH compounds. The rate of removal of the four are not the
same; the half-distances (distance required for the waterborne PAH concentration to drop to 50% of the initial level) for naphthalene, anthracene,
benz(a)anthracene, and benz(a)pyrene, respectively, are 5.8, 3.0, 4.3, and
1.6 km. Several points are apparent from Figure 4. First, microbial
transformation in the water column is predicted to be unimportant for all four
compounds. Sorption to bedded sediment comprises 20 to 25% of the removal for
all compounds smaller than benz(a)pyrene (for which it is a negligible
process). Volatilization, while dominating the behavior of naphthalene,
rapidly decreases in significance as PAH increase in size. Finally, photolysis
is unimportant for naphthalene, but dominates the transformation behavior of
the larger PAH. If photolytic degradation products do not undergo further
rapid removal of other processes, therefore, they would be expected to increase

ORNL-DWG 79-11677

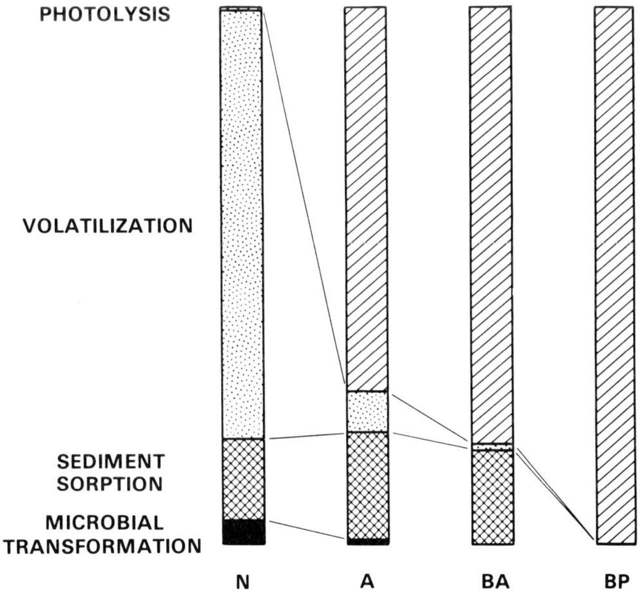

Fig. 4. Predicted contributions of major transport
processes to PAH removal from water in a shallow,
rapidly flowing stream.

downstream in this type of stream system because the bulk of the PAH contaminant load would be expected to undergo photolytic transformation.

EFFECTS OF ENVIRONMENTAL VARIABLES

Environmental variables which change with season, time of day, and location may dramatically alter the transport behavior of PAH (and other contaminants). An obvious example is the anticipated difference between day and night on the rate of benz(a)pyrene breakdown in water: because photolysis in Figure 4 accounted for approximately 99% of the total removal rate, the removal rate would be predicted to be about 100-fold slower at night.

The influences of six major environmental variables on rates of four transport processes are summarized in Table 6. In several cases, a change in an environmental variable (e.g., increasing temperature) will cause one process to increase in rate (e.g., microbial degradation), while another will decrease (as does sedimentation, when higher temperatures cause a lower fraction of waterborne PAH to sorb). In such a case the increasing rate of one process may counteract the decreasing rate of the other, and the overall rate of removal of the compound may remain relatively constant, although the relative contributions of the individual processes change.

TABLE 6

QUALITATIVE EFFECTS OF ENVIRONMENTAL PARAMETERS ON RATES OF TRANSPORT PROCESSES

Increase in:	Causes process rate change:			
	Photolysis	Volatilization	Sedimentation	Microbial degradation
Temperature	--[a]	Up or down	Down	Up
Turbidity	Down	Down	Up	--
Water velocity	--	Up	Down	--
Depth	Down	Down	Down	--
Sunlight	Up	--	--	--
Wind speed	--	Up	--	--

[a] No significant effect.

The predicted effect of varying environmental variables may be demonstrated by consideration of the transport behavior of a single PAH compound in several aquatic systems. The representative compound in this comparison is benz(a)anthracene. Representative aquatic systems are a clear river, a turbid channelized river, and a reservoir, whose hydrological characteristics are outlined in Table 7. All were assigned the same flow rate (50 m^3/sec); thus, an effluent entering each system would experience the same dilution factor. Major differences between the three are water depth, flow velocity, and turbidity (suspended solids concentration).

TABLE 7

HYDROLOGICAL CHARACTERISTICS OF REPRESENTATIVE AQUATIC SYSTEMS

	Clear river	Channelized river	Reservoir
Flow (m^3/sec)	50	50	50
Depth (m)	1	5	10
Width (m)	100	200	1000
Velocity (m/sec)	0.5	0.05	0.005
Turbidity (mg/liter)	5	50	30

The predicted behavior of benz(a)anthracene in the three systems is shown in Figure 5. The half-life increases 23- and 17-fold from the clear river to the channelized river and the reservoir, respectively. However, because the velocity decreases 100-fold over the three systems, the predicted half-distances in the two river systems are relatively similar, and both are considerably longer than in the reservoir. The dominant process similarly vary. While photolysis is important in all three areas, it becomes less important in the two more turbid systems than in the clear river. Due to slower water flow, microbial transformation (both in water and as a motivating force for direct movement into sediment) is somewhat more important in the channelized river and reservoir. Sedimentation, which does not occur as a net process in rivers during constant water flow, becomes significant under the extremely slow flow conditions postulated for the reservoir. In all three cases, transformational processes (photolysis and microbial alteration) account for approximately

126

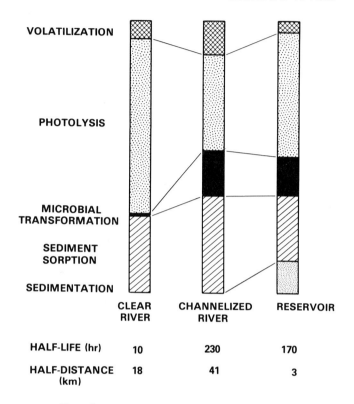

ORNL-DWG 79-11676

Fig. 5. Predicted transport behavior of benz(a)anthracene in several representative aquatic systems.

one-half of the PAH removed, which suggests that PAH degradation products (if not further degraded) may be present at significant concentrations.

FIELD VERIFICATION OF PREDICTIONS

The hypotheses raised by the transport process rate measurements are being tested in our laboratory by measuring concentrations of PAH in water and sediment downstream from a large coal coking wastewater discharge in Bethlehem, Pennsylvania[10]. Until these data are fully evaluated our predictions of PAH transport remain unverified. Initial results from the field site indicate that PAH are at least as persistent as we predict, and may in fact be more slowly degraded than we anticipated. Other data indicate that concentrations of PAH in sediment are several thousand-fold higher than waterborne PAH levels, as predicted from measurements of sorption coefficients in laboratory studies. Additional conclusions must await further sample collection and analysis.

SUMMARY

An understanding of the transport processes affecting the persistence and fate of waterborne contaminants is important in fully assessing their potential hazard to humans. Despite quantitative uncertainties due to lack of sufficient validation data at present, the questions posed at the beginning of the paper may be addressed in summary:

PAH may persist for periods of days to weeks in surface waters, while traveling distances of dozens of kilometers from effluent sources. Water turbidity and depth, sunlight intensity, and flow velocity may change predicted half-lives by an order of magnitude or more.

PAH are largely present in the dissolved state in clear waters although four- and five-ring compounds may distribute roughly equally between dissolved and particulate forms. The particulate fraction, being less amenable to breakdown by sunlight and nonvolatilizable, is more persistent.

PAH may accumulate several thousand-fold in sediments and biota.

Photolysis products (and to a lesser extent, microbial transformation products) of PAH are generated in surface waters, and may accumulate if not degraded further.

Because some PAH are more persistent than others, the relative composition of a PAH mixture will vary with distances from the source. To determine how the relative composition will vary requires knowledge of the dominant processes acting on PAH in a particular water body.

ACKNOWLEDGEMENTS

We thank C. P. Allen for excellent technical help in measurement of microbial transformation rates and sorption equilibrium constants. R. V. O'Neill and E. A. Bondietti provided valuable comments on the manuscript. Research sponsored by the Office of Health and Environmental Research, U.S. Department of Energy, under contract W-7405-eng-26 with Union Carbide Corporation. Publication No. 1379, Environmental Sciences Division, Oak Ridge National Laboratory.

REFERENCES

1. Andelman, J. B. and Suess, M. J. (1970) Bull. W. H. O., 43, 479-508.

2. Daudel, P. and Daudel, R. (1966) Chemical Carcinogenesis and Molecular Biology, Wiley Interscience, New York. pp. 34-35.

3. Chouroulinkov, A. G. and Guerin, M. (1967) Bull. Cancer, 54, 67-78.

4. Southworth, G. R. (1979 in press) Proceedings of Second Annual Symposium on Aquatic Toxicology, ASTM, Philadelphia, Pennsylvania.

5. Zepp, R. G. and Schlotzhauer, P. F. (1979 in press) Polynuclear Aromatic Hydrocarbons (Jones, P. W. and Lever, P., eds.), Ann Arbor Science Publishers, Ann Arbor, Michigan. pp. 141-158.

6. Herbes, S. E. and Schwall, L. R. (1978) Appl. Environ. Microbiol., 35, 306-316.

7. Karickhoff, S. W., Brown, D. S., and Scott, T. A. (1979 in press) Water Res.

8. Neeley, W. R., Branson, D. R., and Blau, G. E. (1974) Environ. Sci. Technol., 8, 1113-1115.

9. Southworth, G. R., Beauchamp, J. J., and Schmieder, P. K. (1978) Water Res., 12, 973-977.

10. Herbes, S. E, Southworth, G. R., and Griest, W. H. (1979 in press) Potential Health and Environmental Effects of Synthetic Fossil Fuel Technologies: Proceedings of First Annual Life Sciences Symposium, CONF-780903, Technical Information Center, Oak Ridge, Tennessee.

© 1980 Elsevier/North-Holland Biomedical Press
The Scientific Basis of Toxicity Assessment
H. Witschi, editor.   129

METABOLIC ACTIVATION OF CARCINOGENS: AN ERROR IN DETOXIFICATION[*]

J. K. Selkirk, M. C. MacLeod, and G. M. Cohen[†]

Biology Division, Oak Ridge National Laboratory,

Oak Ridge, Tennessee 37830

INTRODUCTION

The last decade has witnessed the greatest expansion of chemical carcinogenesis research since the discovery of benzo(a)pyrene in coal tar. Investigators from virtually all scientific disciplines are now involved in attempts
to understand and explain some facet of why certain classes of chemicals
cause cancer. Some of the major reasons for this phenomenal increase in research
effort lie in the development of more sophisticated analytical techniques which
ensure rapid and reproducible separation and isolation of the metabolic intermediates[1] and an intensive synthesis program that has produced large varieties
of test substances for carcinogenesis and metabolic studies[2]. In addition,
there has been significant increase in the variety and types of biological
systems, both mammalian and bacterial, used for chemical carcinogenesis
studies[3,4,5]. These in turn have enabled researchers to select out those
species, tissues, or cells that have been most effective for studying the mechanism of action of chemical carcinogens, including those types that are closest
to humans.

As with any xenobiotic, the detoxification response of the organism toward
chemical carcinogens is to transform these potentially toxic compounds into
more polar, less lipid soluble substances that are readily excretable, and
therefore rendered harmless. However, it would appear that nature has made a
serious mistake in the case of chemical carcinogens. This concept can be
stylized by superimposing the steps in metabolic activation upon a chemical
energy activation diagram (Figure 1). It is generally assumed that the parent
molecules of an environmentally prevalent chemical carcinogen are structurally

---

[*]Research sponsored jointly by the Environmental Protection Agency under Inter-
agency Agreement 40-516-75, the National Cancer Institute under Interagency
Agreement 40-5-63, and the Office of Health and Environmental Research, U.S.
Department of Energy, under contract W-7405-eng-26 with the Union Carbide
Corporation.

[†]Permanent Address: Department of Biochemistry, University of Surrey,
Guildford GU2 5XH, Surrey, England.

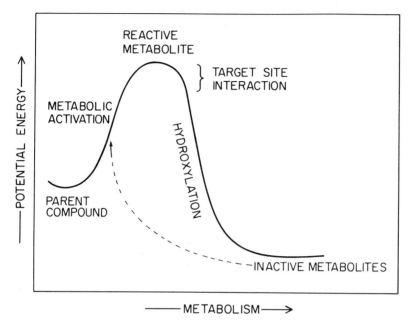

Fig. 1. Diagrammatic representation of the steps in metabolic activation super-
imposed upon a cheimcal energy-of-activation curve. In order for an unreacted
chemical to be metabolized it must be raised to a higher energy state during
which it is thought to be carcinogenically active.

stable and relatively inactive metabolically. This is not unreasonable from a
teleological point of view since one would expect labile chemical substances to
be rapidly degraded or oxidized if released in the open environment due to sunlight and weather. This is seen by the fact that synthetically prepared activated carcinogens, such as polyaromatic epoxides and nitrosamines, have been
shown to possess very short half-lives under physiological conditions[5]. Therefore, the parent compound undergoes a decrease in entropy to increase its
potential energy for subsequent metabolic degradation. This requires enzymatic
transformation into a reactive intermediate antecedent to further catabolism.
Current evidence shows that all known carcinogenic chemicals are electrophilic
reagents that seek out nucleophilic sites inside the cell[6]. The peak of the
curve in Figure 1 is the zone where the electron-deficient reactive metabolite
is thought to interact with nucleophilic target sites which are hypothesized to
begin the process of malignant transformation. If no such interaction takes
place, the most common reaction is hydroxylation to form a metabolically inactive polar structure that is more hydrophilic and can be readily excreted.
Therefore, the major thrust of the detoxification process is to render the

parent compound into a structure of greater entropy and consequently less potential to exert a toxic effect. All of the major carcinogenic chemicals, including polyaromatic hydrocarbons, aflatoxins, aromatic amines and nitrosamines
follow the same biochemical scheme and must pass through this highly reactive
state during metabolism. Presumably all types of chemical carcinogens possess
some common physical-chemical relationship that provokes the same type of disruption to cellular homeostasis that transforms it from a normal cell into a
cancer cell. The burgeoning of research in all these classes of carcinogens
has produced a host of new biochemical data that more clearly describes the
mode of activation, the sites of interaction, and the various types of detoxification products formed. Yet, the complete mechanism of maligant trans-
mation, for any of these carcinogens, remains obscure. It is possible
that the problem of carcinogenesis must now be approached through a kinetic
mechanism which exploits the knowledge of resistant and susceptible species,
strains, and cells that has accumulated from the numerous model systems
developed in recent years. The rationale behind relative resistance and
susceptibility may be viewed through a hypothesis that deals with the net
accumulation and spatial orientation of the reactive carcinogenic intermediate
within the cell. If it is assumed that the qualitative nature of the carcinogen
metabolite profile is common to both susceptible and resistant cells, then it
may be possible that a susceptible cell is producing an active metabolite at a
rate faster than the hydroxylating and conjugating enzymes can remove it.
Similarly, this same cell may produce the reactive metabolite at a rate
equivalent to a resistant cell, but possess a reduced capacity to hydroxylate
or conjugate carcinogenic intermediates. In either case, the net result would
be a longer half-life for the reactive intermediate with a concomitant increase
in the probability that the activated intermediate will interact with a critical
target site for malignant transformation. Therefore it becomes necessary to
attempt to separate the various metabolic components as they occur within the
cell and to observe any compartmentalization or segregation of metabolites which
may alter the relative probability for a given metabolite to reach cellular
macromolecules such as chromatin.

Benzo(a)pyrene Metabolism

Benzo(a)pyrene has been the prototype chemical carcinogen for tumorigenesis
and metabolic studies in recent years. This chemical, which is a potent laboratory carcinogen _in vivo_[7] and _in vitro_[8], and is suspected, based on epidemiological evidence, as a human carcinogen,[9] is a major pollutant of air, water and
soil[10]. B(a)P and other polyaromatic hydrocarbons are formed as pyrolysis prod-

132

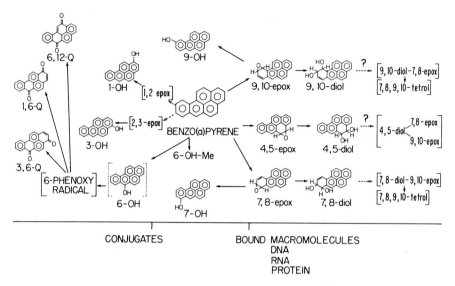

Fig. 2. Known and suspected metabolites of benzo(a)pyrene. Structures in brackets have not been directly isolated due to chemical instability. The 7,8-diol-9,10-epoxide is thought to be the major carcinogenic intermediate for benzo(a)pyrene.

ucts in the incomplete combustion of carbonaceous material such as fossil fuel. A number of metabolic products have been isolated and identified, including the hydration product of the reactive intermediate presumed to be responsible for malignant transformation[11]. Figure 2 shows a large number of known and suspected metabolites of benzo(a)pyrene. The most cogent generalization that has become apparent during recent years concerning the metabolism of benzo(a)pyrene is the qualitative identity of metabolites in all eukaryotic species studied. While there can be marked variations in the amount of metabolism between species and tissues as a function of the relative ability to induce the microsomal mono-oxygenase enzymes, it would appear that both susceptible and resistant species, tissues, and cells, form an identical metabolite profile. Therefore, it would seem unlikely that there is a unique reactive intermediate which is specific to susceptible cells and tissues. Therefore, it becomes necessary to study complete metabolism kinetics from the moment the carcinogen enters the cell and at various stages of activation and detoxification until the deactivated compound is excreted.

If benzo(a)pyrene is incubated with hamster embryonic fibroblasts for 24 hr and the medium and cells extracted with organic solvent and analyzed by high-pressure liquid chromatography, typical results are seen in Figure 3[12]. Under

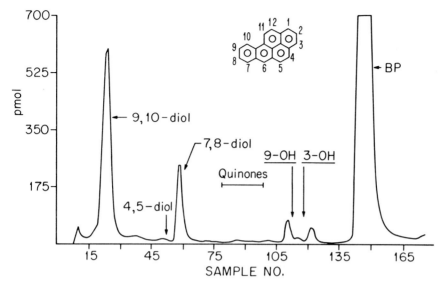

Fig. 3. Organic-Solvent Soluble. Benzo(a)pyrene metabolites formed by hamster embryonic fibroblasts during a 24 hr incubation. Analysis by high-pressure liquid chromatography.

these conditions the major products are the 9,10- and 7,8-diols. The phenol yield is negligible and the quinones are essentially absent, while the 4,5-diol is in trace amounts. This metabolite profile is markedly different than that observed from tissue homogenates[13], where 3-OH is the major product, usually comprising over 30% of the total metabolites. The one similarity that exists between cell-free and intact cell metabolism is the relatively large amount of the 9,10-diol.

These major differences can be observed if one realizes that preparation of subcellular fractions completely disrupts the normal cellular homeostatis, and after incubation with B(a)P presents a metabolite profile that does not corre-spond to an intact cell situation where there exists a full complement of micro-somal and cytoplasmic enzymes. The metabolite profile seen in Figure 3 can be further resolved into intracellular and extracellular components by analyzing the medium separately after 24 hr incubation (extracellular) and then lysing the cells with detergent and analyzing the metabolite profile confined within the cytoplasm[14]. Figure 4 represents the partitioning of benzo(a)pyrene metabo-lites by the cell between the intracellular compartment and the medium. The 9,10-diol is completely removed by the cell into the extracellular space while the 7,8-diol appears to be able to cross the cell membrane as it is observed both inside and outside the cell. Although the quinones are somewhat reduced,

134

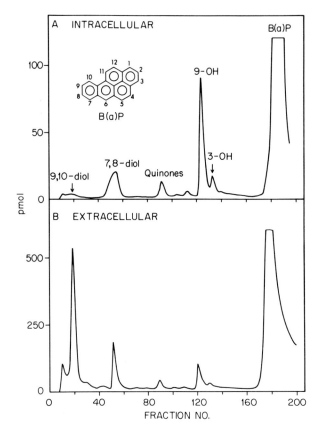

Fig. 4. Partition of Benzo(a)pyrene Metabolites Between Cytoplasm and Surrounding Medium. 9,10-Diol is not retained within the cell. The free phenols and quinones are largely intracellular while the 7,8-diol appears on both sides of the cell membrane.

they are able to remain within the cell as in the case with the phenol fraction. This metabolite profile then represents a situation where the cell, for reasons yet obscure, is able to discriminate between two very similar dihydrodiols and exclude quantitatively the 9,10-diol into the extracellular medium.

Conjugation of the various hydroxylated products to glucuronic acid appears to be a final detoxification step that may be important to in vivo metabolism and detoxification of benzo(a)pyrene. It further reduces the chances of remetabolism of hydroxylated intermediates into even more reactive electrophiles. The 9,10-dihydrodiol has been shown to be carcinogenically[8] and mutagenically[15] inactive and as seen in Figure 5 is a poor substrate for subsequent conjugation to water-soluble products. Treatment of the aqueous phase with β-glucuronidase

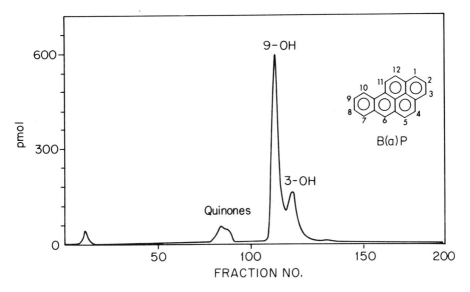

Fig. 5. Water-Soluble Metabolites. Water-soluble radioactivity treated with β-glucuronidase freed phenols and quinones. Diol conjugates were not detectable in hamster embryonic fibroblasts, however, glucuronides are formed in tracheal tissue[18].

failed to produce any 9,10-dihydrodiol[16], and also confirms earlier reports which indicate that the cell forms glucuronic acid conjugates with benzo(a)pyrene phenols and quinones by means of microsomal transglucuronylase and cytoplasmic UDPGA. Benzo(a)pyrene diols were not substrate for glucuronic acid conjugation in these cells.

The structural isomer of benzo(a)pyrene, benzo(e)pyrene (Figure 6) displays,

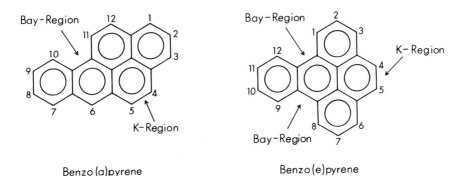

Fig. 6. Structures of Benzopyrene Isomers. Both isomers possess K-region and bay-region descriptors that have been used to predict carcinogenic activity. Bay-region calculations predict the non-carcinogenic benzo(e)-pyrene to be almost as tumorigenic as carcinogenic benzo(a)pyrene.

at best, marginal carcinogenic activity[7]. This is most unusual since benzo(e)-
pyrene contains two equivalent bay-regions which have been postulated as a major
stru tural requirement for a polyaromatic hydrocarbon to display carcinogenic
activity, and bay-region calculations have predicted benzo(e)pyrene to be
almost as carcinogenic as benzo(a)pyrene[17].

    Using identical incubation conditions, benzo(e)pyrene was incubated with
hamster embryonic cells. As can be seen in Figure 7, the metabolite profile
consists almost totally of the K-region, 4,5-diol with no demonstrable metabolism in the bay-region area (D_1; carbons 9, 10, 11 or 12). In addition, it
appears that there is a single extracellular metabolite which is also the
K-region 4,5-diol (Figure 7) suggesting that the cell does not maintain any
special intracellular partitioning of this diol metabolite. Peaks labeled P1
and P2 may be phenolic compounds based on their chromatographic retention time

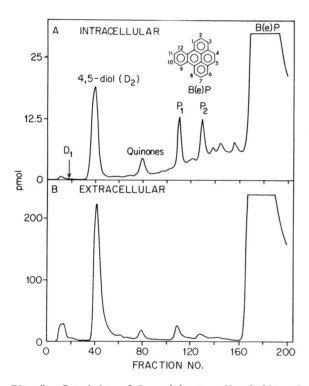

Fig. 7. Partition of Benzo(e)pyrene Metabolites Between Cytoplasm and
Surrounding Medium. A Single Major Metabolite; the K-region 4,5-diol.
Bay-region metabolism is not favored for this isomer by hamster embryo
cells. Peaks P_1 and P_2 chromatograph in the phenol region but are yet
not identified.

with the methanol-water gradient. Figure 8 shows the results of ß-glucuronidase
treatment of the radioactivity remaining in the water residue after ethyl-
acetate extraction, and the K-region 4,5-diol and the peak P_2 were both
shown to be substrates for glucuronide conjugation.

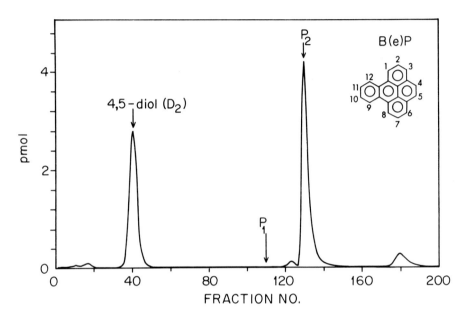

Fig. 8. Water-Soluble Metabolites. Water-soluble radioactivity treated with
ß-glucuronidase freed the 4,5-diol and the P_2 peak. No bay-region diols were
observed.

Thus these results suggest a metabolic basis for the relative lack of carcinogenic activity of B(e)P. Hamster embryonic fibroblasts do not form significant amounts of the non-K-region dihydrodiol [B(e)P-9,10-dihydrodiol] under
these conditions, and, therefore, are not producing the diol substrate in the
proper position for subsequent formation of a bay-region diol-epoxide. The
reason why little or no B(e)P-9,10-dihydrodiol is formed is not clear but may
be due to physical or chemical factors such as membrane solubility or stereo-
chemical requirements of the active site of the enzyme. The bay-region theory
of PAH carcinogenesis predicts that carbonium ion formation from B(e)P-9,10-
dihydrodiol-11,12-oxide, if formed, would be energetically favorable[17]. Thus,
the inability of hamster embryonic cells to form B(e)P-9,10-dihydrodiol, the

138

precursor of its potentially highly reactive diol-epoxide, would explain the
reactive inertness of B(e)P in several biological systems.

As the subtle biochemical interactions of the various carcinogen intermediates become clarified, it becomes apparent that susceptibility and resistance
to malignant transformation is based on a complex set of both chemical and
physical parameters. Figure 9 shows the various reactions on the benzo(a)-
pyrene molecule along its route toward tumor formation. The diagram shown
presents a number of reactions designed to reduce the available substrate at
each step along the metabolic activation pathway toward the formation of the
diol-epoxide. Clearly this is an imperfect detoxifying system since susceptible
species, such as Swiss mice, readily form tumors from benzo(a)pyrene. Since
there is no unique intermediate produced by the monooxygenases in these susceptible species, it is becoming clear that metabolism kinetics and membrane interactions help dictate the movements of the carcinogen into and through the cell's
metabolic machinery. As with the case of benzo(e)pyrene, the present calculations cannot accurately predict biochemical or carcinogenic activity since it
is probable that all the biochemical parameters necessary to make accurate
prognostications are not yet known.

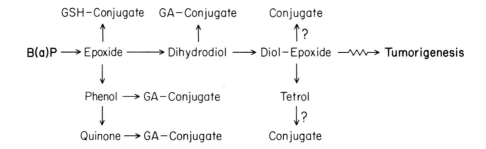

Fig. 9. Competing Reactions for Benzo(a)pyrene Intermediates During Activation
to the Highly Reactive Diol-Epoxide. Those reactions which will reduce the
final amount of diol-epoxide formed may be species-variable and important in
·determining resistance and susceptibility.

REFERENCES

1. Selkirk, J. K. (1978) Advances in Chromatography, Marcel-Dekker, Inc., New York, pp. 1-36.

2. Searle, C. E. (1976) Chemical Carcinogens. ACS Monography, 173.

3. Heidelberger, Charles (1973) Advances in Cancer Research, 18, 317-360.

4. McCann, J. B. and Ames, B. N. (1976) Proc. Natl. Acad. Sci. USA, 73, 950-954.

5. Slaga, T. J., Sivak, A., Boutwell, R. K. (1976) Mechanisms of Tumor Promotion and Co-Carcinogenesis, Raven Press, New York, pp.

6. Miller, J. A. and Miller, E. C. (1977) Origins of Human Cancer, Cold Spring Harbor Symposium, pp. 605-627.

7. Survey of Compounds Which Have Been Tested For Carcinogenic Activity, Public Health Service Publication No. 149.

8. Mager, R., Huberman, E., Yang, S. K., Gelboin, H. V., and Sachs, L. (1977) Int. J. Cancer, 19, 814-817.

9. Cuyler-Hammons, E., Selikoff, Irving J., Lawther, Patrick L., and Seidman, Herbert (1976) Annals of the New York Academy of Science, 271, pp. 116-124.

10. Committee on Biological Effects of Atmospheric Pollutants, Particulate Polycyclic Organic Matter. (1972) The National Academy of Sciences, Washington, D.C.

11. Weinstein, I. B., Jeffrey, A.M., Jennette, K. W., Blobstein, S. H., Harvey, R.G., Harris, C., Autrup, H., Kasai, and Nakanishi, K. (1976) Science, 193, 592-595.

12. Selkirk, J. K., Croy, R. G., Wiebel, F. J., and Gelboin, H. V. (1976) Cancer Res., 36, 4476.

13. Selkirk, J. K., Croy, R. G., and Gelboin, H. V. (1974) Science, 184, 169.

14. MacLeod, M. C., Cohen, G. M., and Selkirk, J. K. Cancer Research, in press.

15. Huberman, E., Sachs, L., Yang, S. K., and Gelboin, H. V. (1976) Proc. Natl. Acad. Sci. USA, 73, 607-611.

16. Baird, W. M., Chern, C. J., and Diamond, L. (1977) Cancer Res. 37, 3190-3197.

17. Jerina, D. M., Lehr, R., Schaefer-Ridder, M., Yagi, H., Karle, J. M., Thakker, D. R., Wood, A. W., Lu, A. Y. H., Ryan, D., West, S., Levin, W., and Conney, A. H. (1977) Origins of Human Cancer, Cold Spring Harbor Laboratory, pp. 639-658.

18. Cohen, G. M., Marchok, A. C., Nettesheim, P., Steele, V. E., Nelson, F., Shilling, H., and Selkirk, J. K. (1979) Cancer Res., 39, 1980-1984.

METABOLIC ACTIVATION OF TOXINS IN EXTRAHEPATIC TARGET ORGANS AND TARGET CELLS

M. R. BOYD, A. R. BUCKPITT, R. B. JONES, C. N. STATHAM, J. S. DUTCHER, and N. S. LONGO

Molecular Toxicology Section, Clinical Pharmacology Branch, Clinical Oncology Program, Division of Cancer Treatment, National Cancer Institute, National Institutes of Health, Bethesda, Maryland 20205

INTRODUCTION

Whereas the overall quantitative contribution of extrahepatic metabolism to the disposition of a particular chemical compound *in vivo* may be small in comparison to hepatic metabolism, the toxicologic consequences of extrahepatic metabolic transformations leading to irreversible or cumulative cellular changes may be profound. This is an especially important consideration in view of the greater cellular heterogeneity of many extrahepatic tissues compared to the liver. It is unlikely that xenobiotic-metabolizing activities in extra-hepatic tissues are randomly distributed throughout all cells in these organs; it is more probable that these activities are restricted to a relatively few cell types. Extrahepatic tissues, and specific cell types contained therein, which possess enzyme systems required for the metabolic activation of xeno-biotic substances therefore might be extraordinarily susceptible to toxicities involving reactive metabolites. For these reasons, studies of the metabolic activation of protoxins and/or procarcinogens by extrahepatic tissues and cells should provide useful information not only as to what kinds of chemicals are likely to damage these tissues but also as to what types of pathological changes are likely to occur in specific tissues or cells that are exposed to chemicals capable of undergoing metabolic activation. The purpose of this paper is to illustrate our approach to this area of research by our recent studies of pulmonary and renal toxicities by the furan derivative, 4-ipomeanol (1-[3-furyl]-4-hydroxypentanone).

Because of the potential importance of 4-ipomeanol as a naturally-occurring toxicant[1-4], and because of its unique toxicologic properties, the mechanism of toxicity of this compound has been the subject of intensive investigation during the past several years[5-25]. 4-Ipomeanol has proved to be an ideal model toxin for mechanistic studies because of its structural simplicity, its biologic potency, and its capacity for inducing striking, target organ-selective toxici-ties in laboratory animals. The compound can be synthesized readily in large amounts needed for biological studies, and radioactive precursors can be easily incorporated to produce radiolabeled 4-ipomeanol essential for metabolic investigations.

Previous studies on the mechanism of 4-ipomeanol toxicity have led to the view that the tissue-specific damage caused by the compound is due to highly reactive, alkylating metabolites formed primarily *in situ* in the target tissues[10,13,25,26]. For this presentation only certain aspects of this work will be discussed that seem especially relevant to the goals of this symposium on "The Scientific Basis of Toxicity Assessment", and, in particular, to the theme of the present session on "What Makes a Chemical a Threat to Health." Major emphasis will be placed on studies showing that target organ and target cell susceptibilities to a toxin requiring metabolic activation can vary considerably (1) among different animal species, (2) in animals of different ages, or (3) in animals previously exposed to inducers or inhibitors of xenobiotic-metabolizing enzymes.

METABOLIC ACTIVATION OF 4-IPOMEANOL AND ITS RELATIONSHIP TO TOXICITY

Some features of the metabolic activation of 4-ipomeanol by tissue preparations *in vitro*. Without prior metabolism, 4-ipomeanol is not capable of covalently binding to tissue macromolecules. Therefore, studies of the *in vitro* metabolic activation of 4-ipomeanol in subcellular tissue preparations have been useful for characterizing enzymatic activities which mediate the formation of alkylating metabolites of the compound. These studies also have provided a basis for the design of appropriate *in vivo* studies to evaluate the role of metabolism in the *in vivo* toxicity of 4-ipomeanol.

Activities capable of mediating the covalent binding of 4-ipomeanol to tissue macromolecules are present in the microsomal fractions from potential target organs for 4-ipomeanol toxicity[14-20,26]. Where such activities are present, they share several common characteristics. The covalent binding reaction occurs only in the presence of oxygen and requires NADPH as a cofactor. The presence of the furan ring of 4-ipomeanol is essential for covalent binding to occur. Analogs of 4-ipomeanol in which the furan group was replaced by phenyl or methyl substituents underwent little or no NADPH-dependent covalent binding in microsomal preparations from rat lung or liver[20]. The covalent binding reaction is strongly inhibited by the presence of carbon monoxide, indicating the probable participation of a cytochrome P-450 in a mixed-function oxidation leading to the production of alkylating metabolite(s) of 4-ipomeanol[20].

Studies[20] showing decreases in the *in vitro* covalent binding of 4-ipomeanol by mixed-function oxidase inhibitors, including SKF-525A and piperonyl butoxide, are consistent with this view. NADPH-cytochrome *c* (P-450) reductase also is an important component of mixed-function oxidase systems, and an antibody prepared against this enzyme was found to strongly inhibit the metabolic activation of 4-ipomeanol in rat lung and liver microsome preparations[16,18].

Nucleophilic sulphydryl compounds such as glutathione (GSH) and cysteine react with the electrophilic, alkylating metabolites of 4-ipomeanol and form water-soluble conjugates. These reactions thereby prevent the covalent binding of 4-ipomeanol metabolites to tissue macromolecules *in vitro*, and they do so without altering the rate of formation of the alkylating metabolites[20,24]. Evidence has been presented that the conjugation of reactive 4-ipomeanol metabolites with GSH may be an important detoxification pathway for 4-ipomeanol *in vivo*[23]. A method has recently been developed for the qualitative and quantitative analysis of GSH conjugates of 4-ipomeanol metabolites[24]; at least two different conjugates were formed in incubation mixtures containing rat lung or liver microsomes, NADPH, 4-ipomeanol, and GSH[24].

The alkylating metabolites of 4-ipomeanol appear to be extremely reactive and short-lived in biological media, and they have not been directly isolable. Nevertheless, the measurement of the covalent binding of 4-ipomeanol to protein (or sulfhydryl compounds) has proved to be a valuable approach to detecting and quantitating the formation of highly reactive 4-ipomeanol metabolites *in vitro* and *in vivo*. It is possible that the covalent binding of 4-ipomeanol metabolites to macromolecules other than protein may be of considerable biologic significance. However, we routinely have measured binding to protein since it adequately reflects reactive metabolite formation and since the amount of metabolite bound to protein quantitatively far exceeds binding to other macromolecules, such as the nucleic acids.

While the microsomal activities mediating the covalent binding of 4-ipomeanol in various tissues and among various animal species share several common features, some major differences, both qualitative and quantitative, have been found[16,18,20,26]. Some of these *in vitro* differences provide interesting correlations with patterns of *in vivo* target organ alkylation and toxicity to be discussed in the following section. In rats, high activities were found in preparations from both the lungs and the livers; rat kidney microsomal preparations, on the other hand, had little, if any, capacity to catalyze the covalent binding of 4-ipomeanol. In mice, relatively high activities also were found in the pulmonary and hepatic microsome preparations. However, in contrast to renal microsomes from other species we have studied (rat, rabbit, guinea pig, hamster, bird), microsomes from the kidneys of adult mice were extremely active in mediating the formation of alkylating metabolites from 4-ipomeanol[14,26]. Studies with avian species (Japanese quail and chickens) have illustrated another interesting contrast; formation of reactive 4-ipomeanol metabolites by bird lung and kidney microsomal preparations was relatively very low (and virtually absent in chicken lungs) in comparison to the very high activities in avian liver microsomes[17].

While these striking quantitative differences in activities suggest a potential basis for different patterns of tissue-specific covalent binding of 4-ipomeanol in different species *in vivo* (i.e., activities are either high, or low or absent in potential target tissues), qualitative differences in the activation pathways also may be important. For example, although the maximal rates of covalent binding of 4-ipomeanol were similar in rat lung and liver microsomes, the K_M for the metabolism and covalent binding in lung microsomes was more than 10-fold lower than in hepatic microsomes[20]. The fact that maximal rates of metabolism and covalent binding of 4-ipomeanol in microsomes from certain extrahepatic tissues are comparable in magnitude to the corresponding rates in hepatic microsomes is striking, considering the relatively low levels of cytochrome(s) P-450 present in these extrahepatic tissues[20,26]. Indeed, although there appears to be an obligatory requirement for a cytochrome P-450 in the metabolic reactions leading to the covalent binding of 4-ipomeanol, there is poor correlation between total microsomal cytochrome P-450 content and the capacity of the microsomes to metabolize 4-ipomeanol[20,26]. For example, rat kidney microsome preparations contain cytochrome(s) P-450, but they are virtually incapable of mediating the covalent binding of 4-ipomeanol[26].

It is now generally appreciated that tissues capable of metabolizing xenobiotics may contain multiple types of cytochrome(s) P-450 and that these different types may show very different substrate specificities for mixed-function oxidations. It therefore seems likely that only certain forms of cytochrome P-450 are capable of supporting the metabolic activation of 4-ipomeanol, and that this could be an important determinant of tissue-specific metabolism of the compound. It is also possible that factors other than cytochrome P-450 are responsible for differences in the kinetic characteristics of extrahepatic vs. hepatic microsomal activities involved in 4-ipomeanol metabolism. This possibility was suggested by recent studies undertaken in collaboration with Drs. Sasame and Gillette[16,18]. An antibody prepared against purified cytochrome b5

was found to inhibit almost completely the metabolism of 4-ipomeanol by rat
pulmonary microsomes, but the antibody had little effect on 4-ipomeanol metabolism by rat hepatic microsomes. These experiments were viewed as consistent
with a mechanism of 4-ipomeanol activation involving a cytochrome P-450-
dependent mixed-function oxidase in which the transfer of the second electron
involved in the reaction sequence occurred via cytochrome b_5 and that this step
was rate-limiting in rat lung microsomes[18].

Aside from these complexities, however, results from *in vitro* experiments
with microsome preparations have illustrated some intriguing correlations with
tissue specificities of the *in vivo* covalent binding and toxicity of 4-ipomeanol.
They have also established the important point that high levels of *in vivo*
covalent binding and toxicity of 4-ipomeanol occur only in tissues which can be
shown to metabolically activate the compound *in vitro*.

Target organ alkylation and toxicity of 4-ipomeanol *in vivo*; species
differences. *In vivo* studies of species differences in the target organ alkylation and toxicity by 4-ipomeanol[15,17,26] support the view that target organ
toxicities produced by the compound result from the generation of highly reactive metabolites *in situ* in the target tissues. Such investigations also have
identified several new *in vivo* models that seem to be of potential value for
further studies of metabolic and dispositional factors underlying the target
organ specificity of 4-ipomeanol. In rats, the levels of covalently bound
4-ipomeanol were highest in the lungs when compared to the liver and kidneys.
The amounts of material covalently bound in other tissues of the rat were
either very low or nondetectable. 4-Ipomeanol also was covalently bound preferentially to the lungs of rabbits and guinea pigs. In adult mice, the levels
of pulmonary alkylation were relatively high, but in this species, in contrast
to all other species we have studied, the amount of renal alkylation also was
exceedingly high. Another unique pattern of tissue specificity was seen in
birds; both the pulmonary and the renal alkylation levels were very low in comparison to the exceedingly high levels of covalent binding of 4-ipomeanol in
the livers.

In sharp contrast to these species differences, the patterns of tissue alkylation in different strains of a given species are highly consistent[15,26]. For
example, three different strains of rats (Sprague-Dawley, Lewis, and Fisher 344)
all showed the pattern of organ-specific covalent binding of 4-ipomeanol typical
for rats. Likewise, six different strains of mice (Swiss, C57BL/6J, DBA/2J,
A/J, C3H/HeJ, and BALB/cJ) all showed the same pattern typical of adult mice.

Studies with two kinds of birds (quail and chickens) gave tissue alkylation patterns that were very similar[17].

Target organ alkylation by 4-ipomeanol *in vivo*; age-related differences. It is important to emphasize that the previously discussed target organ specificity of 4-ipomeanol covalent binding in mice represents a highly characteristic pattern that consistently is obtained in the adult animals (20-30 g). However, in this species there are very striking age-related differences in the patterns of target organ alkylation by 4-ipomeanol[21]. In young mice (8-10 g) there is relatively little alkylation of the kidneys; but in adult mice (20-30 g) renal alkylation levels are very high and, in fact, exceed the levels occurring in all other tissues, including the lungs. Tissue alkylation patterns obtained with 4-ipomeanol in mice of intermediate ages have demonstrated a definite age-related transition from the "young mouse" pattern to the "adult mouse" pattern of binding. All of these characteristic patterns of binding specificity are consistent over a wide range of doses of 4-ipomeanol. Preliminary *in vitro* studies indicate that these differences in the *in vivo* renal alkylation levels are due to age-related differences in the renal microsomal enzyme activities required for metabolic activation of 4-ipomeanol. Renal slice preparations from kidneys of adult mice actively metabolized 4-ipomeanol to alkylating metabolites, while similar slice preparations from kidneys of young mice showed only very low activity.

Target organ toxicity of 4-ipomeanol *in vivo*; species and age differences. The major target organs for 4-ipomeanol toxicity *in vivo* in different species closely parallel the respective organ specificities of *in vivo* covalent binding of the compound. Thus, in rats, rabbits, and guinea pigs the lungs were the primary site of damage by 4-ipomeanol[19,26]. Likewise, in young mice the lungs were the primary target organ for 4-ipomeanol toxicity, and the kidneys usually appeared normal[21]. However, in older mice both the lung and the kidneys consistently were severely damaged by 4-ipomeanol[21]. In the Japanese quail the liver was the major site of damage by 4-ipomeanol, and there was little or no evidence of renal or pulmonary damage[17].

Effects of 3-methylcholanthrene pretreatment on target organ metabolism, covalent binding, and toxicity of 4-ipomeanol. Further evidence for the role of *in situ* metabolic activation. The patterns of preferential extrahepatic tissue alkylation such as those found in rats and mice would be difficult to explain by a mechanism in which alkylating metabolites binding to the extrahepatic tissues were formed primarily in the liver and reached tissues such as the lungs and kidneys via the circulation. Indeed, the studies with birds offered an interesting contrast in which very high levels of alkylating metabolite production in the liver were accompanied by relatively low levels of extrahepatic tissue alkylation. Moreover, in all of these species, relatively little or no alkylation occurred in extrahepatic tissues incapable of metabolically activating 4-ipomeanol (e.g., blood, heart, skeletal muscle). Thus, a more satisfactory explanation for these characteristic patterns of tissue alkylation is that the major portion of the reactive metabolite of 4-ipomeanol that becomes covalently bound in extrahepatic tissues such as the lungs and kidneys, and which leads to damage to those tissues, is actually formed *in situ* in those organs.

Results of studies with animals pretreated with the inducer, 3-methylcholanthrene (3MC), also are consistent with a mechanism of extrahepatic target organ alkylation and toxicity primarily involving the *in situ* generation of highly reactive 4-ipomeanol metabolites. *In vitro* studies demonstrated that the 4-ipomeanol covalent binding activity was markedly enhanced in liver microsome preparations from both Sprague-Dawley rats[20] and C57BL/6J mice[14] pretreated with 3MC, but covalent binding was not significantly altered in hepatic microsomes from the "noninducible" DBA/2J mouse strain treated with 3MC[14]. The 3MC pretreatment did not significantly increase the *in vitro* covalent binding of 4-ipomeanol in microsome preparations from rat lungs[20] or from mouse lungs or kidneys[14].

Coordinate with these alterations measurable *in vitro*, the 3MC pretreatment caused marked alterations in the target organ specificity for covalent binding and toxicity of 4-ipomeanol *in vivo*. For example, in the 3MC-induced rats, the relative proportion of covalent binding of the toxin to liver was markedly increased, whereas it was decreased in the lung, over a wide range of doses of 4-ipomeanol[19]. Consistent with these alterations in binding patterns, toxic doses of 4-ipomeanol frequently caused severe centrilobular hepatic necrosis in 3MC-pretreated rats (no liver damage occurs in control rats). Lung toxicity was relatively less pronounced when compared to controls[19]. Similarly, in comparison to nonpretreated controls, the *in vivo* covalent binding of 4-ipomeanol was markedly elevated in the livers of 3MC-pretreated C57BL/6J mice, while the binding was actually decreased in the lungs and the kidneys[14]. 4-Ipomeanol frequently caused hepatic necrosis in the pretreated mice (but not in controls), and renal and pulmonary toxicity was less than in controls[14]. In contrast, 3MC pretreatment had no sifnificant effect on target organ alkylation and toxicity by 4-ipomeanol in "noninducible" DBA/2J mice[14].

Thus, the findings that 3MC could greatly increase the formation and covalent binding of reactive 4-ipomeanol metabolites in the liver, without increasing the amount of 4-ipomeanol binding in extrahepatic tissues, argues strongly against the possibility that a major proportion of alkylating metabolites formed in the liver could escape that organ and covalently bind to tissues such as the kidney and lung. In fact, the 3MC pretreatment invariably caused a decrease in the levels of alkylation in the kidneys and the lungs[14,19]; it is possible that these decreases are due to an increased rate of hepatic clearance and shortened biological half-life of the 4-ipomeanol in the induced animals[10,19].

Target cell specificity for covalent binding and toxicity of 4-ipomeanol in kidney and lung, and the effects of inhibitors of 4-ipomeanol metabolism. Autoradiographic studies[11,12,14] have shown that metabolites covalently bound in susceptible extrahepatic tissues after administration of toxic doses of 4-ipomeanol are highly localized in specific cell types, and that these cells are major targets for 4-ipomeanol toxicity. Thus, covalently bound 4-ipomeanol metabolite was located almost exclusively in proximal cortical tubular cells of the kidneys from adult mice[14]. Likewise, the proximal renal tubular cells were the major site of damage (necrosis) by 4-ipomeanol; there was little or no covalent binding of 4-ipomeanol in renal medullary cells, and these cells did not become necrotic[14].

Similarly, after the i.p. administration of toxic doses of 4-ipomeanol, the covalently bound 4-ipomeanol metabolite was found to be present primarily in the nonciliated bronchiolar (Clara) cells of the pulmonary airways in the lungs of rats, mice, and hamsters[11,12]. 4-Ipomeanol also was capable of preferentially damaging pulmonary Clara cells in these species[11,12] as well as others that were tested, including rabbits and guinea pigs[26]. Considering the previously discussed finding that there was relatively little covalent binding or toxicity of 4-ipomeanol in bird lungs, it is interesting that lungs of avian species are somewhat unique in structure and physiologic functions[27]. They are devoid of airway cells analogous to the Clara cells and the ciliated bronchiolar cells typically found in many other vertebrate species[27].

By pretreating animals with piperonyl butoxide, a potent inhibitor of 4-ipomeanol metabolism[20], it was possible to completely block the alkylation and destruction of Clara cells in rats[12] and mice[14] and of renal tubular cells in mice[14]. These results provided further evidence that these target cell toxicities were due to highly reactive 4-ipomeanol metabolites formed in these target cells.

The pulmonary cellular specificity for the metabolic activation of 4-ipomeanol recently was studied *in vitro* in systems containing intact lung cells[22]. 4-Ipomeanol was actively metabolized and covalently bound in incubation mixtures containing mouse lung slices and in isolated whole mouse lungs suspended in, and perfused intratracheally with, oxygenated Kreb's solution. The covalent binding reaction was time-dependent and was concentration-dependent up to 0.25 - 0.50 mM 4-ipomeanol, at which concentrations the maximal rates of binding were achieved. Heat-denatured tissues did not mediate the covalent binding of 4-ipomeanol. The *in vitro* covalent binding reaction was markedly decreased in lung preparations from animals pretreated *in vivo* with the inhibitor of 4-ipomeanol metabolism, piperonyl butoxide. In lung tissue preparations from animals pretreated *in vivo* with diethylmaleate (an agent which depletes lung glutathione), the *in vitro* covalent binding of 4-ipomeanol was markedly enhanced. Autoradiographic studies showed that the 4-ipomeanol covalently bound in these *in vitro* systems was located primarily in the nonciliated bronchiolar (Clara) cells. Thus, all of these *in vitro* results are fully consistent with previous *in vivo* studies which indicated the involvement of *in situ* metabolic activation in the preferential damage to pulmonary Clara cells by 4-ipomeanol.

IMPLICATIONS FOR STUDIES OF TOXICITIES BY REACTIVE METABOLITES

Possible importance of species differences, age differences, and the effects of prior exposure to drug metabolism inducers or inhibitors in studies of extrahepatic target organ and target cell toxicities by reactive metabolites. The biologic factors determining whether a given reactive metabolite produces an acute cellular change such as necrosis, or a more latent response such as neoplastic transformation, are not known. However, it is clear that both kinds of responses can be caused by otherwise inert chemicals that must be metabolized *in vivo* to produce the active cytotoxic or carcinogenic materials. These materials usually are highly reactive, electrophilic metabolites. Therefore, the precise characterization of the metabolic "machinery" involved in the production of alkylating metabolites is of fundamental importance.

4-Ipomeanol has proved to be an extremely useful tool with which to investigate metabolic factors that may have direct relevance for other kinds of compounds that are oxidatively metabolized to cytotoxic or carcinogenic metabolites. The highly reproducible, acute target organ cytotoxicities of 4-ipomeanol have provided rapid and reliable biological "end-points" for studies on the metabolic activation of the compound. Moreover, the toxic metabolite(s) of 4-ipomeanol

is extremely reactive, and covalently binds predominantly in the immediate
vicinity of its formation, and this has greatly facilitated studies of the
organ- and cell-specific metabolism and toxicity of the compound.

As illustrated vividly by the studies described herein, activities of monooxygenase enzymes that probably are involved in the metabolic activation of a
variety of potentially toxic and/or carcinogenic chemicals can vary widely among
extrahepatic tissues of different animal species. Moreover, these variations
seem to be reflected by the striking species differences in patterns of *in vivo*
target organ alkylation by 4-ipomeanol which we have observed. Also, even within
a particular species, relatively subtle factors such as differences in age or
prior exposure to other chemicals (e.g., inducers or inhibitors) apparently can
alter enzymatic activities that are reflected *in vivo* by profound differences in
extrahepatic target organ alkylation patterns. Therefore, all of these factors
which can markedly influence the target organ specificity of the covalent binding and toxicity of 4-ipomeanol should be considered as potential variables
influencing the biologic responses (particularly those in which extrahepatic
target tissues are involved) to other toxic or carcinogenic chemicals that are
activated by enzymatic systems that are the same or similar to those involved in
the metabolic activation of 4-ipomeanol.

Potential importance of cell-specific metabolic activation in extrahepatic
tissues. The finding that reactive 4-ipomeanol metabolites became covalently
bound and caused damage preferentially to pulmonary Clara cells of several
species, and also to the proximal renal tubular cells of adult mice, raised the
possibility that 4-ipomeanol was metabolically activated preferentially in these
cells.

The cellular localization of mixed-function oxidase activity in the lung is an
issue of particular interest, especially because of the increasing incidence of
lung disease of environmental origin, and the realization that many chemical
toxins and carcinogens require mixed-function oxidase-mediated activation.

Studies indicating that 4-ipomeanol was preferentially metabolized to alkylating metabolites in pulmonary Clara cells led to the conclusion that these
cells are an important site of cytochrome P-450-dependent mixed-function oxidase
activity in lung[12]. It therefore was predicted that these cells might be important targets for other cytotoxic or carcinogenic agents requiring metabolic activation by monooxygenase enzymes. Consistent with this view are studies[28,29] of
the bronchiolar metabolism and toxicity of 3-methylfuran, a naturally occurring
potential atmospheric contaminant, and also studies[30] showing pulmonary Clara
cell damage by carbon tetrachloride.

Recent studies by Reznik-Schüller[31] indicated that a carcinogenic nitrosamine derivative, nitrosoheptamethyleneimine, was irreversibly bound preferentially in pulmonary Clara cells of hamsters after oral administration. Morphologic similarities were noted between Clara cells and cells of tumors resulting from administration of this and related nitrosamine derivatives[32,33] and such tumor cells also appeared capable of binding the nitrosamine[31] *in vivo*. It therefore seemed likely that the tumors were derived from Clara cells[31-33]. Unfortunately, definitive metabolic evidence is not available to indicate that the cellular binding or the pulmonary tumorigenicity of nitrosamines such as nitrosoheptamethyleneimine is due to a metabolite of these compounds formed *in situ* in Clara cells. Moreover, there presently is no direct evidence that the lung-toxic furans, such as 4-ipomeanol and 3-methylfuran, are pulmonary carcinogens. Taken together, however, the research on these two classes of compounds provides strong evidence that the pulmonary Clara cell indeed is a potential site of oxidative metabolic activation of carcinogens. Therefore, not only is it likely to be a potential cell of origin for tumors induced by certain classes of chemical agents, it also seems possible that other bronchiolar or bronchial cell types could be targets for carcinogenic metabolites having sufficient stability to pass from one cell to another following formation in Clara cells.

Important areas for future investigations include (1) the further elucidation of the role that the Clara cell plays in the pulmonary metabolism of xenobiotics, (2) further investigations of the possible xenobiotic-metabolizing capacities of other lung cell types, and (3) the potential importance of these activities to the pathogenesis of environmentally associated acute and chronic pulmonary diseases in man.

REFERENCES

1. Wilson, B.J., Yang, D.T.C. and Boyd, M.R. (1970) Nature, 227, 521-522.
2. Boyd, M.R. and Wilson, B.J. (1972) J. Agric. Food Chem., 20, 428-430.
3. Boyd, M.R., Wilson, B.J. and Harris, T.M. (1972) Nature New Biol., 236, 158-159.
4. Boyd, M.R., Burka, L.T., Harris, T.M. and Wilson, B.J. (1974) Biochim. Biophys. Acta, 337, 184-195.
5. Boyd, M.R., Burka, L.T., Wilson, B.J. and Sastry, B.V.R. (1974) Toxicol. Appl. Pharmacol., 29, 132.
6. Boyd, M.R., Burka, L.T., Neal, R.A., Wilson, B.J. and Holscher, M.M. (1974) Fed. Proc., 33, 234.
7. Boyd, M.R. (1975) Toxicol. Appl. Pharmacol., 33, 132.

8. Boyd, M.R., Burka, L.T., Osborne, B.A. and Wilson, B.J. (1975) Toxicol. Appl. Pharmacol., 33, 135.

9. Boyd, M.R., Burka, L.T. and Wilson, B.J. (1975) Toxicol. Appl. Pharmacol., 32, 147-157.

10. Boyd, M.R. (1976) Environ. Hlth. Persps., 16, 127-138.

11. Boyd, M.R. (1977) Proc. Am. Assoc. Cancer Res., 18, 246.

12. Boyd, M.R. (1977) Nature, 269, 713-715.

13. Nelson, S.D., Boyd, M.R. and Mitchell, J.R. (1977) Drug Metabolism Concepts (D.J. Jerina, Ed.), American Chemical Society, Washington, D.C., pp. 155-185.

14. Boyd, M.R. and Dutcher, J.S. (1978) Toxicol. Appl. Pharmacol., 45, 229.

15. Dutcher, J.S. and Boyd, M.R. (1978) Toxicol. Appl. Pharmacol., 45, 267.

16. Sasame, H.A. and Boyd, M.R. (1978) Fed. Proc., 37, 464.

17. Buckpitt, A.R. and Boyd, M.R. (1978) The Pharmacologist, 20, 181.

18. Sasame, H.A., Gillette, J.R. and Boyd, M.R. (1978) Biochem. Biophys. Res. Commun., 84, 389-395.

19. Boyd, M.R. and Burka, L.T. (1978) J. Pharmacol. Exp. Ther., 207, 687-697.

20. Boyd, M.R., Burka, L.T., Wilson, B.J. and Sasame, H.A. (1978) J. Pharmacol. Exp. Ther., 207, 677-686.

21. Jones, R., Allegra, C. and Boyd, M. (1979) Toxicol. Appl. Pharmacol., in press.

22. Longo, N. and Boyd, M. (1979) Toxicol. Appl. Pharmacol., in press.

23. Boyd, M., Statham, C., Stiko, A., Mitchell, J. and Jones, R. (1979) Toxicol. Appl. Pharmacol., in press.

24. Buckpitt, A., Dutcher, J. and Boyd, M. (1979) Fed. Proc., 38, 692.

25. Boyd, M.R. (1979) Mechanisms in Respiratory Toxicology (H. Witschi and P. Nettesheim, Eds.), CRC Press, West Palm Beach, Florida, in press.

26. Boyd, M.R., Dutcher, J.S., Buckpitt, A.R., Jones, R.B. and Statham, C.N. (1979) Proceedings of the 9th International Symposium of the Princess Takamatsu Cancer Research Fund, Tokyo, Japan, in press.

27. Fedde, M.R. (1976) Avian Physiology (P.D. Sturkie, Ed.), Springer Verlag, New York, pp. 122-145.

28. Boyd, M., Statham, C., Franklin, R. and Mitchell, J. (1978) Nature, 272, 270-271.

29. Statham, C.N., Franklin, R.B. and Boyd, M.R. (1978) Toxicol. Appl. Pharmacol., 45, 111.

30. Longo, N., Statham, C., Sasame, H. and Boyd, M.R. (1978) Fed. Proc., 37, 505.

31. Reznik-Schüller, H. and Lijinsky, W. (1979) Cancer Res., 39, 72-74.

32. Reznik-Schüller, H. (1976) Am. J. Pathol., 85, 549-554.

33. Reznik-Schüller, H. (1977) Am. J. Pathol., 89, 59-65.

© 1980 Elsevier/North-Holland Biomedical Press
The Scientific Basis of Toxicity Assessment
H. Witschi, editor.

THE INTERACTION OF PLATINUM COMPOUNDS WITH THE GENOME: CORRELATION BETWEEN DNA BINDING AND BIOLOGICAL EFFECTS*

R. O. RAHN, N. P. JOHNSON[†], A. W. HSIE, J. F. LEMONTT, W. E. MASKER, J. D. REGAN, and W. C. DUNN, JR., Biology Division, and J. D. HOESCHELE, Health and Safety Research Division, Oak Ridge National Laboratory, Oak Ridge, Tennessee 37830; D. H. BROWN, Medical and Health Sciences Division, Oak Ridge Associated Universities, Oak Ridge, Tennessee 37830 (U.S.A.)

INTRODUCTION

As pointed out by several participants at this symposium, there is a need to make toxicology a more predictive science and to search for mechanisms which explain cytotoxicity at the molecular level. In particular, there is a need to quantitate dose as the amount of a given toxic substance at or near the site of action within the cell and not as the extracellular concentration. It is necessary, therefore, to measure the binding of chemicals to cellular components and to follow the kinetics of uptake and disappearance. Such results should reflect metabolic activation as well as repair and help provide a better understanding of potential targets and molecular mechanisms.

A great deal of information has been obtained on the pharmacology and toxicology of platinum anticancer drugs (a comprehensive bibliography of publications in this field containing 950 entries has been prepared in the laboratory of B. Rosenberg, Michigan State University). The biological effects that apparently arise from reactions between cis-Dichlorodiammine Pt(II) (cis-Pt) and DNA have been the subject of a recent review article by Roberts and Thompson[1]. Evidence exists that the toxicity of cis-Pt is a result of inhibition of DNA synthesis[2,3]. Presumably its antitumor activity arises from the greater sensitivity of rapidly dividing cells such as cancer cells to agents which inhibit DNA synthesis.

cis-Pt offers many advantages to the investigator interested in the molecular mechanism of its toxicity. It can be radioactively labeled with ^{195m}Pt ($t_{1/2}$ = 4d) and, since it binds irreversibly to DNA, the in vivo DNA binding

*Research sponsored by the Office of Health and Environmental Research, U.S. Department of Energy, under contract W-7405-eng-26 with the Union Carbide Corporation.

[†]American Cancer Society Postdoctoral Fellow, supported in part by a Carcinogenesis Training Grant (#CA05296-03) awarded to The University of Tennessee by the National Cancer Institute.

can be quantitated. In addition, the trans isomer [trans-Dichlorodiammine
platinum(II) (trans-Pt)] is biologically inactive and can be used in comparative
studies. A number of investigations are underway in our laboratory to compare
various biochemical and biophysical parameters of these two compounds in order
to identify the variables important for the biological activity of cis-Pt.

Binding to DNA

The notion that DNA is the target molecule when cis-Pt interacts with cells
has prompted a number of studies on the mode of binding of Pt to DNA. In
general, these studies support the idea that binding to all of the bases can
occur but that the preferred order of binding is G > A > C > T. One model
proposed by Goodgame et al.[4] assumes that bidentate binding of cis-Pt to two
neighboring guanines at the N(7) position is the most likely mode of binding
to DNA. Another model proposed by Macquet and Butour[5] involves binding of
cis-Pt to guanine in a bidentate fashion involving the O(6) and N(7) positions
of individual guanine bases. Hopefully, better knowledge of the actual
lesions formed in DNA will permit a clearer understanding of how various Pt
compounds exert different effects at the biological level. The most detailed
binding studies to date (see review by Harrison and McAuliffe[6]), however,
have mainly considered interactions with the components of DNA rather than
with DNA itself.

We have attempted to follow the kinetics of binding of ^{195m}Pt-labeled cis-
and trans-Pt to DNA in vitro and have proposed[7] the following scheme in order
to account for the observed binding data.

$$Pt(II)(NH_3)_2Cl_2$$

$$
\begin{array}{c}
\downarrow \quad 8\text{ h (c)} \\
2\text{ h (t)}
\end{array}
$$

Aquated species
$$
\left\{
\begin{array}{l}
[Pt(II)(NH_3)_2Cl(H_2O)]^+ + Cl^- \xrightarrow{\begin{subarray}{c}6\text{ h (c)}\\2\text{ h (t)}\end{subarray}} \\[2ex]
\downarrow \begin{array}{l}6\text{ h (c)}\\>4\text{ h (t)}\end{array} \\[2ex]
[Pt(II)(NH_3)_2(H_2O)_2]^{2+} + 2\,Cl^- \xrightarrow{0.8\text{ m (c)}}
\end{array}
\right\}
$$
Reaction with DNA

[1]

A chloride ligand must be replaced by a water in order for Pt to bind to
DNA. The monoaquo species can either react directly with DNA or can subsequently react as the diaquo species after losing a second chloride ligand in

a rate-limiting step. Shown in the scheme are the half-reaction times for the _cis_ (c) and _trans_ (t) isomers. These times are all on the order of hours (except for reaction of the diaquo species with DNA which is on the order of minutes) and were obtained at 25°C in 0.005 $\underline{M}$ NaClO$_4$ (pH < 7) and with a DNA concentration of 10^{-4} $\underline{M}$. Obviously, the addition of chloride would shift the equilibrium in favor of the neutral species and binding to DNA would be inhibited. Ligands involving nitrogen are considered to be stable enough so that neither the amino ligands nor the bonds involving ring nitrogens of the bases can be dissociated. Hence, when these Pt complexes are added to cells, the presence of chloride is expected to inhibit the formation of the reactive mono- and diaquo species but that once binding to DNA occurs, the Pt is attached in an irreversible fashion. These studies indicate both _cis_- and _trans_-Pt should bind to DNA _in vivo_.

Inhibition of DNA synthesis

The most convincing evidence that DNA is the target molecule in cells treated with _cis_-Pt is the observed subsequent inhibition of DNA synthesis. For example, Howle and Gale[2] demonstrated persistent and selective inhibition of DNA synthesis _in vivo_ by _cis_-Pt. Mice containing the transplantable Ehrlich ascites tumor were treated with _cis_-Pt and after various times the tumor was removed and the amount of RNA, DNA and protein synthesis was measured in cell suspensions. All macromolecular synthesis was initially inhibited, but after 72-96 hours RNA and protein synthesis had returned to normal; DNA synthesis on the other hand remained suppressed.

The inhibitory effects on DNA, RNA and protein synthesis of _cis_-Pt along with several other platinum antitumor compounds was studied by Harder and Rosenberg[3] in human amnion AV$_3$ cells. It was found that DNA synthesis was more sensitive to the antitumor drugs than was either protein or RNA synthesis. Platinum complexes that did not show antitumor activity did not show any inhibitory effects on DNA synthesis.

The effect of bound Pt on the ability of DNA to act as a template for DNA synthesis has also been studied in several _in vitro_ model systems. Harder et al.[8] examined the ability of DNA polymerase α and β from human lymphocyte cell lines to synthesize DNA using as template primers DNA treated with either _cis_- or _trans_-Pt. The amount of bound platinum needed to achieve 50% inhibition of synthesis varied from R_b = 0.01 (_cis_) to R_b = 0.02 (_trans_), where R_b is the molar ratio of bound platinum per DNA nucleotide.

The effects of Pt on the _in vitro_ replication of T7 DNA have been examined by Johnson et al.[9] DNA is copied by a mechanism that closely mimics _in vivo_

156

DNA replication. The DNA products of this reaction are biologically active
and the inhibition of in vitro DNA synthesis in this system presumably results
from interference with any of the steps involved in the movement of the replication fork. DNA templates were prepared containing a known number of either
cis- or trans-Pt lesions. As shown in Fig. 1 at an R_b of 2 x 10^{-4}, cis-Pt
reduces the rate of synthesis by 50%. The trans isomer is 5-fold less
effective.

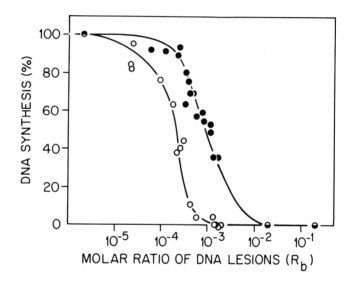

Fig. 1. Relative percent DNA synthesized in vitro from T7 DNA templates
containing various amounts of either cis- (O) or trans-Pt (●) lesions.

Cytotoxicity and mutagenicity in yeast

Cytotoxic effects of cis-Pt in the haploid yeast Saccharomyces cerevisiae
were found to depend upon both physiological and genetic factors. Table 1
shows that cells harvested from growing cultures lose colony-forming ability
much more rapidly than those harvested from stationary cultures. Moreover,
cis-Pt sensitivity is greater in strains carrying mutations in genes controlling DNA repair; rad3 causes defective pyrimidine dimer excision repair, while
rad5 and rad6 are involved in the pathway of error-prone repair of UV damage[10].
These and other rad mutations also influence mutagenesis and repair following
treatments with a variety of chemical mutagens[11]. Thus, our results suggest
that cis-Pt cytotoxicity in yeast is caused by repairable damage to cellular
DNA.

Table 2 shows that cis-Pt is also mutagenic in wild-type (repair-proficient) yeast. Log-phase cells appear to be more mutable than stationary cells, and, in addition, the number of mutants increased after posttreatment cell division prior to mutant selection on agar.

TABLE 1

CYTOTOXICITY OF cis-Pt IN WILD-TYPE AND rad STRAINS OF YEAST

Strain	Survival (%)	
	Stationary phase	Log phase
RAD	61	62
rad3	0.8	8.6
rad5	26	0.3
rad6	50	0.5

Cells harvested from either stationary- or log-phase cultures were treated with 100 µg/ml cis-Pt in distilled water at 30°C for 3 h or 0.5 h, respectively.

TABLE 2

MUTAGENICITY OF cis-Pt IN WILD-TYPE YEAST

Cells	Concentration[a] (µg/ml)	Survival (%)	Mutants per 10^7 viable cells[b]	
			Without posttreatment	With posttreatment
Stationary phase	0	100	12	19
	100	73	26	52
Log phase	0	100	11	15
	100	22	26	216

[a]Treatments were for 50 min at 30°C after which cells were washed and resuspended in distilled water.

[b]Recessive forward mutations at a single genetic locus, from CAN1 (canavanine sensitivity) to can1 (canavanine resistance) were selected on agar with or without a prior period (24 h) of posttreatment cell division in growth medium.

Mutants resistant to the arginine analogue, canavanine, arise by mutational alteration of the structural gene for the arginine-specific permease[12,13]. It should be emphasized that, unlike the loss of a soluble enzyme activity (like HGPRT in CHO cells) which must be diluted out during expression, mutant arginine permease can be expressed without posttreatment cell division, presumably due to a high turnover rate of this gene product. Mutations are vigorously induced and expressed without posttreatment following exposure to a variety of physical and chemical mutagens. Hydrazine mutagenesis in this system is an exception, however, in that it requires posttreatment DNA replication[14]. Previous studies in yeast[14,15] and in Haemophilus[16,17] have strongly suggested that hydrazine-induced DNA lesions lead to mutation by base mispairing at replication. The similar mode of expression observed with cis-Pt tentatively suggests a similar replicative error mechanism.

With the use of [195m]Pt-labeled cis-Pt, cellular uptake and numbers of DNA lesions formed and removed can be monitored and potentially correlated with genetic effects exhibited by wild-type and repair-defective yeast strains[18].

DNA repair

The persistence or lifetime of a particular type of DNA lesion obviously influences the ability of the lesion to induce a biological response. Therefore, DNA repair capacity is an important parameter in determining the ability of a cell to cope with various forms of damage. Previous studies[19] have shown that Chinese hamster V79-397A cells respond to cis-Pt-induced DNA damage by means of a postreplication repair mechanism.

In order to test for DNA excision repair, human skin fibroblasts exposed to cis-Pt were assayed, using the bromodeoxyuridine (BrdUrd) photolysis method described by Regan et al.[20] Briefly, cells were labeled in Eagle's minimal essential medium supplemented with 10% calf serum (E-90/cs), containing either [^{3}H] or [^{14}C]thymidine (dT), for 24 hours. Cells were treated with unlabeled E-90/cs for 2 hours to deplete radioactive pools. The medium was replaced with Hanks' balanced salt solution containing 25 μM cis-Pt. Following a 90 min exposure period, the cells were washed with E-90/cs and allowed to undergo a 20 hour repair period in E-90/cs containing either 100 μM BrdUrd (^{3}H-labeled cells) or 100 μM dT (^{14}C-labeled cells). Cells were washed and suspended in ice-cold saline-0.02% EDTA, and ^{3}H- and ^{14}C-labeled cells were mixed together at a concentration of 2×10^5 cells/ml prior to exposure to increasing fluences of 313 nm light from a Hilger monochromator. DNA weight average molecular weights (M_w) were determined from alkaline sucrose sedimentation profiles. M_w's of photolyzed (BrdUrd containing) DNA were compared to M_w's of control DNA (repaired in the presence of dT) in order to calculate the number of single-strand DNA breaks/10^8 daltons.

The results (as shown in Fig. 2) suggest that DNA damage by cis-Pt is repaired by an incision repair mechanism. The lack of curve saturation in strand break accumulation following 313 nm doses of up to 12×10^4 J/m^2 suggests repair by an X-ray-type mechanism (few nucleotides inserted per repaired region). However, quantitation is difficult due to the presence of high molecular weight DNA caused by apparent cross-linking of the DNA by cis-Pt. Preliminary results with trans-Pt indicate no evidence of excision repair.

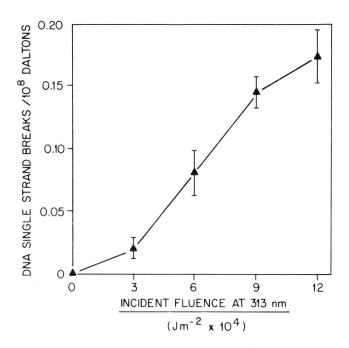

Fig. 2. Formation of DNA strand breaks following 313 nm photolysis of cells exposed in culture to cis-Pt and allowed to undergo DNA repair synthesis in the presence of BrdUrd.

Mutagenicity and cytotoxicity in the CHO/HGPRT system

This system is a quantitative mutational assay which selects for 6-thioguanine-resistant variants of Chinese hamster ovary (CHO) cells[21]. The cytotoxicity and mutagenicity of cis- and trans-Pt per platinum bound to DNA are compared in Table 3. Survival and DNA binding was measured after Pt treatment for 16 hours and mutants were selected after 8-10 days posttreatment incubation. These data indicate that both isomers bind to DNA during treatment, but cis-Pt is 9 times more toxic and 50 times more mutagenic per DNA lesion than the trans isomer. Subsequent expression and/or repair of these DNA lesions must account for the different biological potencies of these molecules.

TABLE 3

INFLUENCE OF cis- AND trans-Pt ON SURVIVAL AND MUTAGENICITY IN CHO CELLS[a]

	cis	trans
Platinum/nucleotide necessary for 50% killing	4×10^{-5}	36×10^{-5}
(Mutants per 10^6 clonable cells)/μM	57.6	0.35
(Platinum per nucleotide)/μM[b]	2.8×10^{-5}	0.87×10^{-5}

[a] Johnson et al.[22]

[b] Less than 1% of the total Pt added became bound to the DNA.

Uptake and DNA binding studies in rats

ACI rats were injected with either cis- or trans-Pt labeled with ^{195m}Pt[23].
Uptake and DNA binding studies revealed no differences in the amount of Pt
present in normal liver or implanted Reuber H-35 hepatoma[24]. The results are
shown in Table 4 from which it is clear that cellular uptake of the cis and
trans isomers occurs to the same extent but that the amount of binding to the
DNA is up to 10-fold greater for the cis than the trans isomer.

TABLE 4

UPTAKE AND DNA BINDING OF ^{195m}Pt-LABELED cis- AND trans-Pt IN RATS[24]

Animal	Organ	Molar concentration of platinum relative to the molar concentration of DNA nucleotide (± 40%)[a]					
		Tissue		Cell		DNA	
		cis	trans	cis	trans	cis	trans
Normal	Liver	4.1×10^{-3}	4.7×10^{-3}	4.0×10^{-3}	3.3×10^{-5}	13×10^{-5}	1.3×10^{-5}
Tumored	Liver	4.5×10^{-3}	4.2×10^{-3}	1.5×10^{-3}	5.7×10^{-3}	15×10^{-5}	10×10^{-5}
	Tumor	5.8×10^{-3}	3.8×10^{-3}	4.7×10^{-3}	1.2×10^{-3}	11×10^{-5}	1.0×10^{-5}

[a] Animals were injected with known amounts of Pt varying from 1-4 mg/kg
trans-Pt and 2-7.5 mg/kg cis-Pt. Because uptake and DNA binding varied linearly
with dose, it was possible to estimate by extrapolation what the binding would
be for a dose of 7.5 mg/kg. Hence all data were normalized to this dose for
comparison purposes. The data shown are for 24 hours following injection,
although similar figures were obtained for the cell and DNA following 2 hours.

Cytotoxicity

One of the main purposes of this work is to relate cytotoxicity to the
amounts of Pt bound to DNA. Table 5 summarizes the available toxicity data for
cis- and trans-Pt in several different biological systems. Of particular

interest in Table 5 is the relative difference in sensitivity expressed as the R_b ratio of trans to cis necessary to achieve equivalent reduction of survival. This ratio, which varies from 5- to 8-fold, resembles that presented previously for inhibition of DNA synthesis (Fig. 1) and suggests that the relative cytotoxicity per DNA lesion of cis- and trans-Pt is a consequence of their different ability to inhibit DNA synthesis.

TABLE 5

LEVELS OF Pt BINDING EXPRESSED AS R_b FOR REDUCING SURVIVAL TO 1/e (37%)

System	R_b		
	cis-Pt	trans-Pt	trans/cis
T7 phage[a]	5×10^{-5}	3.5×10^{-4}	7
HeLa cells[b]	2×10^{-5}	1×10^{-4}	5
CHO cells[c]	4.5×10^{-5}	4×10^{-4}	9
V79 cells[d]	1.3×10^{-5}	--	--

[a]Shooter et al.[25] These are estimated values presumably based on concentrations relative to measured values of R_b obtained using [^{14}C]dichloro-ethylene-diammine platinum(II).

[b]Pascoe and Roberts.[26]

[c]Johnson et al.[22] Trans data are a projection based on binding data obtained at lower concentrations of Pt.

[d]van den Berg and Roberts[27].

Summary

Evidence has been presented as to how cis-Pt binds to DNA and causes mutations and cell killing. Inhibition of DNA synthesis is thought to be the major reason why cells treated with cis-Pt die. Because cis-Pt binds to DNA in rat cells up to 10-fold more effectively than trans-Pt and since the cis isomer inhibits DNA synthesis 5-fold more effectively than the trans isomer, then from a simplistic point of view it is relatively easy to see how the cis isomer might be more toxic to an animal cell than the trans isomer. Furthermore, if inhibition of DNA synthesis initiates cell killing, then fast-growing tumor cells are more likely to be affected by Pt than normal nondividing cells.

REFERENCES

1. Roberts, J. J. and Thomson, A. J. (1978) Progress in Nucleic Acid Research and Molecular Biology, Vol. 22. W. E. Cohn, ed. Academic Press, New York, pp. 71-133.

2. Howle, J. A. and Gale, G. R. (1970) Biochem. Pharm. 19, 2757-2762.

162

3. Harder, H. C. and B. Rosenberg (1970) Int. J. Cancer 6, 207-216.

4. Goodgame, D. M. L., Jeeves, I., Phillips, F. L. and Skapski, A. C. (1975) Biochim. Biophys. Acta 378, 153-157.

5. Macquet, J. P. and Butour, J. L. (1978) Biochimie 60, 901-914.

6. Harrison, R. C. and McAuliffe, C. A. (1978) Inorganic Perspectives in Biology and Medicine 1, 261-288.

7. (a) Johnson, N. P., Hoeschele, J. D. and Rahn, R. O. (1979) Manuscript in progress. (b) Aprile, F. and Martin, D. S., Jr. (1962) Inorg. Chem. 1, 551-557.

8. Harder, H. C., Smith, R. G. and Leroy, A. F. (1976) Cancer Res. 36, 3821-3829.

9. Johnson, N. P., Hoeschele, J. D., Kuemmerle, N. B., Masker, W. E. and Rahn, R. O. (1978) Chem. Biol. Interactions 23, 267-271.

10. Cox, B. S. and Game, J. (1974) Mutation Res. 26, 257-264.

11. Prakash, L. (1976) Genetics 83, 285-301.

12. Grenson, M., Mousset, M., Wiame, J. W. and Bechet, J. (1966) Biochim. Biophys. Acta 127, 325-338.

13. Whelan, W. L. Gocke, E. and Manney, T. R. (1979) Genetics 91, 35-51.

14. Lemontt, J. F. (1977) Mutation Res. 43, 165-178.

15. Lemontt, J. F. (1978) Mutation Res. 50, 57-66.

16. Kimball, R. F. and Hirsch, B. F. (1975) Mutation Res. 30, 9-20.

17. Kimball, R. F. and Hirsch, B. F. (1976) Mutation Res. 36, 39-48.

18. Lemontt, J. F., Johnson, N. P., Rahn, R. O. and Hoeschele, J. D. (1979) Paper presented at the Environmental Mutagen Society Meeting, March 8-12, 1979, New Orleans, La.

19. van den Berg, H. W. and Roberts, J. J. (1975) Mutation Res. 33, 279-284.

20. Regan, J. D., Setlow, R. B. and Ley, R. D. (1971) Proc. Nat. Acad. Sci. USA 68, 708.

21. O'Neill, J. P., Brimer, P. A., Machanoff, R., Hirsch, G. P. and Hsie, A. W. (1977) Mutation Res. 45, 91-101.

22. Johnson, N. P., Hoeschele, J. D., Rahn, R. O. and Hsie, A. (1979) Manuscript in preparation.

23. Hoeschele, J. D., Butler, T. A. and Roberts, J. A. (1979) Am. J. Roentgenol., Radium Ther. Nucl. Med. (In press).

24. Hoeschele, J. D., Johnson, N. P., Rahn, R. O. and Brown, D. H. (1978) Paper presented at the Euchem. Conf. of Coordination Chemistry and Cancer Chemotherapy, July 1978, Toulouse, France.

25. Shooter, K. V., Howse, R., Merrifield, R. K. and Robbins, A. B. (1972) Chem. Biol. Interactions 5, 289-307.

26. Pascoe, J. M. and Roberts, J. J. (1974) Biochem. Pharmacol. 23, 1345-1357.

27. van den Berg, H. W. and Roberts, J. J. (1976) Chem. Biol. Interactions 12, 375-390.

MECHANISMS IN ORGAN AND TISSUE DAMAGE
Chairman: Hanspeter R. Witschi

© 1980 Elsevier/North-Holland Biomedical Press
The Scientific Basis of Toxicity Assessment
H. Witschi, editor.

MECHANISMS IN ORGAN AND TISSUE DAMAGE: INTRODUCTION

H. P. WITSCHI

Biology Division, Oak Ridge National Laboratory, Oak Ridge, Tennessee 37830

Environmental agents cause acute and chronic disease in animals and man. It is the great challenge in modern toxicology to identify pathogenetic agents and, even more important, to understand the mechanisms by which they cause cell and tissue lesions. Mechanisms will eventually be understood at the molecular level. Work done in numerous laboratories, some of it presented in this symposium, has given some admirable insight on one problem: what are the metabolic transformations a given chemical must undergo before it produces lesions in a living organism.

To unravel the pathways by which chemicals are metabolized into ultimately toxic compounds covers one aspect only of the problem. It is equally important to understand and eventually to predict the molecular changes chemicals induce in their target and how these alterations relate to the ultimate effects. However, there is one major problem if we focus our attention on molecular mechanisms only: which of the biochemical changes observed, described or quantitated with our most sophisticated, analytical capabilities lies on the main pathways leading to pathologic conditions and which ones are only secondary disturbances or possibly of no relevance at all to the ultimate pathologic outcome (1). The problem is compounded by a simple fact: there are thousands of possibly harmful chemicals. If they interact with the biochemical machinery of the living cell, each one may well produce a very specific initial biochemical lesion. However, a cell, a tissue, or even an entire organism will react only in a few limited ways to such an insult: cell death or cell degeneration, abnormal cell permeability, inflammation, normal or abnormal recovery, or cancer. Many biochemical studies on mechanisms of toxicity provide us with detailed knowledge on inhibition of specific enzymes, disturbances in metabolic pathways, or may define subtle changes in vital tissue constituents. However, it is often not possible to link in an intellectually satisfactory way such changes to the eventual acute or chronic tissue lesion.

It also has become evident that, in a given tissue, different cell types may present different susceptibilities towards a toxic agent. Initially, critical lesions may well be confined to this cell population alone. There is, however, a continuous interplay between

166

all cells in a tissue.   Often methods of biochemical analysis fail to separate changes in a critically affected cell population from overall and possibly irrelevant changes in all the remaining cells or do not allow to make a distinct separation between crucial initial events and secondary disturbances (2, 3).   In other cases, the cells selectively damaged by a specific agent represent such a small fraction that it is not possible, at the moment, to characterize damage with biochemical methods alone (4).   To study mechanisms of toxicity necessitates thus a truly integrated approach, making use of many techniques.   The search for mechanisms should not limit itself to a mere description of events, but should aim at discovering and formulating the pathogenetic principles underlying the biological response.

1.   Judah, J. (1969) Brit. Med. Bull., 25, 272–277.
2.   Smith, L. L. and Rose, M.S. (1977) in Biochemical Mechanisms of Paraquat Toxicity, Autor, A. P., ed., Academic Press, New York, pp. 187–199.
3.   Witschi, H. P., Kacew, S., Hirai, K. I. and Côté, M. G. (1977) Chem.-Biol. Interact., 19, 143–160.
4.   Boyd, M. R. (1977) Nature, 272, 270–271.

© 1980 Elsevier/North-Holland Biomedical Press
The Scientific Basis of Toxicity Assessment
H. Witschi, editor.

MYOCARDIAL TOXICITY

ETHARD W. VAN STEE
National Institute of Environmental Health Sciences, P.O. Box 12233, Research
Triangle Park, North Carolina 27709

INTRODUCTION

A number of reviews of the relationship between chemicals and cardiovascular
disease, principally heart disease, have been published in recent years.
Goldwater[1] in his 1960 review of heart disease related to occupational exposures, tabulated 28 industrial chemicals reported to act on the heart. However,
emphasis on cardiotoxicity as a subdiscipline of toxicology has emerged only
in recent years. Aviado[2] reviewed iatrogenic cardiomyopathies in 1975. Balazs
et al[3] expanded this to include general toxic cardiomyopathies in 1976, and
Deglin et al[4] continued with a review of drug-induced cardiomyopathies in
1977. In 1978 Ghione[5] reviewed the cardiotoxicity of antitumor agents including radiation and chemotherapeutic agents, an effort spurred by the emergence of the peculiar cardiotoxicity of the anthracycline antibiotics. Two
conferences on cardiovascular toxicology have been held recently. Myers and
McGuire[6] edited the proceedings of a conference held in 1977 on methods of
prospective monitoring for anthracycline cardiotoxicity, and Van Stee[7] edited
the proceedings of a target organ conference on cardiovascular toxicology held
in 1978.

Difficulty is encountered in attempting to classify expressions of cardiotoxicity. Balazs and Ferrans[8], for example, chose to divide mechanisms of
cardiotoxicity into those that are essentially extrinsic to the heart, as in
the myocardial necrosis that follows high doses of isoproterenol, and those
that represent true, autonomous cardiotoxic effects that are independent of
the pharmacological action, as in the toxicity of the anthracycline antibiotics.
I have chosen as an alternative, to catalog a variety of chemicals and their
effects on the heart, and to arrange them into several groups having certain
features in common (Table 1). A few topics selected from Table 1 are then
discussed in some detail, followed by comments on problems associated with the
assessment of cardiotoxicity in the research laboratory.

168

TABLE 1

CARDIOTOXIC DRUGS AND CHEMICALS

Electrophysiological Mechanisms

Cardiotonic drugs
Phenytoin
Tricyclic antidepressants
Clofibrate
Lithium
Propylene glycol
Local anesthetics
Emetine
Chlordimeform
Contrast media
Antimalarial drugs
Calcium antagonists

Non-specific Myocardial Depression

Lipid soluble, organic compounds
Myocardial depressant factor
Antimicrobial antibiotics
Carbromide, carbromal

Interference with Nucleic Acid Metabolism, Protein Synthesis

Antineoplastic drugs

Cardiomyopathy

Allylamine
Furazolidone
Ethanol
Cobalt
Adrenergic agonists
Methysergide
Vasodilators

Involvement with Lipid Metabolism

High cholesterol diet
Rapeseed oil
Brominated vegatable oils

Miscellaneous

Phenothiazines

CHEMICAL CARDIOTOXICITY

Tricyclic Antidepressants

   The hallmarks of the clinical cardiotoxicity of the tricyclic antidepressants have been described by Rose[9]. A wide variety of arrhythmias have been monitored in both man and experimental animals following toxic doses of these drugs. Preexisting myocardial disease enhances the apparent cardiotoxicity of the tricyclic antidepressants, an observation common to a variety of cardiotoxic agents. Harvengt et al[10] have examined the possible role of elevated circulating catecholamines induced by the drugs in the precipitation of the arrhythmias, but toxicodynamic interactions are not clear. Whereas activation of β-adrenergic receptors in the cardiovascular system was postulated as a mechanism, β-adrenergic blockade only partially mitigated the toxic effects. Furthermore, the temporal sequence of changes in the concentration of plasma catecholamines did not correlate well with the occurrence of the arrhythmias.

Cardiac rhythm disturbances are likely to accompany marked imbalances within the autonomic regulatory system of the heart. Cholinergic inhibition reinforced by hyperadrenergic activity[11] could be expected to set the stage for cardiac arrhythmias that would lead to cardiodynamic impairment[12], in addition to ECG abnormalities.

Propylene Glycol

The research pharmacologist (or toxicologist) frequently encounters the need to select a vehicle for the administration of a drug. Propylene glycol (PG) often has been selected as the solvent for water-insoluble drugs in preparation for parenteral administration. Pearl et al[13] have reported evidence that corroborated earlier suspicions that PG may possess a significant cardiotoxic potential when given intravenously. The deleterious effects of PG on cardiac rhythm were easily demonstrated against a background of deslanoside-induced ventricular tachycardia (VT). VT was converted to fibrillation by PG when the deslanoside had been given at dosages producing only VT, and time to fibrillation was shortened by PG following fibrillatory doses of glycoside.

The same authors[14] went on to demonstrate why selection of a vehicle should be done with care in drug studies on the heart. They compared polyethylene glycol-500 (PEG-500), dimethylsulfoxide (DMSO), and dimethylformamide (DMF). PEG-500 and DMSO seemed to be harmless enough by themselves in the presence of drug-induced VT, but DMF was lethal. When an experimental antiarrhythmic drug (diazepam) was added to the solvents, the combination with DMSO was lethal. PEG-500 in combination remained innocuous.

The message to the laboratory worker is clear. Practicing veterinarians also might heed the warning to select drugs for administration to their patients with the thought in mind that those preparations in which PG is used as the vehicle e.g., dexamethasone, have the potential to aggravate preexisting cardiac problems, especially in dogs and cats.

Chlordimeform

Chlordimeform is an insecticide of relatively low toxicity to mammals whose mode of action in the target species is other than through the inhibition of cholinesterase[15]. Rats given lethal doses of the chemical become hyperexcitable and succomb within a few hours[16]. Hypotension preceding death suggested that cardiovascular toxicity might have been involved[17].

Chlordimeform (CDM) is unique among insecticides in its ability to inhibit monoamine oxidase (MAO)[15]. All MAO inhibitors have a hypotensive action as does clonidine, a recently introduced antihypertensive agent[18]. Clonidine activates α-adrenergic receptors in the brainstem that inhibit central sympathetic outflow. MAO inhibitors presumably act analogously by elevating local concentrations of α-adrenergic neurotransmitter at these same sites. It would not be unreasonable, therefore, to suspect that CDM might have a similar mechanism of hypotensive action.

Robinson and Smith[16] reported that pretreatment of rats with p-chlorophenylalanine, an indolamine depletor, or α-methyl-p-tyrosine, a catecholamine depletor, were without effect on CDM lethality. This was interpreted to mean that elevations of these amines subsequent to MAO inhibition did not participate in the lethal mechanism.

Lund et al[17] evaluated the toxicodynamics of CDM in dog, rabbit, and cat preparations. They found similarities between CDM and lidocaine. Both agents caused cardiovascular dynamic depression with CNS stimulation. Reflex pressor responses followed initial vasodepression. Both agents decreased contractility in isolated, perfused rabbit hearts similarly, implying a direct myocardial depressant action. Impulse traffic in cervical sympathetic efferents waxed and waned in synchrony with arterial blood pressure supporting the idea that the secondary rise in blood pressure was a consequence of an increased central sympathetic outflow.

These observations, taken together, do not rule out unequivocally the activation of central adrenergic receptors in the brainstem. Indeed, it could be a principal mechanism. The possibility was not excluded by rigorous experimentation and CDM has been shown to inhibit brain MAO. Furthermore, myocardial depression was demonstrated only in anesthetized animals or isolated hearts, both decidedly unphysiological representations of the integrated, functioning organism. Since anesthesia more often than not obscures the cardiovascular actions of chemicals[19], the evaluation of CDM in conscious, unmedicated dogs prepared with implanted instruments for assessing cardiovascular function[20] would be illuminating.

Lipid Soluble, Organic Compounds

A variety of physiological, biochemical, and physicochemical mechanisms of action have been implicated as mediators of the cardiovascular depressant action of a wide variety of organic chemicals that share the general property of being lipid soluble. Many such chemicals have anesthetic properties and have been shown to affect membrane-dependent subcellular activities, e.g., electrophysiological function of excitable cells and electron transfer at the mitochondrial inner membrane. A unifying hypothesis that may bring together many of the observed effects of these agents on myocardium is contained in the modern version of the Meyer-Overton partition theory of general anesthesia[21,22] i.e., cell narcosis occurs when the membrane concentration of lipid soluble chemical reaches 40-60 millimolal (millimoles per kg of membrane, dry weight), although it by no means accounts for all of the observed toxicodynamic effects of this broad group of chemicals. A related rule states that when membranes have expanded by approximately 0.4% as a result of the presence of chemically indifferent molecules distributed to hydrophobic regions of integral proteins and membrane phospholipids, anesthesia occurs. This is the critical volume hypothesis. Support for these hypotheses has been provided by directly measuring the concentrations of anesthetic molecules in erythrocyte membranes at anesthetic concentrations. For example, the membrane concentration of chlorpromazine is 30-60 millimolal at anesthetic concentrations, thus supporting the Meyer-Overton hypothesis[21]. The demonstration by Miller and Wilson[22] of the pressure reversal of anesthesia supports the membrane-expansion correlate.

Unfortunately little, direct experimental support is available for the idea that the preferential distribution of lipid soluble chemicals to hydrophobic subcellular regions contributes to their mechanism of myocardial depression. The universal observation that the degree of depression of cardiovascular dynamics by these chemicals in the absence of neurohumoral modulation is directly proportional to the concentration to which the animal or tissue has been exposed, supports a theory in which non-receptor-specific physiocochemical mechanisms are at work. That these observed effects are usually readily reversible when irreversible, secondary metabolic alterations have been avoided adds further support. Finally, non-ionized, relatively less polar, and larger molecules (to a point) exert the more profound toxicodynamic effects (see, for example, the study by Koerker et al[23] on the toxicity of a series of short-chained alcohols in cultured mouse neuroblastoma cells). Increasing lipid solubility clearly reduces the extramembranal effective concentration supporting the idea that the greater the lipid solubility, the more of the compound that is bound in hydrophobic regions of the cells.

Major interactions between the lipid and protein constituents of membranes according to the fluid mosaic model[24,25] occur between the fatty acid hydrocarbons of the phospholipids and the hydrophobic amino acids of the proteins.

Phospholipids associated with particular membrane functions have a spatial distribution different from that of the bulk-phase phospholipids, a relation-ship particularly susceptible to disruption by "foreign" molecules[26]. The direct, reversible inhibition of plasma membrane-dependent ATPases from rat liver by CCl_4[27] is an example of this. The inhibition of state 3 mitochondrial respiration by a spectrum of inhalational anesthetics and a series of hydro-carbons[28] is another.

Halothane affects the configuration of mitochondrial cristae[29]. The explanation of the consequences of this is dependent on a conformational theory of energy transduction[30]. Along similar lines McNutt et al[31] perfused the hearts of guinea pigs in situ in an atmosphere containing $CBrF_3$ known to cause depression of myocardial contractility in a wide variety of laboratory preparations[32]. Mitochondrial cristae in the hearts of exposed animals were shown by electron microscopy to have assumed an orthodox configuration as compared to the energized configuration of the controls. The orthodox con-figuration is thought to be associated with impaired mitochondrial function in the heart.

Anthracycline Antibiotics

Daunorubicin (Daunamycin) and doxorubicin (Adriamycin) are anthracycline antibiotics that are used in cancer chemotherapy. Soon after their intro-duction reports began appearing of serious clinical cardiotoxicity associated with their use. Gilladoga et al[33] reported that 8 (16%) of 50 children who had received doxorubicin, and 2 (3%) of 60 who had received daunorubicin had severe cardiomyopathy with congestive heart failure. Von Hoff et al[34] in another survey reported that 110 (2%) of 5613 children and adults treated with daunorubicin displayed evidence of cardiotoxicity.

Clinically, anthracycline-induced cardiomyopathy differs little from other congestive cardiomyopathies[35]. Central and peripheral circulatory congestion are accompanied by cardiac dilatation and diminished contractility as decom-pensation supervenes. Echocardiography is useful in evaluating the congestive heart failure but the value of electrocardiography in monitoring the onset of cardiotoxicity is debated[36]. The lack of consistency of electrocardiographic changes during therapy with anthracyclines has been reported to limit its utility in assessing cardiotoxicity.

Chemical injury to the heart by antineoplastic drugs continues to be reviewed regularly[5,37,38,39] and some generalizations may be inferred from these reports. The toxic response of the heart to the anthracyclines may be determined, in part, by the prior state of the organ, i.e., preexisting myocardial pathology may predispose the individual to anthracycline cardiotoxicity. Furthermore, concurrent treatment with other anti-cancer agents such as cyclophosphamide[37] or x-rays[40] may potentiate anthracycline cardiotoxicity.

Evidence points toward 5 possible mechanisms of the cardiovascular toxicity of the anthracyclines. 1) Anthracyclines are able to intercalate with mito- chondrial and nuclear DNA (mtDNA, nNDA)[33,41], 2) they have been shown to inhibit coenzyme Q enzymes[42], and 3) evidence has been reported that they initiate peroxidation of membrane lipids[43]. 4) An immunologic mechanism has been suggested by Fioretti et al[44] and 5) the release of histamine has been reported to contribute to a hypotensive action[45].

Mitochondrial DNA is apparently replicated at all times throughout the eukaryotic cycle[46] and Borst[47] has suggested that this activity is coupled mainly to the synthesis of inner membrane proteins. Current estimates are that about 90% of the mitochondrial protein complement arises from extra- mitochondrial ribosomes and 10% from intramitochondrial synthesis[47]. Since the anthracyclines are able to intercalate with both nDNA and mtDNA which interferes with the template activity of the DNA, protein synthesis is likely to be impaired.

Mitochondrial degeneration in the heart has been reported to occur in man[37], rats[49,50] and rabbits[51] intoxicated with the anthracyclines. Impairment of protein synthesis with the consequential loss of mitochondrial integrity might be sufficient to explain mitochondrial injury, but, in addition, evidence has been presented that electron transport may also be impaired through an inhibition of coenzyme Q (ubiquinone)[42]. On the one hand, this mechanism could turn out to be of more than incidental importance. Combs et al[52] demon- strated that another inhibitor of coenzyme Q, a naphthoquinone analog, mimicked the cardiotoxicity of doxorubicin in the rat. On the other hand, Bier and Jaenke[53] followed the cardiomyopathic progression in the rabbit and observed that, although prominent mitochondrial lesions developed, respiratory control was preserved.

Thus, at least 2 mechanisms may converge at the mitochondrial inner membrane, 1) inhibition of synthesis of inner membrane proteins necessary for a functional respiratory chain, and 2) impairment of electron transport. The combination of these effects would result in the overall impairment of cellular respiration. The clinical observation that the cardiotoxicity of the anthracyclines can be reversible with time could be rooted in the redundancy of mtDNA and the interdependency of mitochondrial and extramitochondrial protein synthesis[48].

Doxorubicin has been shown to have a special affinity for phospholipids[54]. When the drug was added to a 2-phase system composed of chloroform, methanol, and water, most of the drug was found in the aqueous phase. When phospholipids were added a rapid shift occurred and most of the drug moved to the lipophilic phase. The negatively charged phospholipids were able to displace the positively charged anthracycline from the hydrophilic phase. Negatively charged lipids other than phospholipids were ineffective in this regard. This may have relevance to the observation by Myers et al[43] that treatment of mice with doxorubicin resulted in the elevation of the concentration of malondialdehyde in cardiac tissue. The detection of lipid peroxides following treatment with doxorubicin suggested that this mechanism may play an important role in the cardiotoxicity of the anthracyclines, a third possible mechanism of injury to, not only mitochondrial membranes, but also other subcellular membranes as well.

Fioretti et al[44] suspected that an immunologic mechanism might participate in the cardiotoxicity of the anthracyclines. They viewed the myocardial damage as possibly the final stage of an immune process that started with the release of autoantigens from myocardial cells. This is an entirely reasonable suggestion, a priori, in view of the foregoing. Their hypothesis was supported by the observation that spleen cells from rabbits treated with doxorubicin lysed rabbit embryonic heart cells, but not similar cultures derived from kidney or skin. Corresponding sera possessed no cytotoxic activity.

A variety of reports support the concept that each of the possible mechanisms of the cardiotoxic action of the anthracyclines that have been discussed may contribute to the overall effect. However, some mechanisms may be more important than others. Zbinden[55] found an amelioration of the cardiotoxic effects of doxorubicin when rats were treated with a combination of doxorubicin and acetyldoxorubicin. Although acetyldoxorubicin is believed to bind to DNA like the other anthracyclines, it is resistant to hydrolysis to the corresponding aglycone. The implication was that the aglycone may have been the proximate toxicant as distinguished from the intercalated form responsible for the chemotherapeutic effect. Competitition by acetyldoxorubicin with doxorubicin for macromolecular binding sites accompanied by limited formation of aglycone may have been responsible for the reduced cardiotoxicity. The conclusion here is that intercalation with DNA may be of less significance in connection with cardiotoxicity than some of the other mechanisms.

Coenzymes Q_9 and Q_{10} have been shown to have a sparing effect on the cardio-toxicity of the anthracyclines in rabbits[56] and (Q_{10}) in rats[57]. But the preservation of respiratory control in the face of evidence of mitochondrial degeneration[53] suggested that the inhibition of coenzyme Q could be of less importance in regard to the structural damage than other possible mechanisms.

Regarding the peroxidation of membrane lipids, Myers et al[58] have reported that α-tocopherol has a sparing effect on the cardiotoxicity of doxorubicin in mice, and finally Herman et al[45] showed that the hypotensive action of doxo-rubicin in the dog was attenuated by antihistamines.

Quite obviously, the final answers are not in concerning the mechanism(s) of the cardiotoxicity of the anthracycline antibiotics. But sufficient infor-mation is becoming available to give direction to efforts to preserve the clinical utility of these drugs while minimizing undesirable side effects.

ASSESSMENT OF CARDIOTOXICITY

Totally satisfactory methods are yet to be established for purposes of the early detection and monitoring of cardiotoxicity in clinical settings[6], or its evaluation in laboratory animals.

Electronmicroscopy provides a powerful tool for the evaluation of structural changes that persist substantially beyond the end of exposure or whose rate of change is slow enough to allow preservation by in vivo perfusion and fixation[31]. The latter procedure, for example, allows the fixation of mitochondria with cristae in altered configurations.

The ultrastructural correlates of myocardial function have been discussed recently by Sommer and Waugh[59]. Reports by McNutt, Weinstein, and Fawcett have created an atlas of myocardial ultrastructure including descriptions of the nexus[60], atrial muscle[61], ventricular papillary muscle[62], and myocardial sarcolemma[63].

The normal postnatal growth of cardiac muscle has been reviewed by Zak[64]. Although the rate of myocardial cell proliferation declines rapidly toward the end of gestation, it does continue through early postnatal life. At birth 1-2% of rat myocardial nuclei contain mitotic figures. This percentage declines to very low levels by 3-4 weeks of age. Thus, heart weight changes during the first 3 weeks of postnatal life, can be a reflection of myocardial cell pro-liferative capacity, e.g., see the report of Myers et al[58] on the cardiotoxicity of doxorubicin.

Special staining procedures may be used to advantage in the assessment of cardiotoxicity using frozen sections or fixed preparations. For example, evidence of myocardial ischemia does not become readily apparent by light microscopy in sections stained with hematoxylin and eosin until the tissue becomes frankly necrotic. The method of Lie et al[65] using the hematoxylin-basic fuchsin-picric acid (HBFP) stain is reported to allow the detection of evidence of early myocardial ischemia prior to the onset of necrosis.

The uses of electrocardiography (ECG) and the monitoring of cardiovascular dynamic variables are mentioned at this point only for the sake of completeness. The ECG is indispensible for the evaluation of cardiac rhythm disturbances in the intact animal, but space does not permit a comprehensive discussion of the topic. Monitoring conventional variables is implied within special contexts later in this review.

Swimming to exhaustion has been suggested informally as of possible potential value in cardiotoxicity testing. Such a test might have some crude diagnostic value in regard to cardiopulmonary reserve, but, in my opinion, has little place in a comprehensive cardiotoxicity assessment program. However, the documentation of death as the final consequence of some element of cardio-vascular failure, e.g., ventricular fibrillation, asystole, congestive heart failure, cardiogenic shock, etc., in an unstressed (or stressed) animal would be of research significance.

Misleading information can arise through attempts to interpret functional data acquired from anesthetized animals. Although it is technically demanding to prepare experimental animals for the later acquisition of functional data in the absence of anesthesia, the quality of the results and the reliability of their interpretation is worth the effort when the necessary facilities are available. Vatner[19] recently reviewed the effects of anesthesia on cardio-vascular control mechanisms in order to emphasize that pitfalls may be encoun-tered when attempting to interpret pharmacodynamic data obtained from anes-thetized animals. Harris et al[20] described their canine model in which 35 variables were either measured directly or computed from measured variables on conscious, unmedicated dogs in which instruments had been surgically implanted earlier. A complete profile of cardiovascular dynamic and myocardial metabolic function was obtained from each set of measurements, which, in their hands, was acquired within 5 minutes per set.

A variety of in vitro technics are useful in routine functional cardio-toxicity testing and do not require an inordinate capital outlay. Adams et al[66] recently described how the isolated, superfused guinea pig atrium may be

used to assess the effects of antimicrobial antibiotics on mechanical function.
Toy et al[67] used isolated, perfused rabbit hearts to assess the effects of
certain halogenated alkanes on myocardial electromechanical activity. This
basic approach was further modified later in the author's laboratory. The
perfusate was sampled just before it enters the coronary circulation and a
fraction of the coronary effluent collected. When the rate of perfusion is
known, extraction of the various components of the perfusate by the myocardium
perfused may be computed.

The use of cultured heart cells in cardiotoxicology represents a technology
of more recent origin than those just discussed. Sperelakis[68] reviewed the
technic of using cultured heart cells as a model system for studying the
physiology, pharmacology, biochemistry, and toxicology of myocardial cells.
The general technics and types of culture preparations commonly used were
given, and some of the advantages and disadvantages of working with cultured
heart cells were summarized.

The scientist's inclination traditionally has been to select the most
robust examples of the young male of the species for the preparation of model
systems. That the population at risk may not always be the human analog of
this model gives rise to the need to consider what, for lack of a more precise
term, we might refer to as "special purpose models" for toxicity evaluation.
The breadth of the spectrum of possibilities is illustrated by A Handbook:
Animal Models of Human Disease from the Armed Forces Institute of Pathology[69]
and the proceedings of a series of symposia published in the Federation
Proceedings during recent years, entitled "Animal Models for Biomedical
Research." The variety is limited only by ones imagination, but some special
examples are worth mentioning.

Lee et al[70] described the pathophysiology of the atherosclerotic rabbit.
The disorder may be induced easily by feeding the rabbits a diet containing 2%
cholesterol for 7-25 weeks. The severity of the lesions is proportional to
the length of time that the animals are maintained on the special diet.
Stressing these animals with drugs or by right atrial pacing elicits S-T
segment depression as evidence of myocardial ischemia. This could become a
useful model in studies of the cardiovascular toxicity of chemicals.

Like atherosclerosis, obesity is a ranking public health problem in the
United States and elsewhere and experimental models for the study of obesity
was the subject of a recent symposium[71]. Of special interest was the gold
thioglucose obesity syndrome[72]. Gold thioglucose enters the ventromedial
hypothalamus causing destruction of cells involved in the regulation of food

intake resulting in hyperphagia and obesity. By comparison, the Zucker-fatty rat[73] is one of a group of animals that inherit obesity as an autosomal Mendelian recessive trait. The genetic model of obesity[73] differs from the hypothalamic model[72], but both exhibit hyperinsulinemia and hyperphagia. Such models could prove to be useful in cardiovascular toxicology studies, particularly in connection with the pharmacokinetic aspects of lipid soluble compounds.

The need for established procedures for the screening of drugs and chemicals with known or suspected cardiotoxic potential is well recognized. Discussions of this matter were held in early 1979 in Pinehurst, North Carolina in prepa-

TABLE 2

METHODS OF ASSESSMENT OF CARDIOTOXICITY

A. Endpoint Analysis

    1. Structure

        Gross Pathology
        Histopathology
        Ultrastructural Evaluation

    2. Organ Weight

        Absolute Weight
        Organ/Body Weight

    3. Histochemistry

        Fat Stain
        Hematoxylin-Basic Fuchsin-Picric acid (HBFP)

B. Functional Assessment

    1. In Vivo

        Electrocardiogram
        Blood Pressure (MAP, CVP)
        Stressed and Unstressed Survival Studies
        Dog, Baboon Implanted with Instruments for Monitoring CV
          System Without Anesthesia

    2. In Vitro

        Paced, Guinea Pig Left Atrium
        Isolated, Perfused Heart
        Cultured Heart Cells

    3. Serum Enzyme Activity

C. Special Purpose Models

    1. Atherosclerotic Rabbit
    2. Obesity Model
    3. Infarcted Myocardium
    4. Drug Interaction Models
    5. Cardiomyopathic Hamster
    6. Functional Deprivation of Neural Influences

ration for activating the National Toxicology Program[74]. The problem was vexing and its solution elusive. The conclusion that must be reached, however, is that protocols must be designed with some prior knowledge in mind. A comprehensive and exhaustive evaluation will not always be practical for every compound of interest. The breadth of the swath must be dictated by a realistic goal. A distillation of the final recommendations from the meeting is contained in Table 2. The ideas should be interpreted only as one place to start and should remain flexible and adaptable to changing research needs, as well as amenable to improved methodology.

Zbinden and Brandle[75] have reported an example of how such research may be targeted. They screened a series of analogs of the anthracycline antibiotics in rats. Their prior knowledge was information on the general cardiotoxicity of the class of chemicals. Their goal was to compare the drugs in the group in the rat model to assist in making a rational selection among them for further clinical evaluation in man. Mettler et al[76] responded to the same need, i.e., the need for a "standardized, accurate, reproducible, and cost-effective system for cardiotoxicity testing." The prior knowledge was the same as for Zbinden and Brandle. The goal was as quoted. They compared their results from the rat with results of others derived from other model systems and found that the rat model yielded results that correlated well with those observed in man. Their discussion is well worth the reading.

CONCLUDING STATEMENT

Mettler et al[76] observed that the selection of an animal model for cardio-toxicity testing must be done with the understanding that significant differences in response may occur among the various species. Nowhere is this more vividly illustrated than by the example of the refractoriness of rat myocardium to the actions of the cardiac glycosides. This observation has led to the uncovering of the anomalous physiology of the rat myocardium[77,78,79]. Had William Withering used the rat as his model system for predicting the cardiotoxicity of the leaves of Digitalis purpurea, he surely would have been led astray, and possibly to the detriment of his patients. Rattus norvegicus has survived the test of time and his continued utility for selected research purposes remains assured. But, although the histopathological consequences of cardiotoxicity often may be well-represented, the investigator would do well to be wary of interpretations of functional data acquired from this species.

REFERENCES

1. Goldwater, L.J. (1960) A.M.A. Arch. Indust. Hlth. 21, 509-513.

2. Aviado, D.M. (1975) J. Clin. Pharmacol. 15(10), 641-655.

3. Balazs, T. and Herman, E.H. (1976) Annals Clin. Lab. Sci. 6(6), 467-476.

4. Deglin, S.M. et al (1977) Drugs 14, 29-40.

5. Ghione, M. (1978) Cancer Chemother. Pharmacol. 1, 25-34.

6. Myers, C.E. and McGuire, W.P., Ed. (1978) Cancer Treat. Reports 62, 855-982.

7. Van Stee, E.W., Ed. (1978) Environ. Health Persp. 26, 149-285.

8. Balazs, T. and Ferrans, V.J. (1978) Environ. Health Persp. 26, 181-191.

9. Rose, J.B. (1977) Clin. Tox. 11(4), 391-402.

10. Harvengt, C. et al (1978) Tox. Appl. Pharmacol. 44, 115-126.

11. Hollister, L.E. (1978) New England J. Med. 299, 1106-1109.

12. Robinson, D.S., and Barker, E. (1976) JAMA 236(18), 2089-2090.

13. Pearl, D.S. et al (1978) Tox. Appl. Pharmacol. 44, 643-652.

14. Pearl, D.S. (1978) Tox. Appl. Pharmacol. 44, 653-656.

15. Maitre, L. et al (1978) J. Agric. Food Chem. 26(2), 442-446.

16. Robinson, C.P. and Smith, P.W. (1977) J. Tox. Environ. Hlth. 3, 565-568.

17. Lund, A.E. (1978) Tox. Appl. Pharmacol. 44, 357-365.

18. Pettinger, W.A. (1975) New England J. Med. 293, 1179-1180.

19. Vatner, S.F. (1978) Environ. Hlth. Persp. 26, 193-206.

20. Harris, A.M. et al (1975) AMRL, AMD, AFSC, Wright Patterson AFB, OH, AMRL-TR-75-125, 227-241.

21. Seeman, P. (1972) in Cellular Biology and Toxicity Anesthetics (Fink, B.R., ed.), Williams and Wilkins, Baltimore, pp. 149-159.

22. Miller, K.W. et al (1978) Anesthesiology 48, 104-110.

23. Koerker, R.L. et al (1976) Tox. Appl. Pharmacol. 37, 281-288.

24. Singer, S.J. and Nicolson, G.L. (1972) Science 175,720-732.

25. Singer, S.J. (1974) Ann. Rev. Bioch. 43, 805-833.

26. Jackson, R.L. et al (1974) New England J. Med. 290(1), 24-29.

27. Dorling, P.R. and LePage, R.N. (1972) Bioch. Pharmacol. 21, 2139-2141.

28. Nahrwold, M.L. et al (1975) in Progress in Anesthesiology, Molecular Mechanisms of Anesthesia, (Fink, B.R., ed.) Raven Press, New York, 1, pp. 431-438.

29. Taylor, C.A. et al (1972) in Cellular Biology and Toxicity of Anesthetics, (Fink, B.R., ed.) Williams and Wilkins, Baltimore, pp. 117-127.

30. Green, D.E. (1972) in Cellular Biology and Toxicity of Anesthetics, (Fink, B.R., ed.) Williams and Wilkins, Baltimore, pp. 79-92.

31. McNutt, N.S. et al (1973) AMRL, ASD, AFSC, Wright-Patterson AFB, OH, AMRL-TR-73-125, 101-115.

32. Back, K.C. and Van Stee, E.W. (1977) Ann. Rev. Pharmacol. Toxicol. 17, 83–95.

33. Gilladoga, A.C. et al (1976) Cancer 37, 1070–1078.

34. Von Hoff, D.D. et al (1977) Amer. J. Med. 62, 200–208.

35. Ewy, G.A. et al (1976) Arizona Med. 33(4), 274–278.

36. Weaver, S.K. et al (1978) J. Electrocardiology 11(3), 233–238.

37. Buja, L.M. and Ferrans, V.J. (1975) in Pathophysiology and Morphology of Myocardial Cell Alteration (Fleckenstein, A. and Rona, G., eds.) University Park Press, Baltimore, pp. 487–497.

38. Lenaz, L. and Page, J.A. (1976) Cancer Treat. Rev. 3, 111–120.

39. Bristow, M.R. et al, 1978 Amer. J. Med. 65, 823–832.

40. Fajardo, L.F. et al (1976) Lab. Invest. 34(1), 86–96.

41. Shafer, R.H. (1977) Bioch. Pharmacol. 26, 1729–1734.

42. Iwamoto, Y. et al (1974) Bioch. Biophy. Res. Comm. 58(3), 633–638.

43. Myers, C.E. et al (1977) Science 197, 165–167.

44. Fioretti, A. et al (1976) Cancer Res. 36, 1462–1469.

45. Herman, E. (1978) Agents and Actions 8(5), 551–557.

46. Pardee, A.B. et al (1978) Ann. Rev. Biochem. 47, 715–750.

47. Borst, P. (1972) Ann. Rev. Bioch. 41, 333–376.

48. Schatz, G. and Mason, T.L. (1974) Ann. Rev. Bioch. 43, 51–87.

49. Olson, H.M. and Capen, C.C. (1977) Lab. Invest. 37(4), 386–394.

50. Olson, H.M. and Capen, C.C. (1978) Tox. Appl. Pharmacol. 44, 605–616.

51. Jaenke, R.S. (1976) Cancer Res. 36, 2958–2966.

52. Combs, A.B. et al (1976) Res. Comm. Chem. Pathol. Pharmacol. 13(2), 333–339.

53. Bier, C.C. and Jaenke. R.S. (1976) J. Natl. Cancer Inst. 57(5), 1091–1093.

54. Duarte-Karim, M. et al (1976) Bioch. Biophy. Res. Comm. 71(2), 658–663.

55. Zbinden, G. (1975) Experientia 31(9), 1058–1060.

56. Ghione, M. and Bertazzoli, C. (1977) in Biomedical and Clinical Aspects of Coenzyme Q (Folkers, K. and Yamamura, Y., eds.) Elsevier, Amsterdam, pp. 183–199.

57. Zbinden, G. et al (1977) in Biomedical and Clinical Aspects of Coenzyme Q (Folkers, K. and Yamamura, Y., eds.) Elsevier, Amsterdam, pp. 219–228.

58. Myers, et al (1976) Cancer Treat. Rpts. 60(7), 961–962.

59. Sommer, J.R. and Waugh, R.A. (1978) Environ. Hlth. Persp. 26, 159–167.

60. McNutt, N.S. and Weinstein, R.S. (1970) J. Cell. Biol. 47(3), 666–688.

61. McNutt, N.S. and Fawcett, D.W. (1969) J. Cell Biol. 42(1), 46–67.

62. Fawcett, D.W. and McNutt, N.S. (1969) J. Cell. Biol. 42(1), 1–45.

63. McNutt, N.S. (1975) Circ. Res. 37, 1–13.

64. Zak, R. (1973) Amer. J. Cardiology 31, 211–219.

65. Lie, J.T. et al (1971) Mayo Clinic Proceed. 46, 319-327.

66. Adams, H.R. et al (1978) Environ. Hlth. Persp. 26, 217-223.

67. Toy, P.A. et al (1976) Tox. Appl. Pharmacol. 38, 7-17.

68. Sperelakis, N. (1978) Environ. Hlth. Persp. 26, 243-267.

69. Animal Models of Human Disease (Jones, T.C. et al, eds.) The Registry of Comparative Pathology, Armed Forces Institute of Pathology, Washington, DC, Fascicles 1-7.

70. Lee, R.J. et al (1978) Environ. Hlth. Persp. 26, 225-231.

71. Bray, G.A. (1976) Fed. Proc. 36, 137-158.

72. Debons, A.F. et al (1977) Fed. Proc. 36, 143-147.

73. Bray, G.A. (1977) Fed. Proc. 36, 148-153.

74. Carter, L.J. (1979) Science 203, 525-528.

75. Zbinden, G. and Brandle E. (1975) Cancer Chemother. Rep. 59, 707-715.

76. Mettler, F.P. et al (1977) Cancer Res. 37, 2705-2713.

77. Nayler, W.G. and Dunnett, J. (1975) Recent Adv. Studies Cardiac Structure Metab. 5, 171-175.

78. Langer, G.A. et al (1975) Circ. Res. 36, 744-752.

79. Langer, G.A. (1978) Environ. Hlth. Persp. 26, 175-179.

© 1980 Elsevier/North-Holland Biomedical Press
The Scientific Basis of Toxicity Assessment
H. Witschi, editor.

ROLE OF METABOLISM IN HEXACARBON NEUROPATHY

G. D. DIVINCENZO, W. J. KRASAVAGE and J. L. O'DONOGHUE

Health, Safety and Human Factors Laboratory, Eastman Kodak Company, Rochester,
New York 14650 (USA)

INTRODUCTION

Several outbreaks of occupationally related polyneuropathy were reported
during the mid to late 1960's and early 1970's in the United States, Europe and
Asia. [1,2,3] Most outbreaks of neuropathy occurred during the winter and spring
in occupational settings marked by poor ventilation. Classical neurotoxins,
such as acrylamide and tri-orthocresolphosphate, were usually excluded as probable causative agents. Epidemiologic evidence suggested that these outbreaks
may be related to prolonged exposure to organic solvents among workers in the
shoe, leather, paint, and fabric coating industries and among individuals con-
sciously inhaling vapors from commercial products. The hexacarbon solvents n-
hexane and methyl n-butyl ketone (MnBK) have been implicated as probable causative agents in 1971 and 1974, respectively; although at the time of these
observations, the phenomenon did not appear to be causally related.

In 1973, over 80 cases of polyneuropathy were reported in a coated fabrics
plant in Columbus, Ohio. [3] The onset of neuropathy followed the introduction
into the workplace of the solvent MnBK as a surrogate for the previously used
methyl iso-butyl ketone (MiBK). This substitution was made because plants
operated by the parent company in other states had changed over to MnBK in order
to comply with community air standards. MiBK, a branch chain ketone, is photo-
chemically reactive while MnBK, a straight chain ketone, is not. For several
years the Columbus, Ohio printing process had continued uneventfully using a
solvent mixture containing 90% methyl ethyl ketone (MEK) and 10% MiBK.

Prior to 1974, MnBK was considered to be low in toxicity and was without any
previous history of neurotoxicity. [4] After 1974 the potential neurotoxic behavior of MnBK was of particular interest because of its relative inertness
compared to classical neurotoxins such as acrylamide or tri-orthocresolphosphate. In addition, no neurotoxic activity had been reported for other widely
used aliphatic ketones. This suggested that the neuropathy produced by MnBK may
not be intrinsic, but may arise from one or more metabolites not formed by
isomeric or homologous ketones. Thus, the metabolism and pharmacokinetics of
MnBK was investigated to clarify the role of metabolism in MnBK neuropathy.

Certain structural features common to MnBK and n-hexane, a known neurotoxin, prompted us also to investigate the metabolism of n-hexane.

This paper describes the studies which led to the characterization of the principal metabolites of MnBK and n-hexane, and elucidates the role of metabolism in the neurotoxicity of these compounds.

EXPERIMENTAL STUDIES

The studies described herein were carried out in guinea pigs, rats and humans.

Studies in Guinea Pigs. Male guinea pigs, ranging in weight from 250 to 400 grams, were dosed with either MnBK or n-hexane. All chemicals were reagent grade and were used without further purification with the exception of commercial grade MnBK which was greater than 97% pure. Guinea pigs were maintained on Purina Lab Chow. Water was available ad libitum. The test compounds were dissolved in corn oil and were administered intraperitoneally in a single dose. Blood was collected by heart puncture at regular intervals after dosing. Whole blood was centrifuged and the serum was collected. Serum was placed in sealed culture tubes, refrigerated and analyzed within 48 hours. The concentration of the test compounds and their metabolites was determined by gas chromatography by direct on column injection of undiluted serum. A LKB-9000 GC-MS was utilized for structure confirmation. Compounds were identified on the basis of their mass spectra and by comparison with the spectra of authentic samples. [5]

Methyl n-Butyl Ketone. Three major peaks and one minor peak were noted upon gas chromatography of serum from guinea pigs dosed with MnBK. Comparision of GC retention times and mass spectra with authentic samples showed these to be MnBK, 5-hydroxy-2-hexanone (5H2H), 2,5-hexanedione (25HD) and 2-hexanol (Table 1). 5H2H undergoes dehydration and cyclization in the GC inlet during analysis and was thus detected as 2,5-dimethyl-2,3-dihydrofuran. Both 5H2H and 2,5-dimethyl-2,3-dihydrofuran had identical retention times and mass spectra, viz. 2,5-dimethyl-2,3-dihydrofuran. The mass spectrum of 2,5-dimethyl-2,3-dihydrofuran is shown in Figure 1. A strong peak at m/e = 98 corresponds to the molecular weight of 2,5-dimethyl-2,3-dihydrofuran. The peaks at m/e = 45 and 55 show fragmentation consistent with the structure proposed in Figure 1.

The principal metabolite of MnBK in serum was 25HD. 2-Hexanol was identified as a minor metabolite. The serum elimination time for MnBK was 6 hours. The metabolites, 5H2H and 25HD, however, were eliminated in 12 hours.

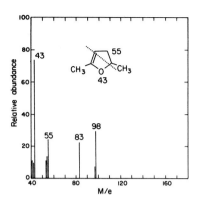

Fig. 1. Mass spectrum of
2,5-dimethyl-2,3-dihydrofuran.

TABLE 1

COMPOUNDS IDENTIFIED IN THE SERUM OF GUINEA PIGS DOSED WITH METHYL n-BUTYL
KETONE

Compound Identified	(M$^+$)	Gas Chromatography-- Mass Spectroscopy Relative abundance of the molecular ion and prominent fragment ions (m/e)
2,5-Dimethyl-2,3-dihydrofuran	98(22%)	97(5%), 83(19)%, 55(20%), 54(11%), 43,(100%)
5-Hydroxy-2-hexanone	98(22%)	97(5%), 83(19%), 55(20%), 54(11%), 43(100%)
Methyl n-butyl ketone	100(14%)	85(10%), 58(87%), 57(19%), 43(100%)
2-Hexanol	102(0%)	87(7%), 84(5%), 45(100%), 43(8%), 41(8%)
2,5-Hexanedione	114(3%)	99(16%), 71(9%), 57(5%), 43(100%)

Fate of MnBK Metabolites. The fate of 5H2H, 25HD and 2-hexanol and of related compounds such as 2,5-hexanediol and n-hexane were also investigated.

5-Hydroxy-2-Hexanone. The serum of guinea pigs dosed with 5H2H contained
25HD and 2,5-hexanediol as metabolites. The major metabolite, 25HD, was formed
rapidly and its concentration in serum was equivalent to, or greater than that

of the parent compound (5H2H) in all samples measured. Serum concentrations of 2,5-hexanediol were markedly lower than those of 25HD.

2,5-Hexanedione. 5H2H was the only metabolite detected in the serum of guinea pigs following the administration of 25HD. The serum elimination time of 25HD was 16 hours.

2,5-Hexanediol. 2,5-hexanediol was rapidly converted to 5H2H and 25HD. 2,5-hexanediol was eliminated from the serum in 8 hours. 5H2H was eliminated from the serum in 16 hours.

2-Hexanol. The following metabolites were identified following the administration of 2-hexanol: MnBK, 5H2H, 25HD and 2,5-hexanediol. 2-hexanol was rapidly converted to MnBK which in turn produced the same metabolites described above. In addition, 2-hexanol was also converted to 2,5-hexanediol which appeared to be a minor pathway. The serum elimination time of 2-hexanol was 6 hours. The metabolites, 2,5-hexanediol and 25HD disappeared from the serum in 12 and 16 hours respectively.

n-Hexane. Since n-hexane was reported to be neurotoxic in man,[2] the metabolism of n-hexane was investigated. 5H2H and 25HD were detected in the serum of guinea pigs injected ip with 250 mg/kg of n-hexane. Subsequent studies were conducted in rats dosed orally with 570 mg/kg of n-hexane and the following metabolites were identified in the serum: 2-hexanol, MnBK, 5H2H, 2,5-hexanediol and 25HD. A common pathway for the metabolism of MnBK and n-hexane is illustrated in Figure 2.

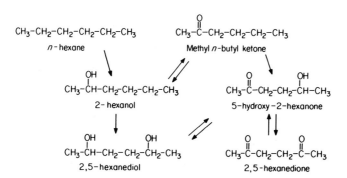

Fig. 2. Partial metabolic pathway for n-hexane and methyl n-butyl ketone.

Studies In Rats. The fate and disposition of $[1-^{14}C]$ MnBK was investigated in the rat to gain further insight in the role metabolism may play in MnBK neuropathy.[6]

Experiments were carried out with groups of four male Charles River CD Rats weighing 200-300 grams. The animals were fasted 24 hours before dosing and were maintained on Purina Rat Chow after dosing. Water was provided ad libitum. [1-^{14}C] MnBK was dissolved in corn oil and administered as a single dose by gavage. Rats were given either 20 or 200 mg/kg of [1-^{14}C] MnBK. Other rats were also pretreated with unlabelled MnBK, sodium phenobarbital or diethylaminoethyl-dithenylpropylacetate (SKF 525A). Unlabelled MnBK (200 mg/kg) was given daily by gavage for 4 days prior to the administration of [1-^{14}C] MnBK. Phenobarbital (50 mg/kg) was injected ip daily for 4 days before dosing with [1-^{14}C] MnBK. SKF 525A (35 mg/kg) was injected ip 30 minutes before the administration of [1-^{14}C] MnBK. The dose of [1-^{14}C] MnBK used to challenge pretreated rats was 200 mg/kg of body weight.

Procedures describing the measurement of radioactivity in body fluids, tissues and excreta and the detection and characterization of metabolites in the urine are described elsewhere. [6]

The excretion of radioactivity by naive and pretreated rats dosed with [1-^{14}C] MnBK is presented in Table 2. Results are expressed as a percentage of the administered dose 48 hours after dosing (mean ± SE for 4 rats). There was little change in the overall rate of excretion of radioactivity by naive rats dosed with either 20 or 200 mg/kg of MnBK. $^{14}CO_2$ and [1-^{14}C] MnBK were the only radioactive compounds detected in the expired air. About 44% of the radioactive dose was eliminated in the breath. The excretion of radioactivity in the urine by rats dosed with 20 or 200 mg/kg was 35.1 and 39.9% respectively. Fecal radioactivity was less than 1.5% of the dose. The amount of radioactivity in the carcass ranged from 13.6 to 17.6% of the administered dose. The overall recovery of the radioactive dose was greater than 97%.

Rats pretreated with MnBK, showed a slight but significant increase in the excretion of $^{14}CO_2$ (42.4 vs. 37.6%) and a decrease in the excretion of radioactivity in the urine (32.2 vs. 39.9%) as compared to naive rats dosed with MnBK. Phenobarbital pretreated rats showed a significant increase ($P < 0.05$) in the breath elimination of $^{14}CO_2$ (43.6 vs. 37.6%) and a decrease ($P < 0.05$) in the excretion of unchanged MnBK (2.4 vs. 6.2). SKF 525A pretreated rats exhibited a significant increase ($P < 0.05$) in the excretion of $^{14}CO_2$ (49.6 vs. 37.6%) and a decrease ($P < 0.05$) of the urinary radioactivity (22.5 vs. 39.9%).

Twenty-four hour urine samples from rats dosed with 200 mg/kg of [1-^{14}C] MnBK were pooled, adjusted to pH 7 and extracted with diethyl ether. The remaining aqueous solution was divided into two equal portions and each was treated with either β-glucuronidase or 3N HCL and subsequently extracted with ether. Approximately 85% of the total radioactivity in the urine was extracted; 15% was

TABLE 2

PERCENT OF DOSE OF TOTAL RADIOACTIVITY DERIVED FROM $1-^{14}C$-METHYL n-BUTYL KETONE RECOVERED IN BREATH, URINE, FECES AND CARCASSES OF MALE CHARLES RIVER CD RATS 48 HOURS AFTER DOSING [a]

Dose (mg/kg)	Pretreatment	Breath Radioactivity			Urine	Carcass	Feces	Total Accounted For
		Unchanged MnBK	CO_2	Total				
20	None	2.2 ± 0.6	41.5 ± 1.4	43.7	35.1 ± 2.3	17.6 ± 1.5	0.8 ± 0.2	97.2 ± 2.0
200	None	6.2 ± 0.7	37.6 ± 1.6	43.8	39.9 ± 2.9	13.6	1.4 ± 0.1	98.7 ± 1.3
200	MnBK[b]	5.8 ± 1.2	42.4 ± 1.8	48.2	32.2 ± 1.1	14.6	1.5 ± 0.2	96.6 ± 0.8
200	PB[c]	2.4 ± 0.2	43.6 ± 1.3	46.0	42.3 ± 2.4	12.5 ± 1.1	1.4 ± 0.1	102.3 ± 1.0
200	SKF 525A[d]	6.6 ± 1.1	49.6 ± 2.6	56.2	22.5 ± 2.5	15.2 ± 0.7	2.5 ± 0.2	96.4 ± 2.0

[a] The results are expressed as mean ± S.E. for 4 rats.
[b] Rats were pretreated with a one dose daily of unlabeled MnBK for 4 days (200 mg/kg po).
[c] Rats were pretreated with a one dose daily of sodium phenobarbital for 4 days (50 mg/kg ip).
[d] Rats were pretreated with 35 mg/kg of SKF 525A, ip, 30 minutes before before the administration of $1-^{14}C$-MnBK.

extracted at pH 7, 28% was extracted after treatment with β-glucuronidase, and 42% was extracted after mild acid hydrolysis. Ether soluble metabolites ident-ified by GC-MS are presented in Table 3.

TABLE 3

URINARY METABOLITES IDENTIFIED BY GAS CHROMATOGRAPHY/MASS SPECTROSCOPY FROM CHARLES RIVER CD RATS DOSED WITH 200 MG/KG OF $1-^{14}C$-METHYL n-BUTYL KETONE [a]

Compound Identified	(M^+)	Gas Chromatography--Mass Spectroscopy Relative abundance of the molecular ion and prominent fragment ions (m/e)
2,5-dimethylfuran	96(100%)	95(83%), 81(38%), 53(47%), 51(14%), 43(80%)
2,5-dimethyl-2,3-dihydrofuran	98(22%)	97(5%), 83(19%), 55(20%), 54(11%), 43(100%)
5-hydroxy-2-hexanone [b]	98(22%)	97(5%), 83(19%), 55(20%), 54(11%), 43(100%)
2-hexanol	102(0%)	87(7%), 84(5%), 45(100%), 43(8%), 41(8%)
2,5-hexanedione	114(3%)	99(16%), 71(9%), 57(5%), 43(100%)
γ-valerolactone	101(9%)	99(5%), 85(53%), 56(100%), 43(33%), 41(47%), 39(12%), 29(53%), 28(60%), 27(27%)

[a] Diluted urine was extracted with diethyl ether at pH 7.0 The remaining aqueous phase was also treated with β-glucuronidase and hydrochloric acid and was then extracted with diethyl ether.

[b] 5-Hydroxy-2-hexanone underwent dehydration and cyclization in the gc inlet and was detected as 2,5-dimethyl-2,3-dihydrofuran.

Three peaks were noted on GC chromatograms upon analysis of the pH 7 ether extract. The first peak had the same GC retention time and mass spectrum as that of an authentic sample of 2,5-dimethylfuran. The other GC peaks had the same retention times and mass spectra as those of two MnBK metabolites previous-ly identified in serum, i.e. 5H2H and 25HD.

GC analysis of the β-glucuronidase ether extract showed 3 peaks which were identified as 2,5-dimethylfuran, 5H2H and 2-hexanol; the latter two compounds have been characterized previously as MnBK metabolites in serum.

GC analysis of ether extracts from urines treated with mild mineral acid showed 5 peaks, 4 of which had been previously characterized, viz., 2-hexanol, 5H2H, 25HD and 2,5-dimethylfuran. The fifth peak had the same GC retention time and mass spectrum as that of an authentic sample of γ-valerolactone.

The relative amounts of radiolabelled metabolites excreted in the urine were estimated by collecting GC effluents. Results expressed as percentage of the radioactivity in urine are shown in Table 4.

TABLE 4

METABOLITES OF $1\text{-}^{14}C$-METHYL n-BUTYL KETONE IDENTIFIED IN THE URINE OF CHARLES RIVER CD RATS (PERCENTAGE IN URINE)

Metabolites Identified	Neutral pH	Diethyl Ether Extracts β-Glucuronidase Treatment	Acid Treatment	Ion Exchange Chromatography	Urease Treatment	Total
2-Hexanol	0	11	11			22
5-Hydroxy-2-hexanone	8	8	5			21
2,5-Hexanedione	6	0	8			14
2,5-Dimethylfuran	1	2	3			6
γ-Valerolactone	0	0	5			5
Amino Acids						
Norleucine				5		5
Unknown				5		5
Urea					4	4
(Recovery)	100%	(75%)	(75%)			82%

Metabolites in urine were characterized by gas chromatography, gas chromatography/mass spectroscopy, thin layer chromatography and ion exchange chromatograpny. Ether soluble metabolites were estimated by gas chromatography by collecting radioactive peaks from the gc column. ^{14}C-Urea was estimated by trapping $^{14}CO_2$ after treatment with urease. Norleucine was identified by TLC and by GLC.

Overall, 3 major and 2 minor metabolites were extracted by diethyl ether, that is, 2-hexanol (22%), 5H2H (21%), 25HD (14%), 2,5-dimethylfuran (6%) and γ-valerolactone (5%). Radioactivity injected in the GC from the pH 7 ether extract was completely recovered. However, only 75% of the injected radioactivity was recovered from the ether extracts following mild acid or β-glucuronidase treatments.

The incubation of urine with urease liberated $^{14}CO_2$ sufficient to account for 4% of the urinary radioactivity, thus indicating that CO_2 derived from $[1-^{14}C]$ MnBK was incorporated into urea. The further analysis of experimental urines indicated that about 10% of the urinary radioactivity was present as two labeled amino acids. One spot was identified as 2-aminohexanoic acid or norleucine. The other amino acid was not characterized. The metabolites described above accounted for about 82% of the urinary radioactivity.

Studies In Humans. Information pertaining to the metabolism of MnBK in man was acquired from inhalation and fate studies.[7]

Inhalation Exposures. Inhalation exposures were performed in a dynamic exposure facility measuring 2.4 x 3.0 x 3.4 meters, equipped with observation windows, and an air supply and exhaust system. MnBK was volitalized and introduced into the ventilation system of the exposure facility. The exposure facility, the method of solvent generation, and the analytical procedures used are described elsewhere.[7]

Three male volunteers, 22, 25 and 53 years in age respectively, were exposed to either 10, 50 or 100 ppm of MnBK vapor. Each person was exposed once. Exposures were carried out for 4 hours to 100 ppm and for 7 1/2 hours to 10 or 50 ppm. The 7 1/2 hour exposures were interrupted after 4 hours for a 1/2 hour period. Volunteers were sedentary during the exposure. Expired air and venous blood samples were collected before, during and after the exposure and were analyzed for MnBK and its metabolites by gas chromatography.[5,8]

Expired air and serum concentrations of MnBK from human volunteers exposed to MnBK vapor are shown in Table 5. Exposures to 10 and 50 ppm for 7 1/2 hours produced mean MnBK breath concentrations of 1.4 and 9.3 ppm respectively. Fifteen minutes after exposure to either 10 or 50 ppm, the expired air concentrations of MnBK were 1.1 and 0.5 ppm respectively. Exposure to 100 ppm for 4 hours produced an average MnBK breath concentration of 22 ppm during the exposure. The above results show that between 75 and 92% of the vapor inhaled by humans was absorbed by the lungs. The post exposure results are of particular interest inasmuch as they show that very little of the absorbed MnBK was eliminated during the post exposure period.

Serum concentrations of MnBK during and after exposure to either 10 or 50 ppm were below the limit of detection but were detectable at 100 ppm. 25HD was not detected in serum of individuals during exposure to 50 or 100 ppm of MnBK, but was detected after the termination of the exposure. No metabolites of MnBK were found in expired air.

TABLE 5

ALVEOLAR BREATH AND SERUM CONCENTRATIONS OF METHYL n-BUTYL KETONE AND 2,5-HEXANEDIONE FROM VOLUNTEERS EXPERIMENTALLY EXPOSED TO METHYL n-BUTYL KETONE VAPOR [a]

Time of Collection (hr)	Concentration of MnBK in Breath (ppm)			Concentration MnBK in Serum (µg/ml)	Concentration of 25HD in Serum (µg/ml)	
	Exposure Concentration (ppm)					
	10	50	100	100	50	100
Exposure						
0	0	0	0		0	0
1	0.8	9.2	24.7	0.3	0	0
2	0.9	10.6	22.0	0.8	0	0
3	1.1	9.5	20.6		0	0
4	1.8	9.8	20.2	1.2	0	0
Lunch						
5	0.6	10.8				
6	0.8	9.2				
7	1.8	8.8				
8	1.4	9.3			0	0
Post-Exposure						
0.25	0.1	0.5	1.0			
0.50	0.1	0.3	0.6		2.0	0.9
1	0	0.1	0.3	0.2		
2		0.1	0.1			
3		0	0	0.2	3.0	0.2
4				0		

[a] Three male volunteers were exposed to MnBK for 7 1/2 hours to concentrations of 10 and 50 ppm and for 4 hours to 100 ppm. Each test subject was exposed once. Alevolar breath was collected in Saran .bags and analyzed by gas chromatography. Blood was collected at regular intervals and serum was analyzed for MnBK and its metabolites.

Oral Administration of [1-^{14}C] MnBK to Humans. The fate of [1-^{14}C] MnBK was studied in two volunteers. Two µCi of [1-^{14}C] MnBK were dissolved in corn oil, placed in a gelatine capsule and swallowed with water. The dose was 0.1 mg/kg of body weight. Expired air was collected for 5 minutes each hour for 14 hours and at regular intervals thereafter. Breath samples were collected through a two-way Douglas valve into a 96 liter Saran bag. The contents of the Saran bag were then passed through 40 ml of 1/2 (v/v) mixture of 2-aminoethanol and 2-

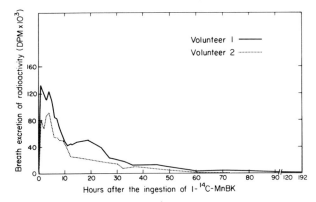

Fig. 3.   Elimination of $^{14}CO_2$ in breath.

methoxyethanol to trap expired CO_2. Urine was collected at 4 hour intervals for
16 hours and a total voiding at irregular intervals thereafter. Shortly after
collection, urine was assayed for radioactivity.

The breath excretion of $^{14}CO_2$ by two volunteers given an oral dose of $[1-^{14}C]$
MnBK is illustrated in Figure 3. The excretion of $^{14}CO_2$ reached a peak within 4
hours after dosing and then decreased slowly over the next 3 to 8 days. It is
noteworthy that MnBK was rapidly converted to CO_2 following ingestion. The
elimination of CO_2 was biphasic. The first phase was rapid and occurred from
the time of ingestion until about 12 hours after ingestion and the second was
more prolonged requiring 8 days before background levels of radioactivity were
reached.

The excretion of radioactivity in the urine is illustrated in Figure 4. The

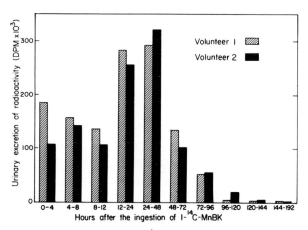

Fig. 4.   Excretion of $[^{14}C]$ in the urine.

194

majority of the radioactivity in the urine was excreted within 48 hours and the remainder was eliminated over the next 6 days.

The breath elimination of $^{14}CO_2$ by two volunteers averaged 39.5% of the dose and the excretion of radioactivity in urine averaged 26.3% of the dose. The overall recovery of $[^{14}C]$ was 65.8%. The remainder of the radioactivity was presumably incorporated into intermediary metabolism (Table 6).

TABLE 6

EXCRETION OF RADIOACTIVITY IN THE BREATH AND URINE BY VOLUNTEERS FOLLOWING THE INGESTION OF 1-^{14}C-METHYL n-BUTYL KETONE

Test Subject	Dose (mg/kg)	Percent of Dose		8 Day Recovery
		Breath	Urine	
1	0.1	49.9	27.6	77.5
2	0.1	29.0	25.0	54.0
Average		39.5	26.3	65.8

Structure Activity Relationships. The identification of the metabolites of MnBK in man and laboratory animals prompted us to test these compounds for neurotoxicity in experimental animals. The chronic intraperitoneal and sub-cutaneous administration of 25HD, the most persistent serum metabolite of MnBK, produced a neuropathy in rats which was indistinguishable from that produced by MnBK.[9-12] These studies suggested that 25HD may itself be an active metabolite of MnBK. Presumably, n-hexane and MnBK metabolites, such as 5H2H, 2-hexanol, and 2,5-hexanediol may also produce neuropathy by a similar mechanism since we have shown that all of the above compounds are all ultimately converted in vivo to 25HD. In view of these findings, the neurotoxic potential of MnBK, n-hexane and their common metabolites was investigated.[11,12]

Male Charles River CD (SD) rats ranging in weight from 220 to 260 g were randomly assigned to 6 test groups of 5 animals each. MnBK, n-hexane, 25HD, 2,5-hexanediol, 5H2H, and 2-hexanol were administered by gavage once daily, 5 days a week over a 90 day period. Each animal was dosed with 6.6 mmol/kg of body weight and doses were adjusted weekly for body weight changes. Purina Laboratory Chow and water were provided ad libitum.

All animals were observed for clinical signs of neuropathy prior to each daily dose. The end point used to terminate treatment of individual animals were clinical signs of neuropathy, that is, severe hind limb weakness or paralysis exhibited by dragging at least one hind foot. Animals not exhibiting clinical signs were terminated at 90 days. At termination, the animals were autopsied and tissues were collected and embedded in plastic for histologic evaluation of 1 μm thick sections.

A separate study was done to determine the time course of 25HD in the serum of rats dosed with each test compound. A single dose of each test compound comparable to those used in the toxicity study was administered to groups of 3 to 5 animals. Serum concentrations of 25HD were measured by gas chromatography at specific intervals for 24 hours after dosing. The analytical procedures were identical to those described previously.[5]

The relative neurotoxicity of MnBK, n-hexane and their common metabolites is summarized in Table 7. 25HD was the most potent neurotoxin tested requiring only 16.8 days to produce clinical signs of neuropathy. The other hexacarbon metabolites, 5H2H, 2,5-hexanediol and 2-hexanol were also neurotoxic presumably due to their conversion to 25HD. A neurotoxic index calculated on the basis of the time to the onset of clinical neuropathy of each compound compared to that of MnBK indicates that 25HD is 3.3 times more potent a neurotoxin than is MnBK and that MnBK is substantially more neurotoxic than is n-hexane.

The onset of neurotoxicity correlated directly with peak serum concentrations of 25HD and with the area under the serum concentration-time curve for 25HD (Figure 5). The time course for the formation and disappearance of 25HD in the serum of rats given equal molar doses of MnBK, n-hexane and their common metabolites is illustrated in Figure 6. These data support the hypothesis that neurotoxic potency of these compounds is related to the animal's ability to convert these compounds to 25HD.

The difference between the neurotoxic potency of MnBK and n-hexane is of interest since it has usually been inferred that these two compounds are of equal neurotoxicity. However unpublished results indicate that 7 times more n-hexane administered over twice the duration is required to produce a neuropathy similar to that seen with MnBK.

DISCUSSION

On the basis of our studies in guinea pigs and rats, MnBK is both oxidatively and reductively metabolized. Oxidation appears to proceed by hydroxylation of ω-1 carbon forming 5H2H. Reduction occurred at the carbonyl group as expected forming a secondary alcohol, 2-hexanol. Studies conducted in our laboratory

TABLE 7

RELATIVE NEUROTOXICITY OF METHYL n–BUTYL KETONE, n–HEXANE AND THEIR COMMON METABOLITES

Compound	Rats with Neuropathy Clinical	Rats with Neuropathy Histologic	Days to Endpoint	Peak Serum Conc. 25HD (μg/ml)	AUC for 25HD[b]	Neurotoxic Index
2,5–Hexanedione	5	5	16.8 ± 1.4 [a]	569 ± 98.0 [a]	4.2	3.3
5–Hydroxy–2–hexanone	5	5	21.8 ± 1.0	318 ± 51.0	2.9	2.6
2,5–Hexanediol	5	5	29.0 ± 1.7	238 ± 59.0	2.0	1.9
Methyl n–butyl ketone	5	5	55.8 ± 4.3	111 ± 12.0	1.0	1.0
2–Hexanol	4	5	82.5 ± 3.2	75 ± 6.5	0.2	< 0.7
n–Hexane	0	0	> 90	24 ± 1.6	0.2	< 0.6
Control	0	0	> 90	-	-	-

a Mean ± S.E.
b Area under the curve (AUC) for 2,5Hxdn was determined by the cut and weigh procedure.

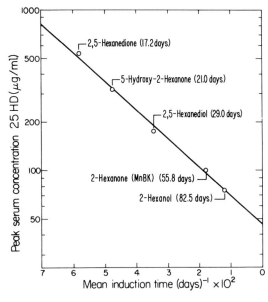

Fig. 5. Correlation between serum concentrations of 25HD and the onset of neuropathy.

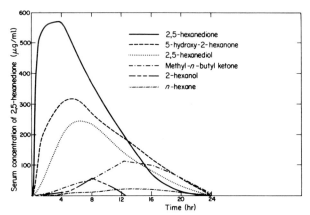

Fig. 6. Time course for 2,5-hexanedione in the serum of rats dosed with 6.6 mmol/kg of each hexacarbon.

with methylethyl ketone, 3-heptanone, di-n-butyl ketone, methyl iso-amyl ketone and di-n-propyl ketone, indicate that ω-1 oxidation and carbonyl reduction are significant routes in the metabolism of aliphatic ketones.

The fate of [1-^{14}C] MnBK in the rat revealed that MnBK is metabolized by a variety of pathways including reduction, α-oxidation, ω-1 oxidation, decarboxylation, and transamination. Radioactively labelled compounds identified in the breath or urine from rats dosed with [1-^{14}C] MnBK were unchanged MnBK, CO_2, 2-hexanol, 5H2H, 25HD, norleucine, 2,5-dimethylfuran, γ-valerolactone, and urea. A proposed scheme for the metabolism of MnBK is shown in Figure 7.

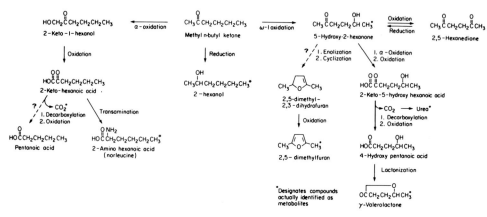

Fig. 7. Proposed metabolic pathway for methyl n-butyl ketone.

Expired $^{14}CO_2$ accounts for the single largest portion of eliminated radio-activity. It is unlikely to be derived from MnBK breakdown to $[1-^{14}C]$ acetate via intermediary metabolism, since urinary acetic acid was unlabelled and there was little incorporation of $[^{14}C]$ into tissue lipids. A likely route of formation of $^{14}CO_2$ from $(1-^{14}C)$ MnBK would be by α-oxidation to α-ketohexanoate followed by decarboxylation to $^{14}CO_2$ and 1-pentanal. 1-pentanal would enter intermediary metabolism after oxidation to pentanoate and would probably be undetected. No radioactive products were detected in the urine that would shed light on this point. The formation of $[^{14}C]$-norleucine from $[1-^{14}C]$ MnBK supports the α-oxidation mechanism since α-ketohexanoate could be available for transamination or decarboxylation. Evidently, the preferred pathway for the metabolism of the hypothetical α-ketohexanoate intermediate is by decarboxylation.

5H2H appears to be a key intermediate in the metabolism of MnBK. Presumably, 5H2H is formed by ω-1 oxidation in the microsomal mixed function oxidase system. It is eliminated partly unchanged and from evidence provided by hydrolysis as a glucuronide and a sulfate. The formation of 25HD, 2,5-dimethylfuran and γ-valerolactone proceeds from 5H2H.

The occurrence of the cyclic metabolite, 2,5-dimethylfuran,is somewhat unexpected, although the potential for cyclization to a furan structure exists for 5H2H. A possible route of formation may involve a hydroxylated precursor eliminated in the urine which would form 2,5-dimethylfuran as an artifact on gas chromatographic analysis. The existence of such a precursor is suggested by the fact that 2,5-dimethylfuran was obtained from urine after acid hydrolysis and β-glucuronidase treatment. Such a precursor could arise from the ω-2 hydroxylation of 5H2H to 2-keto-4,5-dihydroxyhexane which could undergo thermal dehydration and cyclization on gas chromatography to 2,5-dimethylfuran.

The metabolism of MnBK in man appears to be similar to that of the rat inasmuch as MnBK is metabolized by at least two pathways, one forming CO_2 and the other 25HD. The fact that radioactivity derived from $[1-^{14}C]$ MnBK was excreted slowly in the breath and urine of human volunteers suggests that repeated daily exposure to MnBK may lead to a prolonged exposure to neurotoxic metabolites. The relatively slow excretion of radioactivity from $[1-^{14}C]$ MnBK in the breath and urine has further elucidated the important role biotransformation has played regarding the neurotoxicity of MnBK. The major metabolite of $[1-^{14}C]$ MnBK in man and in the rat was expired $^{14}CO_2$.

While the mechanism of MnBK induced neuropathy is unknown, biotransformation evidently plays a significant role. Thus the α-oxidation and decarboxylation pathways evidently yield products handled by intermediary metabolism or excretory products possessing no neurotoxic properties. On the other hand, ω-1 oxidation appears to play a central role in the production of metabolic intermediates which lead to the development of peripheral neuropathy. The metabolic intermediate most frequently implicated in the phenomenon is 25HD. The relative neurotoxicity of MnBK, n-hexane and its metabolites clearly establishes 25HD as the most potent neurotoxin tested. The onset of neurotoxicity can be directly correlated with the amount of 25HD produced from each hexacarbon tested.

The mechanism by which the above hexacarbons can produce neuropathy is still elusive. Ongoing studies conducted in our laboratory suggest that a γ-diketone is required to produce a neuropathy.[13] Structures possessing an α, β or δ-diketone were biologically inactive whereas structures containing a γ-diketone, such as 2,5-heptanedione or 3,6-octanedione produced a neuropathy similar to that produced by 25HD.

The onset of MnBK or n-hexane neuropathy in man and experimental animals may be shortened due to the presence of other aliphatic ketones such as methyl ethyl ketone.[14,15] The mechanism by which this phenomenon occurs is unclear at this time. Conceivably, MEK may alter the metabolism of MnBK or n-hexane to produce more 25HD than would be produced under conditions of single solvent exposure. Further work is needed to clarify the role methyl ethyl ketone plays in the development of neuropathy by MnBK or n-hexane.

REFERENCES

1. Yamada, S. (1964). Jap. J. Ind. Health 6, 192.

2. Herskowitz, A., Ishii, N., and Schaumburg, H. (1971). N. Engl. J. Med. 285, 82-85.

3. Billmaier, D., Yee, H. T., Allen, N., Craft, R., Williams, N., Epstein, S. and Fontaine, R. (1974). J. Occup. Med. 16, 665-671.

4. Patty, F. A (1963). Industrial Hygiene and Toxicology, 2nd Ed., Vol. 2, John Wiley and Sons, New York, pp. 1731-1743.

5. DiVincenzo, G. D., Kaplan, C. J. and Dedinas, J. (1976). Toxicol. Appl. Pharmacol. 36, 511-522.

6. DiVincenzo, G. D., Kapaln, C. J. and Dedinas, J. (1977). Toxicol. Appl. Pharmacol. 41, 547-560.

7. DiVincenzo, G. D., Hamilton, M. L., Kaplan, C. J., Krasavage, W. J. and O'Donoghue, J. L. (1978). Toxicol. Appl. Pharmacol. 44, 593-604.

8. DiVincenzo, G. D., Yanno, F. J. and Astill, B. D. (1971). Amer. Ind. Hyg. Assoc. J. 32, 387-391.

9. Raleigh, R. L., Spencer, P. S. and Schaumburg, H. H. (1975). J. Occup. Med. 17, 286.

10. Spencer, P. S. and Schaumburg, H. H. (1975). J. Neurol. Neurosurg. Psychiat. 38, 771-775.

11. Krasavage, W. J., O'Donoghue, J. L., DiVincenzo, G. D. and Terhaar, C. J. (1979). Toxicol. Appl. Pharmacol. In Press.

12. O'Donoghue, D. L., Krasavage, W. J. and Terhaar, C. J. (1978). Toxicol. Appl. Pharmacol. 45, 251.

13. O'Donoghue, J. L. and Krasavage, W. J. (1979) Toxicol. Appl. Pharmacol. In Press.

14. Saida, K., Mendell, J. R., and Weiss, H. S. (1976) J. Neuropathol. Exp. Neurol. 35, 207-225.

15. Altenkirch, H., Mager, J., Stoltenburg, G. and Helmbrecht, J. (1977) J. Neuol. 214 137-152.

© 1980 Elsevier/North-Holland Biomedical Press
The Scientific Basis of Toxicity Assessment
H. Witschi, editor.

MOLECULAR MECHANISMS OF TOXIC CELL DEATH

JOHN L. FARBER

Department of Pathology and the Fels Research Institute, Temple University

School of Medicine, Philadelphia, Pennsylvania, 19140, U.S.A.

The mechanisms of toxic cell injury have been largely pursued through
an attempt to go from chemistry to biology. Such a "forward" approach is
rationalized by the fact that one is starting with a defined chemical - the
toxin - whose reactivity can be characterized and whose fate in the cell
can be traced. This approach has been widely applied to a number of toxins
acting on a variety of cell systems. The results of these investigations
have generally been quite consistent and have produced two major conclusions
that currently dominate molecular toxicology. First, most toxic chemicals
are not themselves biologically active but must be converted to reactive
metabolites usually by their target cells. Target cell specificity and the
actual extent of cell injury is, in turn, dependent upon this metabolism.
Second the critical metabolite exerts its biological action by virtue of an
ability to covalently bind to cellular macromolecules.

There are limitations to the "forward" approach and inherent difficulties in trying to derive biology solely from chemistry. This approach
has produced very little insight into the nature of those macromolecules
whose interaction with toxic metabolites forms the basis for their toxicity
or of the sequence of events that presumably exists between these interactions and the death of the cells. There is no inherent way to predict
what the ultimate target macromolecule is and what functional consequence
will result from its injury. With cell death there are no a priori guidelines for selecting any particular part of the cellular machinery for study.

Making matters worse is the fact that ultimately all metabolism is going to stop and, therefore, anything chosen to study will eventually become perturbed. How then does one decide if any change is a cause or an effect? The belief that identification of the earliest biochemical or morphological changes will give a lead to the mechanism of cell death is potentially risky, since the fact that a change occurs early in the process does not necessarily indicate that it is causally related to this process.

The alternative to the forward approach is a "backward approach." Here one attempts to go from biology to chemistry by starting at the end of the process and working backward to its beginning. Such an approach has allowed a presumed sequence of events underlying toxic liver cell necrosis to be traced backwards to a point where, in a few cases, they approach the pathway elucidated by the "forward" approach. This has allowed in these specific cases some preliminary understanding of the sequence of chemical and biochemical events that underly toxic cell death. In other cases, this approach has indicated the direction that current research effort should take in achieving a similar degree of understanding.

Our initial concern is with intracellular calcium homeostasis, since there is now some evidence that toxic liver cell death most likely represents a disturbance in this process. All cells in the body are bathed in a fluid very rich in Ca^{2+} ions (10^{-3}M), while intracellular Ca^{2+} concentrations are much lower, on the order of 10^{-7} to 10^{-6}M [1]. The electrical potential across the plasma membrane of these same cells tends to drive Ca^{2+} into the cell. Such a large electrochemical gradient is maintained by the relative impermeability of the plasma membrane to Ca^{2+} and by active extrusion. Damage to the plasma membrane by any one of a number of different mechanisms would disrupt this permeability barrier with a consequent influx of Ca^{2+}. Calcium ions are biologically very active, being capable of considerable disruption of metabolic order.

Although calcium had been known for many years to accumulate in necrotic tissues, a possible active role for Ca^{2+} ions in the production of liver necrosis was first suggested by investigations of Judah and his colleagues[2-7] showing that some anti-inflammatory drugs gave considerable protection to the liver against the action of selected hepatotoxins. These studies showed an early increase in the calcium content of the cells that was prevented by promethazine and that could be related to inhibition of various enzyme activities. Antihistamines like promethazine were known to block ion movements, and it was suggested that the primary lesion is a loss of the semi-permeable properties of the cells with consequent entry of lethal concentrations of Ca^{2+}. Alterations in intracellular calcium homeostasis have since been demonstrated with CCl_4 [8-12], galactosamine[13], dimethylnitrosamine and aflatoxin B_1 [14] as well as the changes just noted with thioacetamide. While consistent with an active role for Ca^{2+} in toxic liver cell death, such accumulations of Ca^{2+} could always be explained, however, as simply a passive equilibration of Ca^{2+} concentrations in cells lethally injured by different and as yet unexplained mechanisms.

In order to explore more directly the role of Ca^{2+} in toxic cell death, we have been studying the Ca^{2+} dependency of the killing of primary cultures of adult rat hepatocytes. We have demonstrated a requirement for extra-cellular Ca^{2+} in the killing of such cells by toxic agents that don't need metabolic activation by the cells and that interact directly with cellular membranes[15]. In Ca^{2+} containing medium each of these agents killed one half or more of the cells as measured by the failure of trypan blue exclusion. In the absence of added Ca^{2+} there was no cell death. A Ca^{2+} gradient across the plasma membrane was, therefore, necessary for the expression of the toxicity of these agents. The simplest interpretation of this Ca^{2+} dependency is that in each case the toxin causes disruption of the permeability barrier function of the plasma membrane allowing a lethal influx of Ca^{2+} down the steep electrochemical gradient that exists between the outside and the inside of the cells. This implies that the killing of rat liver cells in culture by the toxins studied involves, at least, two clearly definable steps. The first represents a disruption of the integrity of the plasma membrane and is independent of extracellular Ca^{2+}. Despite the widely differing mechanisms whereby this injury can be produced, there is a common functional consequence in what follows. The second step is dependent upon extracellular calcium and most likely represents an influx across the damaged plasma membrane and down a steep electrochemical gradient. This influx, then, is a final common pathway by which the cells are killed. Recognition of this pathway indicates that the toxic death of liver cells under the preceding conditions is ultimately a very specific consequence of a disturbance in intracellular Ca^{2+} homeostasis and not some nonspecific slowing down of cellular metabolism or some generalized disruption of membrane function. Since our primary concern still remains the role of Ca^{2+} ions in liver cell necrosis in the intact animal and man, recognition of this pathway in vitro strengthens the hypothesis that disturbances in calcium homeostasis induced by a variety of hepatotoxins are causally related to liver cell death. The model derived from our in vitro studies suggested that an initial approach to the in vivo mechanisms should be to attempt to relate the time course of changes in intracellular Ca^{2+} homeostasis to the time course of changes in the plasma membrane. To date this has been accomplished in intact livers with 2 hepatotoxins, galactosamine and carbon tetrachloride.

A single dose of 400 mg/kg galactosamine produces foci of hepatocellular necrosis scattered throughout the lobules within the first 24 hours. The biochemical basis for this toxicity of galactosamine presumably lies in its metabolism by the liver cells[16]. The formation of UDP-hexosamines functions as a trap for uridine nucleotides, producing a fall in the concentration of uridine nucleotides and UDP-hexoses. Administration of uridine will reverse both the deficiencies of uridine nucleotides and UDP-hexoses.

Administration of galactosamine to rats produces a disturbance in the control of intracellular Ca^{2+} levels within the liver cells[13]. During the first 2 hours there is a significant elevation in the total liver cell calcium, although there is no detectable liver cell necrosis at this point. The calcium content continues to rise, and necrosis is first detectable at 4 hours. If the galactosamine-treated animals are given a single intraperitoneal injection of chlorpromazine, a potent inhibitor of Ca^{2+} fluxes, 2 hours after galactosamine there is no further elevation in the liver cell calcium content over a 48 hour period and virtually no detectable liver cell necrosis[17].

This distrubed calcium homeostasis induced by galactosamine can be directly related to an as yet poorly characterized alteration in the structure of the plasma membrane[13]. Plasma membranes isolated within the first 2 hours from galactosamine-treated rats show a 40% reduction in 5'-nucleotidase activity and a two-fold increase in maximum negative ellipticity determined by circular dichroism. Simultaneous administration of uridine prevents these alterations in the plasma membranes. The membrane alterations are also reversed when uridine is administered for up to 2.5 hours after galactosamine. Uridine will at the same time prevent and reverse the changes in Ca^{2+} content. Uridine given up to 2.5 hours after galactosamine prevents the appearance of liver cell necrosis[18].

These observations suggest that the disturbance in calcium homeostasis induced by galactosamine is a consequence of the plasma membrane injury with an increased passive influx of calcium as suggested for the membrane damage induced in cultured hepatocytes. While the nature of the plasma membrane alteration induced by galactosamine is unknown at present, there are reasons to suspect that it may be related to a disturbance in plasma membrane ganglioside composition. Galactosamine has been shown to inhibit ganglioside synthesis[19], and the absence of any evidence of microsomal membrane injury in galactosamine-intoxicated cells[20] is consistent with the primary localization of gangliosides in the plasma membrane. It might be speculated further that plasma membrane gangliosides may function to gate a physiological calcium channel, which would be opened by disturbances in the composition of these lipids induced by galactosamine.

Carbon tetrachloride also induces a disturbance in the control of intra-cellular Ca^{2+} homeostasis in rat liver cells[8-12], and there is again a correlation between the time course of this change and manifestations of plasma membrane injury[21]. CCl_4 produces a biphasic pattern of altered Ca^{2+} homeostasis. Within the first 2 hours there is a slight increase in the Ca^{2+} content of all of the cells in the liver lobule. By 4 hours the Ca^{2+} has returned to normal and remains low at least through the 8th hour. Between 8 and 12 hours the Ca^{2+} begins to rise and increases dramatically to some 20 times the normal by 48 hours. Liver cell death first becomes evident between 8 and 12 hours and increases in extent in parallel to the increasing Ca^{2+} content. A single injection of chlorpromazine given 2 hours after CCl_4 prevents the late rises in calcium for at least 48 hours. Chlorpromazine prevents the necrosis caused by CCl_4 for, at least, 48 hours.

Plasma membranes isolated from CCl_4-intoxicated livers manifest a pro-gressive loss of 5'-nucleotidase that reaches 85-95% by 12 hours[21]. Liver cell Ca^{2+} content, then, begins to rise and liver cell death begins to be

evident at the time when 5'-nucleotidase inhibition is maximal. This
inhibition of 5'-nucleotidase, however, is not simply a consequence of
liver cell death. Pretreatment of the rats with diethyldithiocarbamate
(DEDTC) prevents this cell death while only reducing the extent without
actually preventing plasma membrane injury[21]. Post-treatment with DEDTC
has no effect on the extent of plasma membrane injury or liver cell viability. Chlorpromazine similarly reduces the extent of plasma membrane
injury produced by CCl4. Accumulation of calcium by the CCl4-injured
cells correlates with the extent of plasma membrane injury as assessed by
5'-nucleotidase, and the reduction in the extent of this injury that
occurs with DEDTC and chlorpromazine is not associated with calcium accumulation or cell death.

Does the destruction of the microsomal membrane by CCl4 catalyzed
lipid peroxidation have anything to do with the liver cell death produced
by CCl4? It is now generally accepted that the toxicity of CCl4 is dependent upon its metabolism by the microsomal membrane. It is also well
known that lipid peroxidation of microsomal membrane phospholipids is
a major consequence of this metabolism. Recently the very interesting
observation was made that some products of microsomal lipid peroxidation
can traverse finite distances and effect membrane damage at other loca-
tions[22] . As yet unidentified compounds - possibly soluble peroxides -
obtained by ultrafiltration of peroxidized microsomal membranes were found
to produce lytic damage to red cell membranes. This observation raises
the critical question as to whether or not the plasma membrane damage and
its accompanying alterations in Ca^{2+} homeostasis seen with CCl4 result
from the action of similar products of the peroxidative decomposition
of the microsomal membrane. If, as seems likely, this is the mechanism
of production of plasma membrane damage, then for the first time a very

consistent picture would begin to emerge of the most likely sequence of
the molecular events responsible for the liver necrosis produced by CCl_4.

The studies with galactosamine and carbon tetrachloride just reviewed
have produced two working models. Many questions, of course, remain, but
the major outline of the events are probably accurate. An important
feature of both models is that the pathogenesis of toxic liver cell necrosis is a multi-step process that can be potentially interfered with
at a number of points.

What is the relevance of these models to the mechanisms of action of
other toxins? In particular we would like to know what the relationship
of the models derived from our so-called "backward" approach is to the
model derived from the "forward" approach . An obvious answer is that
the macromolecules to which reactive metabolites of various toxins covalently
bind are constituents of cellular membranes and of the plasma membrane in
particular. The functional consequence of such an interaction would be
an alteration in permeability property leading to a lethal influx of Ca^{2+}.
While certainly attractive, there are, unfortunately, very little data at
present to support such a unifying hypothesis. We were able to kill cultured hepatocytes with 3 agents whose mechanisms of action are dependent
upon the formation of covalent bonds[15]. This would argue that covalent
binding presumably to the cell membrane can produce the function result
postulated. There are, however, little or no data that relate the time course
of the in vivo covalent binding of reactive, toxic metabolites to plasma membranes with the time course of the appearance of cell death. In addition, there
are little or no data that the death of cells exposed to these same toxic
chemicals is associated with increases in Ca^{2+} content accompanying the
binding of reactive metabolites to membranes, on the one hand, and the

appearance of necrosis on the other. Such studies are badly needed and should be given a high priority. A word of caution, however, is in order. CCl4 is metabolized to a reactive intermediate, presumably the trichlor-methyl free radical, that binds significantly to macromolecules. The extent of this binding correlates with the extent of liver cell necrosis. However, covalent binding of this radical to the microsomal membrane has clearly been shown to be unrelated to the functional damage produced by the metabolism of CCl4 [23], and it is very unlikely, in the light of our preceding discussion, that this binding is related to the liver cell death produced by CCl4. This, of course, doesn't mean that covalent binding produced by other hepatoxins is not related to necrosis, but it does indicate that it isn't necessarily and suggests some caution in the interpretation of such data.

REFERENCES

1. Rasmussen, H. (1970) Science, 170, 404.

2. Gallagher, G.H. et al. (1956) J. Pathol. Bacteriol. 72, 193.

3. Judah, J.D. et al. (1964) in Ciba Symposium in Cellular Injury, ed. de Reuck, A.V.S. and Knight, J. (J.&A. Churchill, Ltd. London) pp. 187-205.

4. McLean, A.E. M et al. (1965) Int. Rev. Exp. Pathol. 4, 127.

5. Rees, K.R. (1962) in Ciba Symposium on Enzymes and Drug Action, ec. Mongar, J.L. and de Reuck, A.V.S. (J.&A. Churchill, Ltd., London) pp.344-358.

6. Rees, K.R et al. (1961) J. Pathol. Bacteriol. 81, 107.

7. McLean, A.E.M. et al. (1964) Ann. NY Acad. Sci. 116, 986.

8. Reynolds, E.S. et al. (1962) J. Biol. Chem. 237, 3546.

9. Reynolds, E.S. (1963) J. Cell Biol. 19, 139.

10. Reynolds, E.S. (1964) Lab. Invest. 13, 1467.

11. Smucker, E.A. (1966) Lab. Invest. 15, 157.

12. Moore, L et al. (1976) J. Biol. Chem. 251, 1197.

210

13. El-Mofty, S.K. et al. (1975) Am. J. Pathol. 79, 579.

14. Farber, J.L. et al. Unpublished results.

15. Schanne, F.A.X. et al. Science. In press.

16. Decker, K. and Keppler, D. (1972) in Progress in Liver Diseases, Vol. IV, ed. Popper, H., and Schaffner, R. (Grune and Stratton, New York) pp. 183-200.

17. Farber, J. L. and Abrams, J. Unpublished data.

18. Farber, J.L. et al. (1973) Am. J . Pathol. 72, 53.

19. Rupprecht, E. et al.(1976) Biochem. Biophys. Acta 450, 45.

20. Farber, J.L. et al. (1977) Arch. Biochem. Biophys. 178. 617.

21. Farber, J.L. et al. Manuscript submitted.

22. Rodgers, M.D. et al. (1977) Science 196, 1221.

23. Glende, E.A., Jr. (et al. (1976) Biochem. Pharmacol. 25, 2163.

© 1980 Elsevier/North-Holland Biomedical Press
The Scientific Basis of Toxicity Assessment
H. Witschi, editor.

ULTRASTRUCTURAL MORPHOMETRIC/BIOCHEMICAL ASSESSMENT OF CELLULAR TOXICITY

BRUCE A. FOWLER

Laboratory of Environmental Toxicology, National Institute of Environmental
Health Sciences, Research Triangle Park, NC   27709

INTRODUCTION

The *in vivo* relationship between physical structure and biochemical functionality of subcellular organelle systems is complex but of potentially great
importance to understanding the mechanisms by which toxicants produce cellular
dysfunction. Ultrastructural morphometry in conjunction with biochemical measurements of isolated organelles provides one approach for identifying and assessing changes in susceptible organelle systems prior to overt organ damage.
This approach, diagrammatically presented in Figure 1, attempts to effectively
combine the inherent advantages of both techniques to quantitatively relate
changes in the structure of sensitive organelle systems within intact cells to
biochemical dysfunction as assessed by a variety of parameters. In effect, this
system of evaluation attempts to delineate the subcellular mechanisms of organelle toxicity by a holistic approach to the cell as the basic organizational
unit of biological function.

In our laboratory, particular emphasis is placed on those biochemical parameters involving organelle structure-function relationships and organelle dependent biological processes with circulating metabolites. Application of this
approach to evaluation of livers and kidneys of rodents exposed to toxic metals
such as arsenic and mercury has proven useful in broadening our knowledge of
the cellular mechanisms of metal toxicity in these organs and permitted development of new biological indicators of toxicity.

Before reviewing some of the ways in which ultrastructural morphometry and
biochemistry have been combined to elucidate information regarding the intracellular effects of a variety of toxicants in several target organ systems, it
would first seem appropriate to examine some of the specific advantages and
limitations involved in applying this approach to understanding mechanisms of
toxicity. As with any scientific technique, the value of combining ultrastructural morphometry with biochemistry to understand cell injury can only be
realized by judicious usuage.

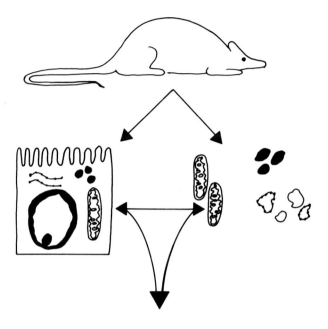

Relationship between biochemical mechanisms
of toxicity and organelle damage.

Development of preclinical biological indicators
of toxicity.

Fig. 1.   Diagrammatic representation of the combined ultrastructural morpho-
metric/biochemical approach to understanding cellular toxicity.

Ultrastructural Morphometry

   The basic assumptions, equations and general correction factors for applications of ultrastructural morphometry to biological systems have been extensively described by several workers[1-8].   The following section is intended
to focus on the specific application of this technique for evaluation of cellular toxicity.

   The primary advantages of ultrastructural morphometry for evaluation of
tissues from target organs are the small amount of tissue required and the
ability to identify organelle changes within specific cell types and to

quantitate changes in those organelle systems so that biochemical evaluation may be focused on the mechanisms of toxicity for these specific organelles.

Biological limitations inherent in the approach are that frequently not all cells or cell types are equally affected by a given toxicant and hence a judgement must be made with regard to the benefits of random or non-random sampling. The former approach tends to be more readily relatable to biochemical changes in homogenized tissues while the latter is useful for quantifying changes in discrete cell populations. Primary technical limitations of the approach are that it is extremely laborious not only in terms of the actual photographic requirements related to electron microscopy but also in terms of the quantitative measurements on the photomicrographs. A typical morphometric evaluation of tissue from an experiment involving a control and 3 treatment groups will involve thin-sectioning of 3-5 tissues blocks from each of 6-10 animals per group (depending on interanimal variation) and then generating 5 micrographs from each tissue block. It is obvious that this sort of approach can easily produce 500 electron micrographs per experiment. Each micrograph must then be individually quantitated and finally subjected to statistical analysis.

The net result of this is that application of ultrastructural morphometry to toxicological problems involves extensive commitments of time and effort, but in return it provides information about the physical state of subcellular organelles within intact cells that is otherwise unobtainable.

Biochemical Evaluation of Subcellular Organelles

The main advantages of biochemical analysis of subcellular organelle systems are that it provides both a means for delineation of toxic mechanisms and an overall assessment of organelle viability.

Primary limitations of this approach for the toxicologist are that homogenization procedures employed for subcellular fractionation mix organelles from different cell types[9] as well as those from both affected and unaffected cells thereby leading to a dilution of measureable biochemical changes. It is hence possible to underestimate severe changes from toxicants in small but important cell populations due to organelle dilution during isolation procedures. Despite this limitation, biochemical analysis is the only available path to understanding mechanisms of toxicant action.

Now that I have hopefully given a brief perspective on these two approaches to understanding toxic mechanisms, I would like to review some of the studies which have attempted to combine both techniques to better understand the relationship between *in vivo* organelle structure and function in livers and kidneys of animals exposed to a variety of biologically active agents and to indicate ways in which information from these studies has helped development of new biological indicators of toxicity.

Liver

Most correlative ultrastructural morphometric/biochemical studies with agents in this organ have examined physical changes in specific compartments directly involved in the metabolism or cellular toxicity of the agent administered. Some of these studies are reviewed below on an organelle basis.

Endoplasmic Reticulum

Administration of phenobarbital to rats has been shown to produce marked *in vivo* increases in the surface density of both rough (RER) and smooth (SER) endoplasmic reticulum which was correlated with concommitant increases in microsomal phospholipid, cytochrome P-450, aminopyrine demethylase and NADPH cytochrome-c-reductase[10-11]. These observed increases in endoplasmic reticulum were found to return to near normal by 5 days following cessation of treatment. These authors concluded that the observed increase in endoplasmic reticulum occurred in two phases which involved first increased synthesis of RER with secondary ribosomal detachment leading to increased amounts of SER. Asynchronous assembly and turnover of proteins in the ER membranes was thought to provide the best explanation for the observed morphometric and biochemical data relating to the induction phenomenon. The observed decreases in SER found 5 days after cessation of treatment were subsequently related to an increase in autophagic vacuoles suggesting preferential removal of unnecessary organelle membranes associated with decreased metabolic activity. Mechanical cholestasis[12] has also been found to cause a 3-4 fold proliferation of both RER and SER surface density but in this case cytochrome P-450 content and the specific activities of glucose-6-phosphatase and several mixed function oxidase enzymes showed decreased specific activities. The point to be derived from these studies is the essential importance of examining biochemical function for this organelle system since the same morphological response to experimental manipulation (increased SER) may involve opposite effects on biochemical functionality.

Mitochondria

Studies with cortisone, vitamin E deficiency, methyl mercury and arsenate in rat liver have illuminated several organelle structure-function relationships. Administration of cortisone[13-14] was found to increase the volume density of hepatic mitochondria with concommitant depression of mitochondrial respiration and ADP:O ratios. Ultrastructural morphometric studies[15] relating dietary vitamin E deficiency to changes in mitochondrial membranes showed that an observed highly specific doubling of the surface density of the inner membrane also doubled calculated distances between cytochrome molecules of the mitochondrial electron transport chain.

Morphometric and biochemical evaluation of liver mitochondria from fetal rats exposed to methyl mercury *in utero*[16] disclosed a decrease in the volume density which was associated with a concommitant decrease in the incorporation of ^{14}C leucine into mitochondrial structural membrane proteins and a corresponding inhibition of respiratory function and membranal marker enzyme activities. Prolonged oral exposure of rats to arsenate[17-22] has been found to increase the overall volume density of hepatocyte mitochondria and the surface density of the inner mitochondrial membrane. These physical effects were associated with depression of NAD-linked substrate respiration, conformational behavior and decreased respiratory control leading to an increase in mitochondrial NAD levels. In addition, the mitochondrial membranal marker enzymes monoamine oxidase, cytochrome oxidase, and Mg^{+2}ATPase were also found to show increased specific activities. The above changes in biochemical function were also found to be associated with increased incorporation of ^{14}C leucine into mitochondrial membranal proteins. Other studies[23] using mice exposed to arsenate for prolonged periods showed similar biochemical perturbations but no measurable change in overall mitochondrial volume density. However, a mild dose-related increase in the nuclear volume density was evident suggesting a more general alteration of overall cellular metabolism. Alteration of the activities of δ-ALA synthetase and ferrochelatase which are key enzymes in the heme biosynthetic pathway localized in the inner mitochondrial membrane was also observed in both rats and mice used in these studies[22]. This disturbance of the heme pathway was found to be associated with markedly increased urinary levels of uroporphyrin and coproporphyrin.

The overall conclusion to be reached from the above studies is that useful correlations between *in situ* mitochondrial structure and biochemical dysfunction are possible particularly with respect to effects of agents or dietary conditions which damage the essential inner mitochondrial membrane and its attendant enzyme activities. Such correlative studies are also of value with respect to expanding interpretation of toxicological significance of urinary porphyrin excretion patterns from heme pathway enzymes localized in this organelle.

Peroxisomes

Correlative ultrastructural morphometric/biochemical studies of peroxisomes have been performed following administration of the peroxisome proliferator SaH 24-348 in rats[24]. These authors reported a 9-fold increase in the volume density of peroxisomes which resulted both from an increase in number and volume of these structures which was found to decrease rapidly following cessation of treatment. The peroxisomal marker enzymes catalase and carnitine acetyl transferase were found to closely follow the same pattern of increase followed by a decease thus providing a good functional correlate for the observed structural changes in this organelle system.

Kidney

Lysosomes

Combined ultrastructural morphometric/biochemical toxicology studies on the kidney have been primarily focused on mitochondria and lysosomes. Prolonged oral exposure to methyl mercury[25] has been found to increase the volume density of both lysosomes and mitochondria in renal proximal tubule cells of rats. Biochemical evaluation of lysosomes from the same groups of animals disclosed increased lysosomal acid phosphatase activity and decreased β-glucuronidase activity. Other studies[26] on renal lysosomes from rats exposed to inorganic mercury for prolonged time periods also showed decreased degradation of labeled proteins by these structures thus confirming the inhibitory effects of this element on the renal lysosome system. A point to be emphasized here is the strong need for measuring several biochemical correlates to morphometric analysis since not all organelle functions may be altered in the same direction or to the same extent.

Mitochondria

Replicate studies[27-28] using the same methyl mercury exposure regimen found to produce mitochondrial swelling and increased mitochondrial volume density were performed to assess mitochondrial function. Results indicated only mild changes in respiratory function and the marker enzymes monoamine oxidase, cytochrome oxidase, and malate dehydrogenase but a marked increased in the specific activity of δ-ALA synthetase and a decrease in that of ferrochelatase which was associated with an attendant porphyrinuria dominated by a 30 fold increase in coproporphyrin and lesser quantities of uroporphyrin. The striking porphyrin excretion patterns and attendant enzymatic changes occurred in the absence of changes in standard tests of renal function[28]. This finding is similar to that reported for elemental interaction studies[29-30] involving lead, cadmium and arsenic which used porphyrin excretion patterns as an index of toxicity in comparison with standard clinical chemistries thus indicating the potential value of porphyrinurias as preclinical indicators.

Concluding Statement

Major points to be derived from these studies are that quantitative *in vivo* changes in the structure of target organelles may be related to pronounced biochemical dysfunctions which may in turn be used to identify new preclinical indicators of toxicity based on an understanding of the mechanisms of the toxicity occurring prior to overt organ damage. Hopefully, expanded future use of this approach will permit a better understanding of the mechanisms by which toxicants at low dose levels exert deleterious effects on tissues and produce pathological changes which ultimately compromise organ function.

REFERENCES

1. Loud, A. V. *et al.* (1965) Lab. Invest. 14, 996-1008.
2. Loud, A. V. (1968) J. Cell. Biol. 37, 24-36.
3. Weibel, E. R. *et al.* (1966) J. Cell. Biol. 30, 23-38.
4. Weibel, E. R. *et al.* (1969) J. Cell. Biol. 42, 68-91.
5. Weibel, E. R. *et al.* (1969) Int. Rev. Cytol. 26, 235-302.
6. Weibel, E. R. and Bolender, R. P. (1973) in Principles and Techniques of Electron Microscopy. Vol. 3 (Hayat, M. A. ed.) Van Nostrand Reinhold Company, New York, pp. 237-296.
7. Bolender, R. P. *et al.* (1978) J. Cell. Biol. 77, 565-583.
8. Weibel, E. R. and Paumgartner, D. (1978) J. Cell. Biol. 77, 584-597.
9. Blouin, A. *et al.* (1977) J. Cell. Biol. 72, 441-455.
10. Staubli, W. *et al.* (1969) J. Cell. Biol. 42, 92-112.
11. Bolender, R. P. and Weibel, E. R. (1973) J. Cell. Biol. 56, 746-761.
12. Denk, H., Eckerstorfer, R. and Rohr, H. P. (1977) Exper. Molec. Pathol. 26, 193-203.
13. Wiener, J. *et al.* (1968) J. Cell. Biol. 37, 47-61.
14. Kimberg, D. V. *et al.* (1968) J. Cell. Biol. 37, 63-79.
15. Frigg, M. and Rohr, H. P. (1976) Exper. Molec. Pathol. 24, 236-243.
16. Fowler, B. A. and Woods, J. S. (1977) Lab. Invest. 36, 122-129.
17. Fowler, B. A. *et al.* (1977) Environ. Health Perspect. 19, 197-204.
18. Fowler, B. A. *et al.* (1979) Lab. Invest. (in press).
19. Schiller, C. M. *et al.* (1977) Environ. Health Perspect. 19, 205-207.
20. Schiller, C. M. *et al.* (1978) Chem. Biol. Interact. 22, 25-33.
21. Woods, J. S. and Fowler, B. A. (1977) Environ. Health Perspect. 19, 209-213.
22. Woods, J. S. and Fowler, B. A. (1978) Toxicol. Appl. Pharmacol. 43, 361-371.
23. Fowler, B. A. and Woods, J. S. (1979) Toxicol. Appl. Pharmacol. (in press).

24. Moody, D. E. and Reddy, J. K. (1976) J. Cell. Biol. 71, 768-780.
25. Fowler, B. A. *et al.* (1975) Lab. Invest. 32, 313-322.
26. Madsen, K. M. and Christensen, E. I. (1978) Lab. Invest. 38, 165-174.
27. Woods, J. S. and Fowler, B. A. (1977) J. Lab. Clin. Med. 90, 266-272.
28. Fowler, B. A. and Woods, J. S. (1977) Exper. Molec. Pathol. 27, 403-412.
29. Fowler, B. A. and Mahaffey, K. R. Environ. Health Perspect. 25, 87-90.
30. Mahaffey, K. R. and Fowler, B. A. (1977) Environ. Health Perspect 19, 165-171.

CHEMICAL STRUCTURE, METABOLIC PATHWAYS, AND TOXICITY

Chairman: Ronald C. Shank

© 1980 Elsevier/North-Holland Biomedical Press
The Scientific Basis of Toxicity Assessment
H. Witschi, editor.

CHEMICAL STRUCTURE, METABOLIC PATHWAYS AND TOXICITY: INTRODUCTION

RONALD C. SHANK

Department of Community and Environmental Medicine, University of California,
Irvine, California 92717

There is increasing pressure from government and the public on the toxicology community
to make frequent, scientifically justified, assessments of the toxicity of chemical contaminants in air, drinking water, food, drugs, cosmetics, and even clothing.   The toxicologist is asked to define the acute and chronic hazards which can result from exposure
to a large and wide variety of chemical agents and to estimate the risks that can be
ascribed to those exposures.   As more knowledge of the science of toxic injury to cells,
tissues, and organisms is obtained, such toxicity assessments can be made with greater
certainty.

Decades of study on the relationships between the structure and biological activity
of a chemical compound have led to greater understanding of mechanisms of toxic action.
These mechanisms must be known to understand why certain chemical structures are toxic
to a particular cell type, and such an understanding may eventually lead to predicting
toxic action based on chemical structure, rather than waiting for results from expensive
animal tests.   Use of structure-activity relationships can help decrease the number of
individual toxicity assessments being requested on thousands of compounds.

Although chemical structure may be the ultimate determinate in toxicity, metabolic
pathways, which can produce or destroy that critical structure, can have great impact
on whether toxic injury will ultimately occur; hundreds of examples exist which demonstrate that the extent to which a compound follows different metabolic pathways is critical
to the toxicity that the compound can bring to bear.   Aflatoxin B_1 itself appears to exert
little toxicity, and most of its several oxidation products seem to cause little direct
toxicity; the proximate metabolite, aflatoxin B_1 epoxide, however, appears to break
down to a highly toxic, mutagenic, and carcinogenic reactant.   Understanding the
relevance of individual pathways to toxicity can lead to studies comparing animal and
human metabolism to determine which test animals are most appropriate for extrapolation
to human risks.   Continued study on chemical structure, metabolism and toxicity promise
to add greatly to the scientific basis of toxicity assessment.

© 1980 Elsevier/North-Holland Biomedical Press
The Scientific Basis of Toxicity Assessment
H. Witschi, editor.

2,3,7,8-TETRACHLORODIBENZO-P-DIOXIN: STUDIES ON THE MECHANISM OF ACTION[+]

ALAN POLAND[‡] AND EDWARD GLOVER

McArdle Laboratory for Cancer Research, University of Wisconsin, Madison,
Wisconsin 53706

2,3,7,8-Tetrachlorodibenzo-p-dioxin (TCDD)[*], a trace contaminant formed
in the commercial synthesis of 2,4,5-trichlorophenol, and one of the most
potent small molecule toxins known, is the prototype of a series of halogenated
aromatic hydrocarbons that all a) produce similar patterns of toxicity, b) are
approximate isostereomers, and c) elicit common biochemical responses.

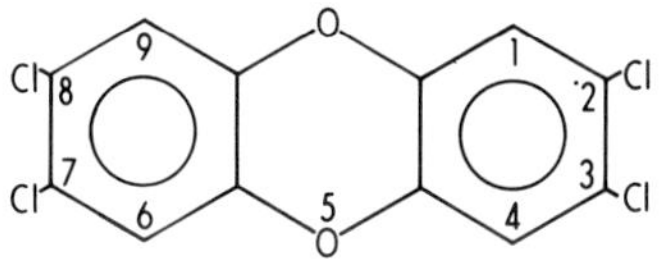

FIGURE 1 - 2,3,7,8 TETRACHLORODIBENZO-P-DIOXIN

TOXICOLOGY - The toxicology of TCDD and related halogenated aromatic hydrocarbons (chlorinated dibenzo-p-dioxins, dibenzofurans, azo- and azoxybenzenes and
biphenyls and brominated biphenyls) have been extensively reviewed elsewhere[1-8]
and the histopathologic responses are not the subject of this review. However
it is essential to briefly summarize the toxicity produced by TCDD, to
appreciate the necessity of resorting to the indirect approach to the
mechanism of toxicity presented in this report.

[+]Supported in part by National Institute of Environmental Health Sciences
Grant R01-ES0-01884, National Cancer Institute Program Project Grant
P01-CA-22484.

[‡]Recipient of Research Career Development Award K04-ES-0017.

[*]Abbreviations: TCDD - 2,3,7,8-tetrachlorodibenzo-p-dioxin; AHH - aryl hydrocarbon hydroxylase; MC - 3-methylcholanthrene; ALAS - δ-aminolevulinic acid
synthetase; ED_{50} - dose which produces one half the maximal response, in
this case induction of hepatic AHH activity; K_D - equilibrium dissociation
constant for binding; TCAB - 3,4,3',4'-tetrachloroazobenzene; TCAOB -
3,4,3',4'-tetrachloroazoxybenzene.

Species differ both quantitatively and qualitatively in their response
to TCDD and its congeners 1) Lethality. The cause of death remains unknown.
Following the administration of a toxic dose of TCDD, animals show a slow
wasting syndrome, with a latent period before death which is species specific.
There is an order of species sensitivity to TCDD and related compounds, with
guinea pigs and chickens being very sensitive, rats intermediate, and mice
being more resistant. 2) Chloracne and hyperkeratosis. This is the most
common and characteristic sign of toxicity observed in humans. Hyperkeratosis
has been reported in rabbits, monkeys and hairless mice. 3) Liver - Hepatocellular necrosis has been reported in rats and rabbits and focal lesions in
mice, but little or no hepatic damage is seen in guinea pigs. Several species
develop disturbances of hepatic porphyrin metabolism. 4) Teratogenicity,
embryotoxicity and fetal wastage. TCDD is a potent embryotoxin and teratogen
in mice, rats, and chicken embryos. 5) Chick edema. Edema, especially hydro-
pericardium, is a characteristic lesion in young chickens. Edema is also seen
in mice. 6) Involution of lymphoid organs. These compound characteristically
produce thymic atrophy and to a lesser degree atrophy of the lymph nodes and
spleen in most species which is accompanied by suppression of the cellular
immune response in young animals.

The early work of Schwetz et al.[9] and the more recent report of McConnell
et al.[10] indicate that each of the chlorinated dibenzo-p-dioxins which is toxic,
will elicit all the responses produced by TCDD, if administered in a sufficient
dose. The data on halogenated dibenzofuran, azo- and azoxybenzene and biphenyl
congeners are more limited, but also suggest that those congeners isosteric
with TCDD, produce the same toxic syndrome.

In spite of the wide spectrum and distinctiveness of the histopathology
produced by TCDD, studies on the mechanism of toxicity have been largely
unrewarded. This is attributable to several factors: 1) The cause of death,
the ultimate "target organ" is unknown, making it difficult to know which
tissue to focus on. 2) If one studies a particular toxic effect (e.g. chloracne, liver damage, chick edema) as a model, the response is often confined
to a particular species; 3) There have been few reports of toxic responses
which are dose-related, easily measured and quantifiable; 4) To date there has
been no report of TCDD toxicity on any cell type in culture, which limits in
vitro studies. 5) Studies on the pharmacokinetics and metabolism of TCDD
have provided little evidence of any reactive metabolite formation or covalent
binding.

We have pursued an indirect approach to the mechanism of toxicity, by examining the biochemical effects produced by TCDD, and then asking how these effects are related to toxicity.

ENZYME INDUCTION - TCDD stimulates the activities of a number of enzymes, the most well studied of these being the hepatic microsomal monooxygenases. Monooxygenase induction by TCDD a) occurs in many itssues and in most species, b) is an extremely sensitive measure of chlorinated aromatic hydrocarbon exposure, and c) gives an easily measured dose-response relationship.

The microsomal monooxygenase system is an enzyme complex embedded in the endoplasmic reticulum consisting of NADPH-cytochrome P-450 reductase and cytochrome P-450, which metabolizes most lipophilic compounds to more polar metabolites. In rat liver several distinct types of cytochrome P-450 have been identified, which differ in the spectrum of substrates they catalyze and which are differentially induced by the administration of various compounds. Aryl hydrocarbon hydroxylase (AHH) activity (measured as the rate of formation of the 3-hydroxy metabolite of benzo[a]pyrene) is a measure of one or two of these cytochrome P-450 species, so called cytochrome P_1-450, induced by TCDD. The studies presented are confined to hepatic AHH activity, but it should be remembered, this enzyme activity is induced in a number of tissues.

INDUCTION OF HEPATIC AHH ACTIVITY IN THE CHICK EMBRYO - The administration of TCDD to chicken embryos produces a dose-related increase in hepatic AHH activity measured in vitro 24 hours later. TCDD produces a 10 to 12 fold increase in AHH activity; the dose which produces one half the maximal induction (ED_{50}) is approximately 3 ng/egg (0.2 to 0.3 nmol/kg). Initially we tested a series of 15 halogenated dibenzo-p-dioxins for their potency to induce AHH activity[11]. The five congeners which induced AHH activity had two common properties: 1) halogen atoms occupied at least three, and for maximal potency, four of the lateral ring positions (positions 2,3,7 and 8) and 2) at least one ring position is nonhalogenated. (The octachlorodibenzo-p-dioxin is inactive, but both heptachloro- analogues are active). The same 15 congeners were tested in the chicken embryo for their capacity to induce hepatic δ-aminolevulinic acid synthetase (ALAS) activity, the initial and rate-limiting enzyme in heme synthesis and an identical structure-activity relationship was observed. A much larger series of halogenated dibenzo-p-dioxins and dibenzofurans have been subsequently examined for their potency to induce AHH activity in the chick embryo liver[12,13] and in a rat hepatoma cell culture[14] and confirmed the above findings.

The most important observation has been that for chlorinated dibenzo-p-dioxins there is an excellent correlation between their potency to induce AHH activity (and ALAS activity) and their toxic potency. The major question to be addressed is: How do we explain this correlation?

GENETIC EXPRESSION OF AHH ACTIVITY IN INBRED STRAINS OF MICE

The classical inducers of AHH activity and cytochrome P_1-450 are the polycyclic aromatic hydrocarbons, such as 3-methylcholanthrene (MC). In a comparison of MC and TCDD for their capacity to induce hepatic AHH activity in the rat, we found MC and TCDD produce parallel dose-response curves, both compounds produce the same maximum response, simultaneous administration of maximally inducing doses of MC and TCDD produces no greater response than that evoked by either drug alone. However, TCDD is 30,000 times as potent as MC, and a single administration produces sustained enzyme induction which lasts over 35 days[15], a reflection of the long biological half-life of the compound[16].

When randomly bred or certain inbred strains of mice are administered MC, they respond with the induction of hepatic AHH activity; certain other inbred strains when challenged with MC fail to respond[17,18]. The prototypical strain responsive to MC is C57BL/6J and prototypical non-responsive strain is DBA/2J. In crosses and backcrosses between C57BL/6J and DBA/2J mice, the trait of responsiveness to aromatic hydrocarbons is inherited in a simple autosomal dominant mode and the genetic locus controlling this trait is called the Ah locus.

The extraordinary potency of TCDD relative to MC prompted us to examine its effects in inbred strains which are responsive and non-responsive to MC. TCDD induced AHH activity in all strains tested regardless of their response to MC[19]. In C57BL/6J mice the enzyme activity and the spectral properties of the cytochrome P_1-450 that were induced by MC or TCDD, or both compunds administered together were found to be similar to those induced in DBA/2J mice by TCDD. These results suggest that the same gene product(s) is induced in C57BL/6J mice by both compounds and in DBA/2J mice by TCDD.

Thus, mice which are nonresponsive to MC, do respond to a more potent stimulus, TCDD, and therefore these mice do have the structural and regulatory genes necessary for the expression of AHH activity. The failure of these mice to respond to MC suggests that they fail to recognize MC as a signal for induction. We postulated that the mutation in nonresponsive mice results in a defective recognition or receptor site for AHH induction, a receptor which has a diminished (or absent) affinity for MC. Consider the hypothesis that TCDD acts at the same receptor as MC, but because of its greater potency, and hence its presumed greater affinity, it is able to saturate this receptor even in nonresponsive mice, and initiate the induction of AHH activity. This hypothesis predicts inbred mice which are nonresponsive to MC, should respond to TCDD, but should be uniformly less sensitive to TCDD, than strains which are responsive to MC.

We administered various doses of TCDD to six inbred strains of mice and 24 hours later measured their hepatic AHH activity[20]. The data are presented in Fig. 2 as the log of the dose versus the fractional response (control activity = 0, maximal activity = 1.0). The three inbred stains which are nonresponsive to MC (DBA/2J, AKR/J, and SJL/J) are less sensitive to TCDD, than are the responsive strains (C57BL/6J, BALB/cJ and A/J) i.e., the log-dose response curves for the nonresponsive strains are shifted to the right. The ED_{50} for AHH induction in responsive strains is approximately $\sim$1 nmole/kg, and for nonresponsive strains the ED_{50} is $\geq$ 10 nmoles/kg. The data support the hypothesis that TCDD and MC act on the same receptor, and that the mutation in nonresponsive strains is due to a receptor with a diminished affinity for inducing compounds.

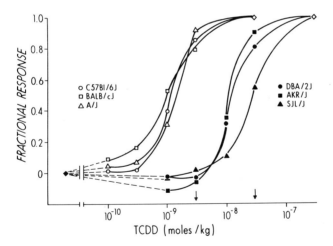

Fig. 2. Log dose-response curves for the induction of hepatic AHH activity by TCDD in six inbred strains of mice. The mice were injected intraperitoneally with varying doses of TCDD dissolved in p-dioxane; 24 hours later the animals were killed and their livers were assayed for AHH activity. The data are expressed as fractional responses to eliminate strain differences in basal and maximally induced enzyme activities (see text). Each point represents the average of four or five animals.

CYTOSOLIC BINDING SPECIES

We next wished to search for a macromolecular species which had the in vitro binding properties one would predict for the hypothesized receptor based on the in vivo biology. Specifically, one would expect such a moiety to have the following in vitro binding properties: 1) reversibly bind TCDD with a high affinity and the binding affinity (K_D) should correspond to the in vivo potency (ED_{50}) for AHH induction; 2) the binding species from mice which are nonresponsive should have a lower affinity for TCDD than the binding species from responsive mice; 3) the rank order of binding affinities of other halogenated dibenzo-p-dioxins, and other chlorinated aromatic hydrocarbons should correspond to their rank order of potencies to induce AHH activity, and 4) other compounds, such as the polycyclic aromatic hydrocarbons, which induce AHH activity, should bind to this moiety.

An initial series of experiments, suggested that there was a moiety which bound ^{3}H-TCDD with a high affinity in the liver cytosol (105,000 xg supernatant fraction).

The binding of ^{3}H-TCDD (specific activity 52.5 Ci/mmole) to liver cytosol was measured by the charcoal-dextran binding assay (for details see reference 13). When hepatic cytosol from C57BL/6J mice was incubated with varying concentrations of ^{3}H-TCDD and ^{3}H-TCDD plus a 200-fold excess of unlabeled 2,3,7,8-tetrachlorodibenzofuran, we observed a small pool of high affinity sites (Fig. 3A) (5). In Fig. 3B the same data for specific binding (displacable, high affinity binding) is presented in a Scatchard plot. The binding affinity for TCDD, K_D, is 0.27 nM which compares quite favorably with the in vivo potency for AHH induction in C57BL/6J mice (ED_{50} = 1 nmole/kg).

The specific binding of ^{3}H-TCDD to liver cytosol from C57BL/6J mice was greater at all concentrations of the radioligand, than was the specific binding to liver cytosol from DBA/2J mice. Unfortunately, the limited aqueous solubility of ^{3}H-TCDD prevents us from achieving a sufficient concentration to saturate the cytosol binding species from nonresponsive mice and estimating the K_D.

Another expectation of the cytosol binding species if it is the receptor, is that the in vitro binding affinity of halogenated dibenzo-p-dioxin congeners should correspond to their in vivo potency to induce AHH activity. The binding affinities of these unlabeled congeners are measured by their capacity to compete with the specific binding of ^{3}H-TCDD, to mouse liver cytocol and the results in Fig. 4 are expressed relative to the binding affinity of TCDD (TCDD = 100). The biological potencies of these congeners to induce hepatic

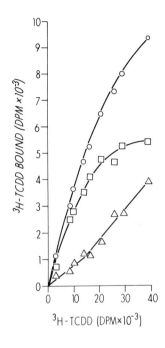
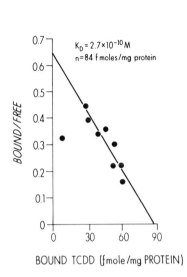

Fig. 3. A) Total, nonspecific and specific binding of (³H)-TCDD to hepatic cytosol from C57BL/6J mice. The cytosolic fraction of liver from C57BL/6J mice at 2 mg protein/ml in buffer was incubated with varying concentrations of (³H)-TCDD and (³H)-TCDD plus a 200 fold excess of 2,3,7,8-tetrachlorodibenzofuran for 2 hours at 0°. Samples were treated with a suspension of charcoal-dextran to remove unbound ligand, and the radioactivity quantified. Total binding - (³H)-TCDD alone (o); nonspecific or nondisplaceable binding - [³H]TCDD plus 2,3,7,8-tetrachlorodibenzofuran (△); specific or displaceable binding (□). B) Scatchard plot of the specific binding in A.

AHH in the chicken embryo (ED_{50}) are also expressed relative to TCDD. As seen in Figure 4, there is a very good correspondence between the rank order of binding affinity and biological potency for these compounds.

We have observed that other compounds which induce AHH activity, such as MC, benzo[a]pyrene and β-naphthoflavone, compete for specific cytosol binding sites, but drugs which induce other types of microsomal monooxygenase activities (e.g. phenobarbital, p,p'-DDT, pregnenolone-16-carbonitrile) and the steroid hormones and their analogues which have liver cytosol binding proteins -- all fail to compete with ³H-TCDD for specific cytosol binding sites.

The cytosolic binding species has all the properties predicted for the induction receptor, most notably, stereospecific recognition of inducing

Structure	RELATIVE BINDING AFFINITY	RELATIVE BIOLOGICAL POTENCY	Structure	RELATIVE BINDING AFFINITY	RELATIVE BIOLOGICAL POTENCY
(dibenzo-p-dioxin congener)	$100^{\dagger}$	$100^{\dagger\dagger}$	(dibenzo-p-dioxin congener)	inactive $(5.4 \times 10^{-7})*$	inactive $(9.4 \times 10^{-8})**$
(dibenzo-p-dioxin congener, C≡N)	167	100	(dibenzo-p-dioxin congener)	inactive (2.7×10^{-8})	inactive (9.4×10^{-8})
(dibenzo-p-dioxin congener, Br)	43	43	(dibenzo-p-dioxin congener)	inactive (5.4×10^{-8})	inactive (9.4×10^{-8})
(dibenzo-p-dioxin congener)	20	22	(dibenzo-p-dioxin congener)	inactive (5.4×10^{-8})	inactive (4.7×10^{-7})
(dibenzo-p-dioxin congener)	16	8	(dibenzo-p-dioxin congener)	inactive (5.4×10^{-8})	inactive (9.4×10^{-8})
(dibenzo-p-dioxin congener, CH_2NH_2)	13	3	(dibenzo-p-dioxin congener)	inactive (2.7×10^{-8})	inactive (9.4×10^{-8})
(dibenzo-p-dioxin congener)	14	0.06	(dibenzo-p-dioxin congener)	inactive (1.1×10^{-8})	inactive (9.4×10^{-8})

Fig. 4. The cytosol binding affinities and biological potencies of dibenzo-p-dioxin congeners relative to TCDD. The binding affinities of the dibenzo-p-dioxin congeners for hepatic cytosol were estimated by the capacity of these compounds to compete with (^{3}H)-TCDD for specific binding sites in C57BL/6J liver cytosol. The binding affinities are expressed relative to TCDD which is assigned a value of 100. For inactive analogues, the highest concentration tested that was judged to be soluble is given in parentheses.

The biological potency (ED_{50}) of each congener was the dose that produced one half the maximal induction of hepatic AHH activity in the chicken embryo, and the potency was expressed relative to TCDD (TCDD=100). For inactive compounds, the highest dose tested (in moles/kg) is given in parentheses. This assumes the weight of an average chicken egg is approximately 50 g.

    a - The absolute value of the K_D for TCDD is 0.27 nM.
    b - The absolute value of the ED_{50} for TCDD induction of hepatic
        AHH activity in the chicken embryo is 0.31 nmoles/kg.
    c - The highest concentration tested that was judged soluble in
        moles/liter.
    d - The highest concentration tested in moles/kg.

compounds. Recent experiments both _in vitro_ and _in vivo_, indicate the cytosol binding species mediates the specific uptake and binding of ^{3}H-TCDD to hepatic nuclei, and the experiments suggest that the ligand-receptor complex in the cytosol translocates to the nucleus[*]. The Ah locus, which determines the trait of responsiveness or nonresponsiveness to polycyclic aromatic hydrocarbons (or greater or lesser sensitivity to TCDD, appears to be structural gene locus for the cytosolic receptor protein. (The biochemical and genetic evidence all suggests, but does not prove this). The mutation in nonresponsive mice appears to result in an altered receptor with a diminished affinity for the inducing compound.[**]

COORDINATE GENE EXPRESSION

The administration of MC or TCDD to laboratory animals stimulates not only AHH activity, but a number of other hepatic enzyme activities. There is evidence for several of these enzymes, that this increase in activity represents true induction, i.e. de novo protein synthesis. MC and TCDD have been shown to induce the following hepatic enzymes: δ-aminolevulinic acid synthetase, UDP-glucuronosyl transferase, glutathione-$\underline{S}$-transferase B, aldehyde dehydrogenase, DT-diaphorase, and ornithine decarboxylase. The induction of several of these enzymes activities have been shown to segregate with the Ah locus in inbred strains of mice, (for a more detailed discussion see ref. 21). It would appear that the Ah locus controls not only the expression of AHH activity, but also the coordinate expression (and perhaps repression) of a number of other enzymes (Fig. 5).

STRUCTURE-ACTIVITY RELATIONSHIP

Considering other classes of halogenated aromatic compounds, we wish to know: 1) if one can generalize about the structure necessary to bind to the cytosol receptor; and 2) whether there is correlation between the potency of congeners to induce AHH activity -- and their toxic potency. Dibenzofurans the structure-activity relationship for the chlorinated dibenzofurans is very similar to that of the dibenzo-p-dioxins for binding to the cytosol receptor and inducing AHH activity with the 2,3,7,8-tetrachloro-analogue being the

[*]Greenlee, W. F. and A. Poland, manuscript submitted.

[**]In this report, we refer to the phenotypes of the Ah locus using the original terminology: responsive or nonresponsive to polycyclic aromatic hydrocarbons with the induction or failure of induction of hepatic AHH activity. Both phenotypes respond to TCDD with induction of hepatic AHH activity and differ only in their sensitivity (responsive mice, ED_{50} = 1 nmole TCDD/kg, "nonresponsive" mice $ED_{50} \geq 10$ nmoles TCDD/kg). Thus, when the nonresponsive phenotype is referred to, it is nonresponsive to MC and relatively less sensitive to TCDD.

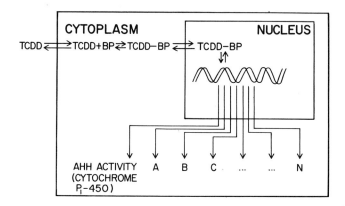

Fig. 5. Schematic representation of the model proposed for the pleiotropic response mediated by the TCDD-receptor complex. BP is the TCDD-binding protein or receptor.

most active. Only this congener has been tested for toxicity, and it was found to produce chloracne and edema in chickens[22].

Azo and Azoxybenzene

3,4,3',4'-Tetrachloroazobenzene (TCAB) and 3,4,3',4'-tetrachloroazoxybenzene (TCAOB) have been reported as contaminants of 3,4-dichloroaniline or herbicides made from 3,4-dichloroaniline and are thought to be responsible for several episodes of chloracne in factory workers[23,24]. TCAOB, TCAB, and 3,4,3',4'-tetrachlorohydrazobenzene are all approximate stereoisomers of TCDD, all bind with a high affinity to the cytosolic binding species, and are all potent inducers of hepatic AHH in the chicken embryo. Congeners such as 3,5,3',5'-tetrachloroazo-, 3,5,3',5'-tetrachloroazoxy-, and 3,5,3',5'-tetrachlorohydrazobenzene, azobenzene or azoxybenzene are inactive as inducers or competitive ligands. TCAOB produced acne in hairless mice, but 3,5,3',5'-tetrachloroazoxygenzene did not.

Halogenated Biphenyls

Of a series of 16 chlorinated and brominated biphenyl congeners, only three (3,4,3',4'-tetrachloro, 3,4,5,3',4',5'-hexachloro-, and 3,4,5,3',4',5'-hexabromo-) induced hepatic AHH activity and competed for the cytosolic binding species[25]. The structural requirements necessary for induction of AHH activity were 1) halogen atoms in at least two adjacent lateral positions on each benzene ring (3,4,3',4' or 3,4,5,3',4',5'); and 2) the lack of halogen substi-

tutions adjacent to the biphenyl bridge (the 2,6,2' or 6' positions) - such
substituions lead to marked nonplanarity. A more extensive investigation of
microsomal monooxygenase induction by chlorinated biphenyl congeners by
Goldstein et al.[26] supports these conclusions. There are a limited number
of investigations on the toxicity of chlorinated biphenyl congeners, but one
report by McKinney et al.[22] is particularly interesting. The authors compared
the toxicity of 5 symmetrical hexachlorobiphenyl congeners in chickens. The
3,4,5,3',4',5'-hexachloro-congener had the greatest toxic potency, and was
the only one to produce thymic atrophy and edema in the chickens, toxic
responses characteristic of the TCDD-syndrome.

We can generalize about the structure-activity relationship of each of
these classes of halogenated aromatic hydrocarbon. Consider a prototype of
each class - TCDD, 2,3,7,8-tetrachlorodibenzofuran, 3,4,3',4'-tetrachloroazo-
xybenzene, and 3,4,3',4'-tetrachlorobiphenyl - depicted in Fig. 6. These
compounds are all approximate stereoisomers and their molecular structures can
be thought of as roughly fitting into a rectangle 3 x 10A with halogen atoms
in the four corners. Planarity or near planarity seems to be essential. In
Figure 6 the in vitro binding affinity for the cytosol binding species and
the potency to induce AHH activity in the chick for each of these compounds,
and for a number of other tetrahalogenated aromatic compound which are approximate stereoisomers, are compared. The toxicity of these latter compounds has
not been tested.

While many points remain to be answered about the chemical features recognized by the receptor, the planar rectangular site depicted in Fig. 6 seems a
good first approximation.

A MODEL FOR THE MECHANISM OF TOXICITY

We have emphasized for chlorinated aromatic hydrocarbon congeners, the
correlation between their potency to induce AHH activity and their toxic
potency. It is difficult to envision how the induction of AHH activity, per
se, is involved in specific organ toxicities such as chloracne or thymic
involution. Therefore, we wish to focus on the receptor - the correlation
between the affinity of congener for the receptor and their toxic potencies.

*We postulate that the toxicity of these chlorinated aromatic hydrocarbons
in mediated through the receptor, that is, the initial event in their toxic
action is the stereospecific recognition and binding to the cytosolic binding
species. It is suggested that the ligand-receptor complex controls a battery
of genes, and the expression (or repression) of one or more of these genes
which are coordinately expressed results in the observed toxic syndrome.*

	Induction of AHH Act. (chick) ED_{50} (nmoles/kg)	Binding Liver Affinity Mouse Liver Cytosol K_D (nm)		Induction of AHH Act. (chick) ED_{50} (nmoles/kg)	Binding Liver Affinity Mouse Liver Cytosol K_D (nm)
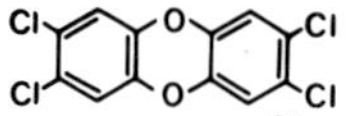	0.31	0.27	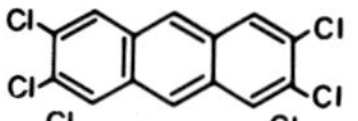	8.9	1.4
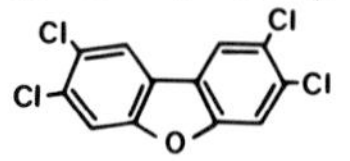	0.46	0.73	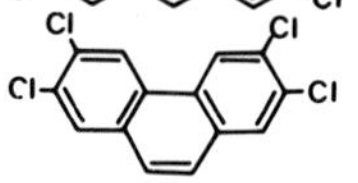	102	3.2
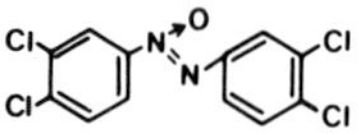	0.45	0.93	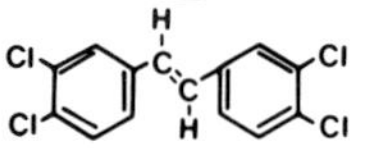	12.6	2.4
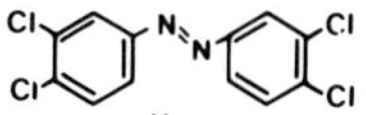	2.0	1.1	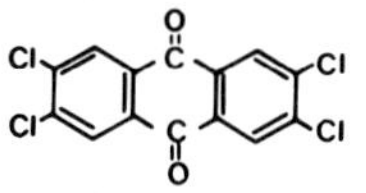	640	>225
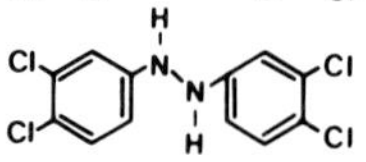	2.9	1.2	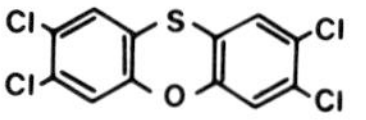	1.6	0.71
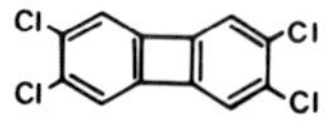	0.28	0.34	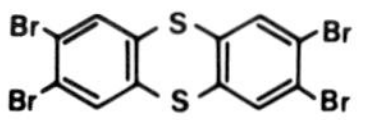	13.2	5.0
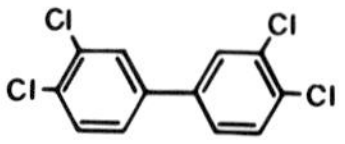	88	15	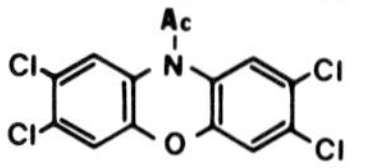	0.3	0.74

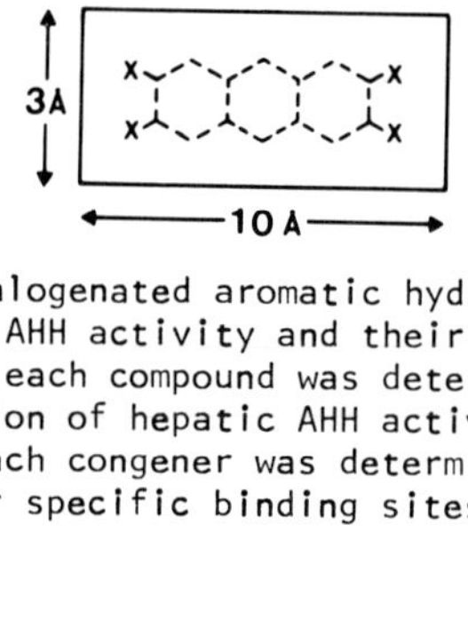

Fig. 6. Isosteric tetrahalogenated aromatic hydrocarbons: Comparison of their potencies to induce AHH activity and their cytosolic binding affinities. The biological potency of each compound was determined from the log dose-response curve for induction of hepatic AHH activity in the chicken embryo. The binding affinity of each congener was determined by its capacity to compete with (^{3}H)-TCDD for specific binding sites in liver cytosol from C57BL/6J mice.

One prediction from this model is immediately obvious. The genetic evidence suggests that the Ah locus determines the receptor protein and its binding affinity. Thus, if the toxicity of TCDD (and related halogenated aromatic compounds) is mediated through the receptor, then inbred strains of mice with a high affinity receptor (and which are sensitive to induction of AHH activity by TCDD) should be sensitive to toxicity from TCDD, and mice with a lower affinity receptor should be less sensitive to the toxicity of TCDD. In short, the toxicity of TCDD should segregate with the Ah locus.

To examine this, we chose the involution of the thymus because 1) we feel this is a "toxic response" - (not just a biochemical response) in that it represents tissue loss and in young animals it is associated with suppression of cellular immunity, and 2) thymic atrophy is dose-related and quantifiable.

C57BL/6J, DBA/2J, and hybrid B6D2F$_1$/J male mice, were given a single intraperitoneal injection of varying dose of TCDD[+]. Six days later the animals were killed, their thymuses dissected out and weighed, and the data expressed as the thymic/body weight ratio (Fig. 7A). TCDD produced a dose related decrease in the ratio of thymus/body weight. The responsive C57BL/6J mice were more sensitive than the nonresponsive DBA/2J mice, and the hybrid mice were intermediate. We than bred B6D2F$_1$/J mice (heterozygous at the Ah locus, Aa) with DBA/2J mice (homozygous nonresponsive, aa) and the resultant offspring were phenotyped as heterozygous responsive (Aa) or homozygous nonresponsive (aa). The animals were dosed with TCDD as above, killed six days later, and their thymus/body weight ratio determined (Fig. 7B). Since sex influences the thymus/body weight ratio in control mice, data from males and females are presented separately. As seen in Fig. 7B, for both males and females, heterozygous responsive mice (Aa) are more sensitive to TCDD, than are homozygous nonresponsive (aa) mice. The data indicate that thymic involution by TCDD segregates with the Ah locus.

Preliminary experiments in inbred strains of mice, suggest that sensitivity to the teratogenic effects of TCDD (cleft palate formation) is determined by the Ah locus, i.e. the responsive strains, those with a high affinity receptor have a greater incidence of fetuses with cleft plates at a given dose of TCDD.

We have reviewed two lines of evidence which suggest that toxicity of TCDD and related halogenated aromatic compounds is mediated by their stereospecific binding to the receptor for AHH induction: 1) the correlation between the binding affinities of these compounds for the cytosolic receptor and their toxic potencies; and 2) for TCDD, the segregation of thymic involution, with the Ah locus. Since the Ah locus controls not only the expression of AHH activity, but several (perhaps many) other genes, it is tempting to postulate that TCDD exerts its toxicity through the expression (or repression) of one or more of the genes controlled by the receptor. However, the genetic evidence only permits us to state that toxicity (thymic involution, and probably cleft palate formation) segregates with the Ah locus.

We do not understand why nonhalogenated compounds, which bind to the induction receptor, such as polycyclic aromatic hydrocarbons and ß-naphthoflavone, do not produce the spectrum of toxic responses characteristic of the chlorinated

[+]Poland, A. and E. Glover, unpublished data.

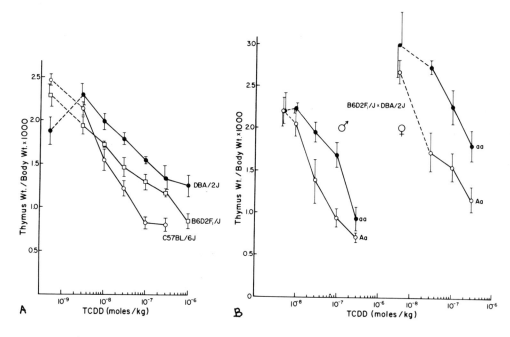

Fig. 7. A) Log dose-response curves for the effect of TCDD on the ratio of thymus/body weight in C57BL/6J, DBA/2J and B6D2F$_1$/J mice. Five week old male mice were given a single intraperitoneal injection of TCDD dissolved in p-dioxane or the solvent alone. Six days later the animals were killed, their thymuses weighed, and the data expressed as the ratio of the thymus/body weight. Each point is the mean ± S.E. of 5 to 8 animals. The solvent injected (control) groups are connected by dashed lines to the rest of the dose-response curves. B) Log dose-response curve of TCDD on thymus/body weight ratio in male and female offspring of the B6D2F$_1$/J x DBA/2J cross. The offspring of the B6D2F$_1$/J x DBA/2J cross were phenotyped as heterozygous responsive - Aa, or homozygous, nonresponsive - aa, at the Ah locus. At five and one half weeks of age the animals were dosed with TCDD as above and killed six days later. The data on males and females are presented separately, because the sex of the mice affected the ratio of thymus/body weight in the solvent injected control groups. Each point is the mean ± S.E. of 4 to 8 animals. The solvent injected (control) groups are connected by dashed lines to the rest of the dose-response curves.

aromatic hydrocarbons. It is possible that toxicity is related to the sustained occupation of the receptor and the relatively long biological half-lives of the halogenated aromatic compounds versus the rapidly metabolized polycyclic aromatic hydrocarbons accounts for the difference.

The model gives no clue to the ultimate biochemical lesions responsible for the toxicity of these compounds, but merely states that toxicity is mediated through binding to the receptor. For a tissue or cell type to develop a toxic response to chlorinated aromatic hydrocarbons the presence of the receptor is essential, but may not be sufficient.

MUTAGENICITY AND CARCINOGENICITY

Recently, several groups have found TCDD to be a potent carcinogen in chronic feeding studies[27-29]. Kociba et al.[27] is a very thorough study maintained rats on diets supplying a daily dose of 0, 1, 10 and 100 ng/kg for two years. Female rats feed the highest concentration of TCDD developed a significant increase in hepatocellular carcinoma, stratified squamous cell carcinoma of the hard palate and nasal turbinate and keratinizing squamous cell carcinoma of the lung. At a dose of 100 ng/kg/day nearly one half the female rats developed one of these neoplasms, suggesting TCDD has a carcinogenic potency comparable to that of aflatoxin B_1, which at lifetime dose of 1 µg/kg/day has been estimated to produce a 50% incidence of hepatocellular carcinoma in the rat[30].

The carcinogenic potency of TCDD is surprising in light of 1) the lack of convincing evidence that TCDD is mutagenic in any in vitro bacterial test systems[31-33], and 2) failure to demonstrate significant covalent binding in vivo. We have recently examined the in vivo binding of ^{3}H-TCDD to rat liver macromolecular fractions. If one assumes unextracted radioactivity is equatable with covalently bound ^{3}H-TCDD, the maximum binding to DNA is 6 pmole of TCDD per mole of nucleotide, 4 to 6 orders of magnitude lower than that of most other chemical carcinogens[34], and equivalent to one molecule of TCDD bound to the DNA in every 35 diploid cells[+]. These results suggest that it is unlikely that the mechanism of oncogenesis is through covalent binding and somatic mutation.

The mechanism(s) by which TCDD produces toxicity and carcinogenicity are unknown. Understanding these processes is important because 1) TCDD is the prototype of a large series of the halogenated aromatic hydrocarbons, many of which are environmental contaminants, 2) the studies to date suggest this series of compounds acts by rather a unique mechanism(s).

ACKNOWLEDGEMENTS

We would like to thank Dr. Andrew Kende and his postdoctoral fellows. Drs. James Wade, Mark DeCamp and John Airey who synthesized all the compounds employed in this work. We also grateful acknowledge the contributions of Drs. Bill Greenlee and Joyce Knutson on the biological aspects of this work.

[+] Poland, A. and E. Glover, manuscript submitted.

REFERENCES

1. Symposium on Chlorinated Dibenzodioxins and Dibenzofurans (1973) Environ. Health Perspect., 5, 1-313.

2. Symposium on PCBs (1972) Environ. Health Perspect., 1, 1-185.

3. Workshop on the Scientific Aspects of Polybrominated Biphenyls (1978) Environ. Health Perspect., 23, 1-369.

4. International Agency for Research on Cancer (1977) IARC Monographs on the Evaluation of the Carcinogenic Risk of Chemicals to Man, 15, pp. 1-354.

5. Chlorodioxins - Origin and Fate, Advances in Chemistry Series, American Chemical Society, Washington, D.C., 120, pp. 1-141. ed. Blair, E.H. 1973.

6. Chlorinated Phenoxy Acids and Their Dioxins, Ecological Bulletins, Swedish Natural Science Research 27, 27, pp. 1-302. ed. C. Ramel.

7. Dioxin: Toxicological and Chemical Aspects, S.P. Medical and Scientific Books, pp. 1-222. 1978. ed. Cattabeni, F. et al.

8. Kimbrough, R. (1974) Crit. Rev. Toxicol., 2, 445-498.

9. Schwetz, B.A., Norris, J.M., Sparschu, G.L., Rowe, V.K., Gehring, P.J., Emerson, J.L. and Gerbig, C.G. (1973) Environ. Health Perspect., 5, 87-99.

10. McConnell, E.E., Moore, J.A., Haseman, J.K. and Harris, M.W. (1978) Toxicol. Appl. Pharmacol., 44, 335-356.

11. Poland, A. and Glover, E. (1973) Mol. Pharmacol., 9, 736-747.

12. Kende, A.S., Wade, J.J., Ridge, D. and Poland, A. (1974) J. Org. Chem., 39, 931-937.

13. Poland, A., Glover, E. and Kende, A.S. (1976) J. Biol. Chem., 251, 4936-4946.

14. Bradlaw, J.A., Garthoff, L.H., Hurley, N.E. and Firestone, D. (1976) Toxicol. Appl. Pharmacol., 37, 119.

15. Poland, A. and Glover, E. (1974) Mol. Pharmacol., 10, 349-359.

16. Rose, J.Q., Ramsey, J.C., Wentzler, T.H., Hummel, R.A. and Gehring, P.J. (1976) Toxicol. Appl. Pharmacol., 36, 209-226.

17. Nebert, D.W. and Gielen, J.E. (1972) Fed. Proc., 31, 1315-1325.

18. Thomas, P.E., Kouri, R.E. and Hutton, J.J. (1972) Biochem. Genet., 6, 157-168.

19. Poland, A., Glover, E., Robinson, J.R. and Nebert, D.W. (1974) J. Biol. Chem., 249, 5599-5606.

20. Poland, A. and Glover, E. (1975) Mol. Pharmacol., 11, 389-398.

21. Poland, A. and Kende, A. (1977) In: Origins of Human Cancer. Eds.: H.H. Hiatt, J.D. Watson and J.A. Winston, Cold Spring Harbor Laboratory, New York, B, pp. 447-467.

22. McKinney, J.D., Chae, K., Gupta, B.N., Moore, J.A. and Goldstein, J.A. (1976) Toxicol. Appl. Pharmacol., 36, 65-80.

23. Poland, A., Glover, E., Kende, A.S., DeCamp, M. and Giandomenico, C.M. (1976) Science, 194, 627-630.

24. Taylor, J.S., Wuthrich, R.C., Lloyd, K.M. and Poland, A. (1977) Arch. Dermatol., 113, 616-619.

25. Poland, A. and Glover, E. (1977) Mol. Pharmacol., 13, 924-938.

26. Goldstein, A., Hickman, P., Bergman, H., McKinney, J.D. and Walker, M.P. (1977) Chem.-Biol. Interactions, 17, 69-87.

27. Kociba, R.J., Keyes, P.G., Beyer, J.E., Carreon, R.M., Wade, C.E., Dittenber, D.A., Kalnins, R.P., Frauson, L.E., Park, C.N., Barnard, S.D., Hummel, R.A. and Humiston, C.G. (1978) Toxicol. Appl. Pharmacol., 46, 279-303.

28. Van Miller, J.P., Lalich, J.J. and Allen, J.R. (1977) Chemosphere, 6, 537-544.

29. Holmes, P.A., Rust, J.H., Richter, W.R. and Shefner, A.M. (1979) Ann. NY Acad. Sci., in press.

30. Wogan, G., Paglialunga, S. and Newberne, P. (1974) Food Cosmetic Toxicol., 12, 681-685.

31. Hussain, S., Ehrenberg, L., Löfröth, G. and Gejvall, T. (1972) Ambio, 1, 32-33.

32. Seiler, J.P. (1973) Experientia, 29, 622-623.

33. Wasson, J.S., Huff, J.E. and Loprieno, N. (1977/78) Mutat. Res., 47, 141-160.

34. Farber, E. (1968) Cancer Res., 28, 1859-1869.

© 1980 Elsevier/North-Holland Biomedical Press
The Scientific Basis of Toxicity Assessment
H. Witschi, editor.

METABOLISM AND MECHANISMS OF TOXICITY OF COMPOUNDS CONTAINING THIONO-SULFUR

ROBERT A. NEAL

Center in Environmental Toxicology, Department of Biochemistry, Vanderbilt University School of Medicine, Nashville, Tennessee 37232

A number of thiono-sulfur containing compounds which find use as pesticides, drugs and in industrial processes, exhibit toxic properties. Figure 1 is the general structure of thiono-sulfur compounds. The central atom (X) to which the sulfur is bound can be either carbon or phosphorus with the groups attached to the carbon and phosphorus (R_1, R_2) being either nitrogen, carbon or sulfur. Also in the case of pentavalent phosphorus containing thiono-sulfur compounds a third group (R_3) would be attached to the X group.

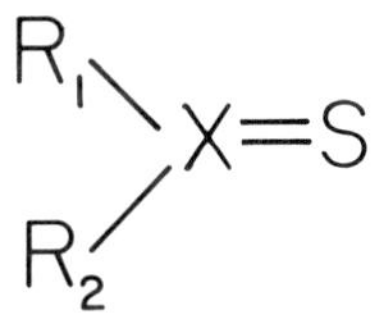

$$R_1, R_2 = \text{Nitrogen, Carbon, Sulfur}$$
$$X = \text{Carbon, Phosphorus}$$

Fig. 1. General structure for thiono-sulfur compounds.

Table 1 is a listing of the adverse biological effects seen on exposure of mammals to thiono-sulfur containing compounds. In our laboratory we have had under way for approximately 10 years studies of the mechanisms of the toxic effects of thiono-sulfur compounds with particular attention to the mechanism by which these compounds inhibit liver and lung monooxygenase enzymes and investigation of the mechanism by which some of these compounds cause liver damage. In the case of liver damage induced by thiono-sulfur containing compounds, the histopathology shows predominantly centrilobular hepatic necrosis.

When a wide variety of thiono-sulfur containing compounds are administered in vivo to rats followed by sacrifice 24 to 48 hours later a decrease in the activity of the hepatic cytochrome P-450 containing monooxygenases is seen as well as a decrease in the concentration of cytochrome P-450 in these hepatic microsomes[1]. If these thiono-sulfur

TABLE 1

BIOLOGICAL EFFECTS OF THIONO-SULFUR CONTAINING COMPOUNDS

---

1.   Inhibition of Thyroid Hormone Synthesis
2.   Carcinogenesis (liver, thyroid, lung, kidney, pituitary, ear duct)
3.   Blood Dyscrasis (leukopenia, agranulocytosis, thrombocytopenea)
4.   Liver Damage
5.   Lung Damage
6.   Teratogenesis
7.   Mutagenesis
8.   Inhibition of Liver and Lung Monooxygenase Enzymes
9.   Inhibition of Copper Containing Enzymes

---

compounds are incubated with hepatic microsomes, in the presence of NADPH, a decrease
in the levels of cytochrome P-450 in the microsomes is also observed. In addition there is
a decrease in the activity of the cytochrome P-450 containing monooxygenases towards
substrates such as benzphetamine (Table 2)[1]. However, if the incubation of the
microsomes with the thiono-sulfur compounds is carried out in the absence of NADPH, no
decrease in cytochrome P-450 or inhibition of monooxygenase activity is seen. When the

TABLE 2

EFFECT OF IN VITRO INCUBATION OF THIONO-SULFUR COMPOUNDS WITH HEPATIC
MICROSOMES FROM PHENOBARBITAL-PRETREATED RATS ON CYTOCHROME P-450
CONCENTRATION AND BENZPHETAMINE METABOLISM[1]

Thiono-Sulfur Compound	Cytochrome P-45 (nmoles/mg Protein		Benzphetamine Metabolism (nmoles/min/mg Protein)	
(1×10^{-3}M)	Plus NADPH	Minus NADPH	Plus NADPH	Minus NADPH
Ethylene Thiourea	1.39±0.17*	2.05±0.02	6.47±0.95*	12.42±1.44
Thiourea	1.16±0.00*	2.07±0.05	7.30±0.63*	13.30±0.58
Thioacetamide	1.87±0.32	2.06±0.11	12.12±0.33	13.32±0.62
Thiouracil	1.36±0.01*	2.12±0.13	4.53±7.39*	11.64±0.86
Propylthiouracil	1.35±0.04*	1.98±0.04	9.42±0.47*	12.23±0.17
Methimazole	1.15±0.12*	2.08±0.06	8.77±0.12*	13.32±1.43
Carbon Disulfide	0.71±0.02*	2.08±0.03	6.45±0.05*	13.09±0.68
Control	1.91±0.33	2.02±0.14	12.50±1.97	13.16±1.09

oxygen analogs of these thiono-sulfur compounds (i.e., uracil in place of thiouracil, urea in place of thiourea, ethylene urea in place of ethylene thiourea, etc.) are administered in vivo or incubated with hepatic microsomes in vitro in the presence of NADPH, no decrease in hepatic cytochrome P-450 or cytochrome P-450 containing monooxygenase activity is seen[1]. These data suggested to us that the ability of the thiono-sulfur coumpounds to inhibit cytochrome P-450 containing monooxygenase activity and to decrease the level of cytochrome P-450 detectable as its carbon monoxide complex, was a result of the action of some metabolite of these thiono-sulfur compounds on the cytochrome P-450 monooxygenase system.

We therefore carried out a series of studies the purpose of which was to examine the structure of metabolites of various thiono-sulfur compounds formed in reactions catalyzed by cytochrome P-450 monooxygenase systems. One of the major purposes of these studies was to identify metabolites which might be responsible for the inhibition of the cytochrome P-450 monooxygenases when these thiono-sulfur compounds were administered in vivo or incubated with the hepatic microsomes in vitro. One of the most extensively studied compounds was the phosphorothionate triester, parathion. Parathion is a widely used insecticide which, when incubated with hepatic microsomes in vitro, leads to an inhibition of cytochrome P-450 monooxygenase activity and to a decrease in levels of cytochrome P-450 analogous to that seen in Table 2[2]. What is known concerning the metabolism of parathion by the rat and other experimental animals is shown in Figure 2[3].

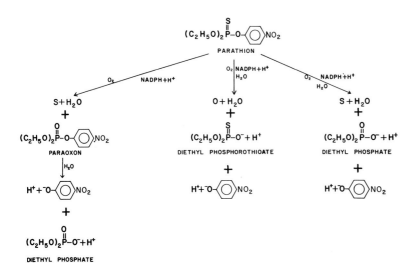

Fig. 2. General scheme for the metabolism of parathion by mammalian hepatic microsomes and reconstituted cytochrome P-450 containing monooxygenase systems[3].

There are five major products of parathion metabolism. One of these is the corresponding phosphate triester, paraoxon, which is formed in a cytochrome P-450 monooxygenase catalyzed reaction in which the sulfur atom of parathion is replaced by an oxygen atom[4]. The other product of this reaction is atomic sulfur[2,5]. The paraoxon is subject to hydrolysis by esterases present in various tissues to diethylphosphate and p-nitrophenol[6]. Parathion is also metabolized to diethyl phosphorothioic acid and p-nitrophenol in a reaction catalyzed by the cytochrome P-450 containing monooxygenases[7,8]. Diethyl phosphate plus p-nitrophenol and atomic sulfur can also be formed from parathion in a cytochrome P-450 monooxygenase catalyzed reaction[3].

Results of studies of the chemical mechanism of metabolism of parathion to paraoxon have led us to propose the sequence of reactions shown in Figure 3[3,5,9]. These studies have indicated that the initial reaction is a transfer of a singlet oxygen atom from the cytochrome P-450 molecule to one of the unshared electron pairs on the thiono-sulfur group of parathion. The resulting S-oxide can assume four resonance forms as shown in Figure 3. Data from these studies suggested that one of these resonance forms of the S-oxide cyclizes to a tricyclic phosphorus-sulfur-oxygen intermediate, a phosphooxathiiran, which can undergo electron rearrangement leading to the formation of paroxon, the predominant product of parathion metabolism by hepatic microsomes, with the other product being atomic sulfur. Atomic sulfur is a highly reactive species of sulfur and would

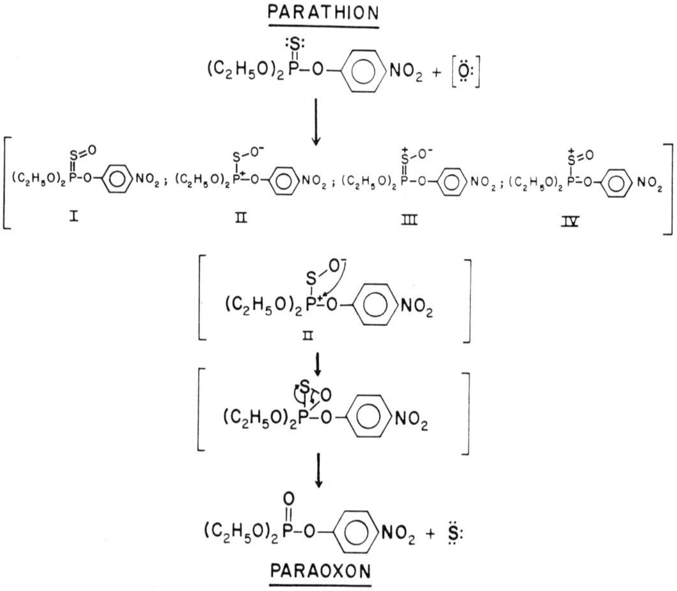

Fig. 3. Chemical mechanism for the metabolism of parathion to paraoxon by a mammalian cytochrome P-450 containing monooxygenase enzyme system[3].

be expected to readily react with nucleophilic groups on macromolecules surrounding the active site of the cytochrome P-450 or participate in carbon-hydrogen insertion reactions. Subsequent studies have indicated[2,10] that, in fact, the sulfur released in the cytochrome P-450 monooxygenase catalyzed metabolism of parathion and other thiono-sulfur containing compounds covalently binds to microsomal macromolecules[2] and to cytochrome P-450 itself[1]. Further studies have indicated that the inhibition of cytochrome P-450 monooxygenase activity and the loss of cytochrome P-450 detectable as its carbon monoxide complex which is seen on administration of thiono-sulfur compounds in vivo or on incubation with hepatic microsomes in vitro is the result of covalent binding of the atomic sulfur to cytochrome P-450[10]. Thus, thiono-sulfur containing compounds can be considered as suicide substrates for the cytochrome P-450 containing monooxygenases. In other words, in the process of the cytochrome P-450 monooxygenase catalyzed metabolism of the thiono-sulfur compounds atomic sulfur is released which covalently binds to cytochrome P-450 and inhibits the enzyme. Studies of the nature of the covalently bound sulfur have shown that 50-70% of the atomic sulfur has reacted with cysteine sulfhydryl groups on cytochrome P-450 forming a hydrodisulfide linkage (Figure 4)[10]. Further studies[11] have revealed that three additional amino acids on the cytochrome P-450 molecule have also reacted with the sulfur atom of parathion released in a cytochrome P-450 monooxygenase catalyzed reaction. It is not clear at this time whether binding of the sulfur atom to all four amino acids or a lesser number is responsible for the loss of cytochrome P-450 detectable as its carbon monoxide complex and to the loss of monooxygenase activity.

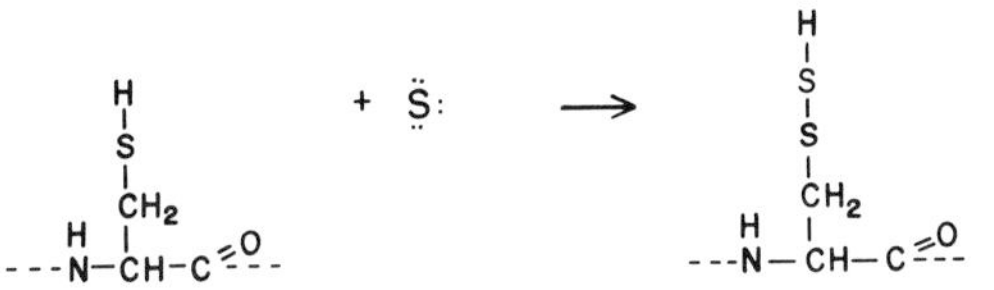

Fig. 4. Proposed mechanism for formation of a hydrodisulfide in a reaction between atomic sulfur and cysteine contained in cytochrome P-450.

One of the most extensively studied hepatonecrotic chemicals is the compound thioacetamide. Figure 5 shows what is currently known about the hepatic microsomal metabolism of thioacetamide[12,13,14]. These data indicate that thioacetamide undergoes a cytochrome P-450 monooxygenase catalyzed conversion to its S-oxide, thioacetamide S-oxide, which in contrast to the S-oxide of parathion (Figure 3) is stable and can be isolated. In a subsequent reaction the thioacetamide S-oxide is further metabolized to an intermediate which cannot be isolated but which we postulate to be the thioacetamide S-dioxide. This intermediate can react by a number of alternate reaction pathways; either

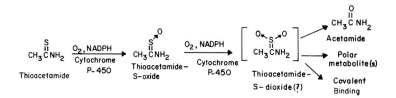

Fig. 5. Proposed metabolic scheme for the cytochrome P-450 containing monooxygenase catalyzed metabolism of thioacetamide.

conversion to acetamide, breakdown to unidentified polar products or covalently bind to liver macromolecules.

We postulate that the reactive intermediate, the intermediate responsible for the hepato-necrotic effects of thioacetamide, is thioacetamide S-dioxide. If this is the case, one would expect the thioacetamide S-oxide to be more toxic to the liver than thioacetamide since in the case of thioacetamide, two sequential reactions would be required to form the toxic intermediate, thioacetamide S-dioxide. Table 3 shows the results of an examination of the relative toxicity of thioacetamide S-oxide and thoacetamide to rat liver[14]. As can be seen, at equal doses of thioacetamide and thioacetamide S-oxide, the S-oxide causes a consistently greater degree of necrosis than thioacetamide. We also examined the time to the appearance of necrosis in rat liver, following administration of thioacetamide-S-oxide and thioacetamide. In the livers of rats given equal doses of thioacetamide and the S-oxide, an earlier onset of necrosis was seen

TABLE 3

HEPATIC NECROSIS PRODUCED IN RATS BY VARIOUS DOSES OF EITHER THIOACET-AMIDE OR THIOACETAMIDE-S-OXIDE

Compound	Dose (mmol/kg)	Extent of Necrosis
Thioacetamide	0.31	+
Thioacetamide-S-oxide	0.31	++
Thioacetamide	0.63	+++
Thioacetamide-S-oxide	0.63	++++
Thioacetamide	1.25	+++++
Thioacetamide-S-oxide	1.25	++++++

+ - single cell necrosis; ++ - single cell thickness of necrosis about central vein; +++ - 2 to 3 cell thickness of necrosis; ++++ - 5 to 6 cell thickness of necrosis; +++++ - 8 to 9 cell thickness of necrosis; ++++++ -> 10 cell thickness of necrosis about central vein.

in animals given thioacetamide S-oxide as compared to thioacetamide. In the case of thioacetamide isolated necrotic cells were detectable at approximately 12 hours following administration of thioacetamide whereas in the case of thioacetamide S-oxide, isolated necrotic cells were evident 6 to 7 hours following administration of this compound[14]. These studies also revealed that the onset of hepatic necrosis occurred at approximately three hours after maximum covalent binding of radioactivity had occurred in the liver.

We next examined the nature of the thioacetamide metabolites covalently bound to liver macromolecules. In these studies thioacetamide S-oxide labeled with tritium in the methyl group, with ^{14}C in the carbonyl group or with ^{35}S were administered to rats. Twelve hours later the animals were sacrificed, the livers removed and the amount of radioactivity covalently bound to the hepatic macromolecules was determined (Table 4). The amount of radioactivity bound to the hepatic macromolecules of the animals administered tritium-labeled thioacetamide S-oxide was nearly equal to the amount of radioactivity bound to the macromolecules in animals given the ^{14}C carbonyl-labeled thioacetamide S-oxide. However, negligible amounts of radioactivity were covalently bound to the liver macromolecules in the animals given ^{35}S-labeled thioacetamide S-oxide. These data indicate that the metabolite of thioacetamide covalently bound to the liver macromolecules contains the methyl group, the carbonyl carbon and perhaps the nitrogen. However, the sulfur group appears to have been displaced in the process of covalent binding.

TABLE 4

RADIOACTIVITY COVALENTLY BOUND TO LIVER MACROMOLECULES 12 HOURS FOLLOWING ADMINISTRATION OF LABELED THIOACETAMIDE-S-OXIDE

Compound	Radioactivity Bound μmol/gm liver
^{3}H(methyl)-Thioacetamide-S-Oxide	2.5 ± 0.3
1-^{14}C-Thioacetamide-S-Oxide	2.4 ± 0.2
^{35}S-Thioacetamide-S-Oxide	0.05 ± 0.0

These and other data suggest that the hepatic necrosis caused by thioacetamide is a result of the cytochrome P-450 catalyzed metabolism of thioacetamide first to thioacetamide S-oxide, which is further metabolized in a cytochrome P-450 monooxygenase catalyzed reaction to an intermediate which we believe to be the S-dioxide. The S-dioxide can break down to acetamide and unknown polar products or is subject to attack by nucleophiles on hepatic macromolecules leading to the covalent binding of the thioacetamide carbon chain. This hypothesis is supported by the fact that inhibitors of the cytochrome P-450 monooxygenases such as SKF 525-A, piperonylbutoxide and pyrazole either eliminate or markedly decrease the degree of necrosis seen on administration of thioacetamide or thioacetamide S-oxide to rats[12]. Shown in Figure 6A and B is the postulated mechanism for covalent binding of thioacetamide S-dioxide to liver macro-molecules. Shown in Figure 6A are the possible charged resonance forms of the thioacetamide S-oxide. An additional neutral form of the S-dioxide is not shown. We

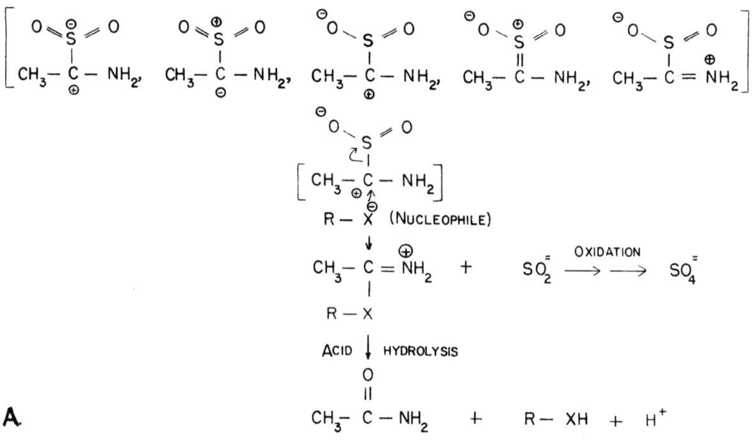

A.

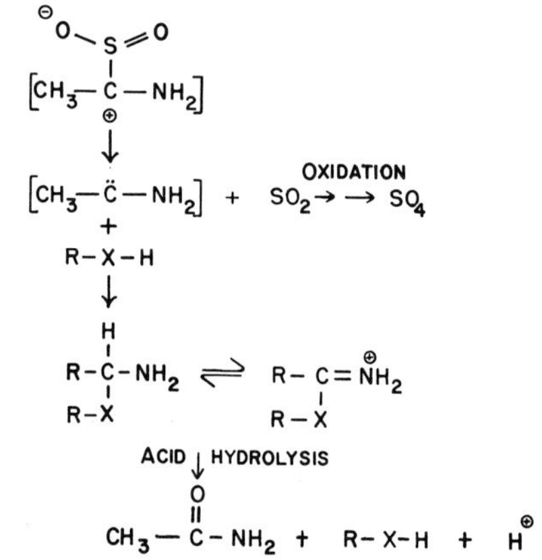

B.

Figs. 6A and 6B. Proposed mechanism for the covalent binding of thioacetamide S-dioxide to hepatic macromolecules.

postulate a nucleophilic attack on the carbonyl carbon of the thioacetamide S-dioxide with displacement of the S-dioxide group as $SO_2^=$ and the resultant covalent binding of the carbon skeleton of thioacetamide S-dioxide to hepatic nucleophiles. Evidence supporting the nature of the covalently bound metabolite being that depicted is derived from acid hydrolysis of liver proteins to which is bound a metabolite of ^{3}H thioacetamide S-oxide. Acid hydrolysis releases the majority of the bound radioactivity as acetamide. Figure 6B shows an alternate mechanism for the formation of a reactive intermediate of the thioacetamide S-dioxide. In this case we propose a cleavage of the carbon sulfur bond to form SO_2 and a carbene intermediate. This carbene intermediate could then engage in carbon-hydrogen or heteroatom-hydrogen insertion reactions or addition across double bonds. In the case of the mechanism proposed in 6B we postulate a carbon-hydrogen or a heteroatom-hydrogen insertion reaction forming the same product shown in 6A. This product on acid hydrolysis would again yield acetamide and release the nucleophile to which the thioacetamide metabolite was bound. We further postulate that the covalent binding of thioacetamide S-dioxide to liver macromolecules leads to hepatocyte disfunction and death.

In summary, thiono-sulfur containing compounds cause a wide variety of toxic effects in mammals. These toxic effects of thiono-sulfur containing compounds appear to be at least partially the result of their metabolism to reactive intermediates by the cytochrome P-450 containing monooxygenase enzyme systems. Covalent binding of atomic sulfur released in the cytochrome P-450 monooxygenase catalyzed metabolism of thiono-sulfur compounds is responsible for the inhibition of monooxygenase activity and the loss of cytochrome P-450 seen on administration of thiono-sulfur compounds in vivo or incubation with cytochrome P-450 monooxygenase enzymes in vitro. Liver necrosis and perhaps the induction of lung edema and neoplasia as well as other effects of these compounds are more likely the result of the covalent binding of the electrophilic S-oxides or S-dioxides or carbene derivatives of these S-oxides and S-dioxides to tissue macromolecules.

ACKNOWLEDGEMENTS

The work described was supported by USPHS Grants ES-00075 and ES 00267. Training support provided by ES 07028 is also gratefully acknowledged.

REFERENCES

1. Hunter, A.L. and Neal, R.A. (1975) Biochem. Pharmacol. 24, 2199-2205.
2. Norman, B.J., Poore, R.E. and Neal, R.A. (1974) Biochem. Pharmacol. 23, 1733-1744.
3. Kamataki, T., Lin, M.C.M.L. and Neal, R.A. (1976) Drug Metab. Dispos. 4, 180-189.
4. Gage, J.C. (1953) Biochem. J. 54, 426-230.
5. Ptashne, K.A., Wolcott, R.M. and Neal, R.A. (1971) J. Pharmacol. Exp. Ther. 179, 380-385.

6. Aldridge, W.N. (1953) Biochem. J. 53, 117-124.

7. Neal, R.A. (1967) Biochem. J. 103, 183-191.

8. Nakatsugawa, T. and Dahm, P. (1967) Biochem. Pharmacol. 16, 25-38.

9. Ptashne, K.A. and Neal, R.A. (1972) Biochemistry 11, 3224-3228.

10. Kamataki, T. and Neal, R.A. (1976) Molecular Pharmacol. 12, 933-944.

11. Halpert, J. and Neal, R.A. Unpublished observations.

12. Hunter, A.L., Holscher, M.A. and Neal, R.A. (1977) J. Pharmacol. Exp. Ther. 200, 439-448.

13. Porter, W.R. and Neal, R.A. (1978) Drug Metab. Dispos. 6, 379-388.

14. Porter, W.R., Gudzinowicz, M.J. and Neal, R.A. (1979) J. Pharmacol. Exp. Ther. (in press).

© 1980 Elsevier/North-Holland Biomedical Press
The Scientific Basis of Toxicity Assessment
H. Witschi, editor.   251

THE METABOLISM OF XENOBIOTICS: A STUDY IN BIOCHEMICAL EVOLUTION

C. F. WILKINSON

Department of Entomology, Cornell University, Ithaca, NY 14853

INTRODUCTION

A major factor in man's success as a species is his ability, through technological innovation, to control and modify the environment to his advantage.
Perhaps nowhere can this be seen more clearly than in the remarkable chemical
revolution which, during the span of a few short decades, has reached such a high
level of sophistication that "virtually all the things that nurture our civili-
zation are made possible by the use of chemicals"[1]. We eagerly accept, enjoy
and even take for granted the enormous benefits we derive from the vast number
of drugs, food additives, pesticides and other synthetic chemicals that have
become an intimate part of our daily lives. These are the types of chemicals
which have been termed "foreign compounds" or xenobiotics; they exist solely as
a result of man's ingenuity, and consequently are alien to the essential life
processes.

As has been the case with other technological advances, however, it now
appears that we have moved too far too fast in utilizing our new-found chemical
expertise. In our enthusiasm for new successes we have often overlooked the
fact that we have caused the serious pollution of our environment and purposely
or inadvertently have exposed ourselves and other forms of life to a multitude of
potentially hazardous chemicals. Currently the pendulum of public opinion is
swinging in an antichemical direction as almost daily we are assaulted with new
environmental horror stories and are continually warned of the potential risks
associated with the continued use of a familiar chemical. It is understandable
that we might become fearful of chemicals and obsessed by the risks their use
entails.

But before we get overly concerned for the ability of man and other organisms to survive in our polluted environment we should not forget that from the
time that life first began, organisms have been engaged in a constant battle to
adapt to changing environmental conditions. In the course of these evolutionary
struggles living organisms have encountered a wide variety of potentially toxic
naturally occurring chemicals of both abiotic and biotic origin. More importantly they have evolved a remarkably effective biochemical defense system which
fortunately for us is as proficient against man's modern synthetic chemicals as

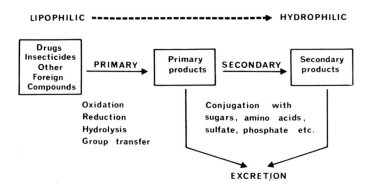

LIPOPHILIC ■■■■■■■■■■■■■■■■■■■■■■■■■■■■▶ HYDROPHILIC

Fig. 1. Metabolism of lipophilic xenobiotics.

it is against the naturally occurring chemicals for which it was selected.
Organisms were consequently forewarned and forearmed to meet the chemical
revolution.

Although many natural and synthetic chemicals are of a highly polar nature,
it is undoubtedly the lipophilic compounds which represent the greatest potential threat to living organisms, since these have the ability to penetrate the
outer protective barriers of the organism and to distribute themselves throughout the tissues. Furthermore, once such chemicals gain access to the tissues
they have a general tendency to accumulate, since their physicochemical
characteristics (fat solubility) preclude their ready removal from the body
in the aqueous or polar media that most organisms employ for their excretory
processes. To overcome this problem organisms have developed a system whereby
lipophilic foreign compounds are transformed into more polar, hydrophilic
materials that can be removed by the normal excretory mechanisms. The process
typically occurs in two major steps, often referred to as primary (phase I) and
secondary (phase II) metabolism (Figure 1). Primary metabolism usually involves
an oxidative, reductive or hydrolytic biotransformation in which a polar, reactive group is either added to or uncovered in the molecule. Sometimes the
products of primary metabolism are excreted directly, but more usually they
undergo one of several secondary reactions that result in their conjugation
with endogenous materials such as glucose, glucuronic acid, sulfate, phosphate
or amino acids. Since the overall process frequently leads to a decrease in
the toxicity or biological activity of the parent compound it is often termed
detoxication. There is, of course, no way in which an organism can prejudge
the potential toxicity of a given compound, and this effect has to be considered
a secondary 'bonus' to the overall function of increasing its hydrophilic character.

Of the several types of reactions through which the primary metabolism of foreign compounds occurs, oxidation has to be considered of maximum overall importance, and is often rate-limiting with respect to both metabolism and toxicity. It is the objective of the remainder of this presentation to examine the basic mechanism by which foreign compounds are oxidized, to examine some of the characteristics of the system that appear to have made it ideally and ubiquitously suited for its role in chemical defense, and finally to take the opportunity to engage in a little speculation into the possible evolutionary development of the system.

MIXED-FUNCTION OXIDATION AND CYTOCHROME P-450

The mammalian liver has long been recognized as the organ primarily (though not exclusively) responsible for the oxidative metabolism of foreign compounds and its functional role in this capacity has been the subject of intense investigation during the past twenty years. Details of all facets of this huge area are available from several sources[2-7] and only a brief overview will be presented here.

The oxidative enzymes involved in xenobiotic metabolism are associated with the microsomal fraction of liver homogenates which is derived from the endoplasmic reticulum of the intact cell. They exhibit an unusual degree of non-specificity and a predilection for lipophilic compounds which they metabolize through reactions involving numerous functional groups[6]. Among these reactions are aromatic, alicyclic and aliphatic hydroxylation, dealkylation of ethers and substituted amines, oxidation of thioethers to sulfoxides and sulfones, epoxidation of double bonds and desulfuration. The majority of these reactions constitute important detoxication pathways for foreign compounds, although (as we have heard in earlier presentations at this symposium) several can lead to biological activity through the formation of a variety of reactive intermediates or products[9]. All of the reactions require NADPH and oxygen, and since in all cases one atom of molecular oxygen is incorporated into the substrate, and the other is reduced to water, they are by definition classified as mixed-function oxidations and can be represented by the general equation:

$$S + O_2 + NADPH + H^+ \longrightarrow SO + H_2O + NADP^+ .$$

The key to the system is a common electron transport pathway (Figure 2) that transfers electrons from NADPH through a flavoprotein, (NADPH-cytochrome $\underline{c}$ reductase, Fp_1) (Figure 2) to a unique cytochrome, cytochrome P-450, which is the terminal oxidase of the chain. Cytochrome P-450 is an unusual $\underline{b}$-type cytochrome that derives its name from the fact that in the reduced form it combines

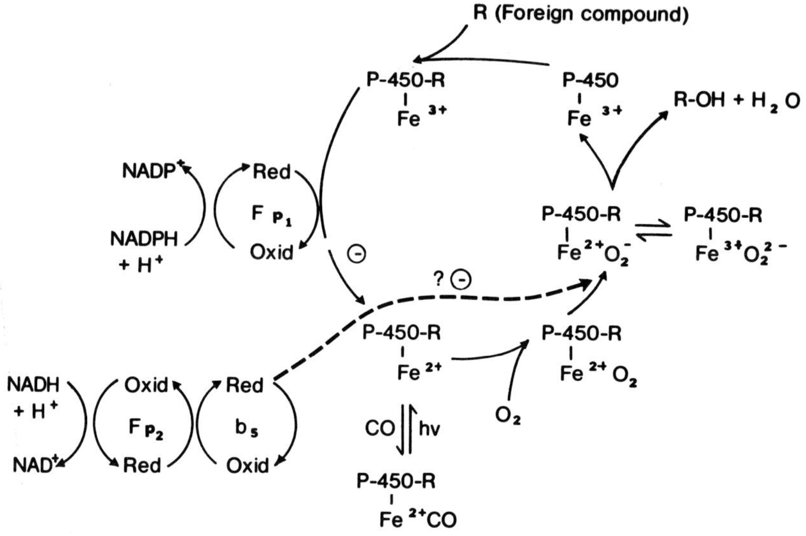

R (Foreign compound)

P-450-R Fe^{3+} → P-450 Fe^{3+} → R-OH + H_2O

NADP / NADPH + H^+ — Red / Oxid — FP_1

$\ominus$? $\ominus$

P-450-R $Fe^{2+}O_2^-$ ⇌ P-450-R $Fe^{3+}O_2^{2-}$

NADH + H^+ / NAD — Oxid / Red — FP_2 — Red / Oxid — b_5

P-450-R Fe^{2+} → P-450-R $Fe^{2+}O_2$

CO ‖ hv O_2

P-450-R $Fe^{2+}CO$

Fig. 2.   Microsomal electron transport pathway.

with CO to form a complex absorbing at 450 nm. The overall mechanism by which
oxidation occurs is now quite well understood[2-9]. The foreign compound first
forms a complex with the oxidized form of cytochrome P-450 which is reduced by
one electron passing down the chain from NADPH. The reduced cytochrome P-450/
substrate complex then reacts with and activates molecular oxygen and the resulting oxygenated complex breaks down to yield the product and water. Reduction, therefore, occurs in two separate one-electron steps. Although the first
of these electrons undoubtedly arises from NADPH, it is still uncertain whether
this is true of the second or whether this originates from NADH and passes through
another microsomal electron transport pathway involving cytochrome b_5 and the
flavoprotein NADH-cytochrome b_5 reductase, Fp_2 (Figure 2).

Despite the accumulation of impressive amounts of data on structural and
mechanistic details of the microsomal electron transport pathway there remain
several intriguing questions concerning the functional role of the system and
its organization in the membrane. One major question relates to the ability of
the system to catalyze such a wide variety of reactions with so many structurally
diverse substrates. This apparent lack of specificity has been largely explained
in recent years by discovery of the existence of multiple forms of cytochrome
P-450 differing from one another in catalytic, spectral, electrophoretic and
immunological properties[10,11].

Initial evidence in support of this was obtained through studies demonstrating the induction of mixed-function oxidase activity following _in vivo_ treatment of animals with a variety of foreign compounds[6,12,13,14]. This phenomenon typically results in a several-fold increase in oxidase activity through enhanced _de novo_ synthesis of cytochrome P-450 and other microsomal enzyme components. However, it has been established that different inducing agents cause the formation of qualitatively different forms of cytochrome P-450. Thus treatment of animals with polycyclic hydrocarbons such as 3-methylcholanthrene results predominantly in the appearance of cytochrome P-448, which differs from the cytochrome P-450 of control or phenobarbital-treated animals not only in spectral characteristics (as indicated by its name), but also in catalytic and structural properties[10].

Detailed comparisons between these different forms of cytochrome P-450 have been made possible in recent years through the development of suitable solubilization and purification techniques and by the successful reconstitution of catalytically active oxidase systems that require only lipoprotein, flavoprotein (NADPH – cytochrome _c_ reductase) and cytochrome P-450 [15]. These studies have clearly established that the functional specificity of the oxidase system resides primarily with the cytochrome P-450 component[16], and there exist immunochemically distinct forms of the cytochrome, not only in different animal species[17], but also within the tissues of the same animal.

Although to date only two major forms of cytochrome P-450 (P-450 and P-448) have been studied in any detail, it is the current general consensus that there are several more[10]. Indeed, the fascinating picture that seems to be emerging is of a common flavoprotein transferring electrons from NADPH to a family of cytochrome P-450s (Figure 3), each catalyzing a limited, perhaps overlapping,

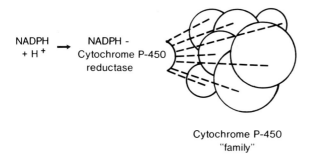

NADPH
+ H⁺ → NADPH -
Cytochrome P-450
reductase

Cytochrome P-450
"family"

Fig. 3. Multiple forms of cytochrome P-450.

spectrum of oxidative reactions with a variety of substrates and each exhibiting varying degrees of sensitivity to different inducing agents. Just how much of the functional specificity is associated with structural differences in the hemoproteins themselves, or how much relates to their location in the lipid environment of the membrane, remains to be seen.

Although the liver is undoubtedly the major site of foreign compound oxidation in mammals, cytochrome P-450-mediated mixed-function oxidases are also found in several other tissues[18] including lung, kidney, small intestine and skin. Compared with those found in the liver, cytochrome P-450 levels and oxidase activities in these tissues are often quite low, but it is probable that they often play a critical role in foreign compound metabolism. The fact that the patterns of microsomal oxidation in extrahepatic tissues frequently are different from those in the liver and that the enzymes often respond differently to inducers, is consistent with the concept of a family of cytochrome P-450s and the existence of qualitatively different pools of cytochrome P-450 in different tissues.

In addition to its role in foreign compound metabolism cytochrome P-450 also participates in several important hydroxylation reactions involved in steroid hormone biosynthesis[19,20,21]. These reactions which include the 11β- and 18-hydroxylations of steroids and the sidechain oxidations of cholesterol leading to pregnenolone and progesterone occur in several tissues including the adrenal cortex, ovary, testis and placenta. In contrast to the cytochrome P-450-mediated oxidases in the liver, those involved in steroid biosynthesis are typically associated with the inner mitochondrial membrane and in keeping with their critical role in steroid hormone regulation are highly specific with respect to the reactions they catalyze. They require NADPH and O_2 and rely on an electron transport pathway similar to that described for hepatic microsomes, but having an additional small-molecular weight iron-sulfur protein component, adrenodoxin, inserted between the flavoprotein and cytochrome P-450.

PHYLOGENETIC DISTRIBUTION OF MIXED-FUNCTION OXIDASES

By the late 1950s or early 1960s when it had become clear that in mammals the mixed-function oxidases were often critical in determining the degree and duration of biological activity of foreign compounds, attention began to turn towards other species. This was stimulated in part by a desire to uncover species differences that might be exploited in the rational design of new, selective biocides (e.g. insect studies) and in part by an increasing concern for the continued well-being of a variety of non-target species exposed to environmental pollutants (e. g. studies with fish, birds, and other wildlife). Since that time comparative studies on the biotransformation of foreign compounds have been conducted with a large number of organisms from widely different habitats and with vastly different lifestyles[22,23,24]. The results of many of these studies are incomplete, sometimes equivocal and in some cases illustrate the dangers of making brief, ill-conceived excursions into the complex world of comparative biochemistry. In some cases oxidase activity has been demonstrated directly through in vitro studies and in others it has been implied by the finding of oxidative metabolites in vivo. Despite these limitations, however, such studies have now firmly established that mixed-function oxidases capable of metabolizing foreign compounds are present in almost every form of life which has been examined.

In considering the comparative aspects of the subject we must try and resist the temptation to generalize and must bear in mind that we have only scratched the surface in terms of the numbers of species which have been studied. Nonetheless, it may prove informative to conduct a brief qualitative survey of what has been uncovered to date.

In the case of the animal kingdom we have data (often incomplete) from perhaps 100 of the 3 million species estimated to exist, and representing only 4 or 5 of the approximately 30 major phyla. Major attention has been given to the phylum Chordata, where in addition to the vast amount of work conducted with common laboratory animals (rats, mice, rabbits, etc.) active mixed-function oxidases have been described and characterized to some extent in most of the major classes including other mammals[25], birds[26,27], reptiles[25,28], amphibia[25,28,29] and fish[30,31].

The Arthropoda, with over one million known species -- by far the largest phylum in the animal kingdom -- has been the object of much interest and investigation in recent years. Mixed-function oxidases·with properties basically similar to those found in vertebrates have been demonstrated in many species of the class Insecta[32] as well as in species representing the Chilopoda (centipedes)[33], Diplopoda (millipedes)[33] and in both terrestrial (sowbugs)[33] and aquatic (lobsters, crabs, shrimp, etc.)[30,34] Crustacea including zooplanktonic forms[35]. Although numerous practical difficulties are encountered in biochemical studies with many of these species[36] it seems reasonable to assume that active mixed-function oxidases occur throughout this large phylum.

Less complete data are available from other invertebrate phyla. Oxidase activity has been reported from several species of earthworms [33,37] (phylum Annelida) and from several representatives of the phylum Mollusca including terrestrial (snails, slugs)[33] and aquatic species; traces of activity have been observed in two echinoderms (starfish)[30,38]. Undoubtedly this list will continue to grow as investigations extend into other corners of the animal kingdom.

However, cytochrome P-450-mediated mixed-function oxidases are not limited to members of the animal kingdom. They have been found in tissues of a variety of species of higher plants[39-43], yeasts[44] and fungi[45] and importantly in several bacteria[46], where detailed studies on the cytochrome P-450 of _Pseudomonas putida_[47] have contibuted greatly to our understanding of the structure and function of the mammalian hepatic system. We will return shortly to consider these enzymes in further detail.

What this brief survey indicates is that mixed-function oxidases based on cytochrome P-450 are distributed throughout the animal and plant kingdoms, as well as in a variety of primitive prokaryotic organisms. This wide distribution immediately suggests the early evolutionary development of cyto-chrome P-450 since it is highly unlikely that it could have developed independ-ently in so many different phyla. But before considering this aspect in more detail, let's briefly compare some of the characteristics of cytochrome P-450s from different sources and see whether any common structural or functional patterns emerge.

The bulk of evidence to date clearly suggests that with the exception of relatively minor differences such as temperature optima, possibly associated with adaptations to a variety of physical environments, the microsomal enzymes from widely different animal sources are remarkably similar to one another in both structure and function. We are reminded once more of the extraordinary uniformity of life at the subcellular metabolic level, in animals of vastly diverse phylogenetic and organic character.

Like the system described for mammalian liver the microsomal mixed-function oxidases of other animals utilize NADPH and O_2 to metabolize a large variety of lipophilic foreign compounds; they all rely on a similar electron transport pathway involving a flavoprotein to transfer electrons from NADPH to cytochrome P-450. The similarities observed at this level appear to extend to the struc-tures of the individual catalytic components. Thus recent studies in our labora-tory (Crankshaw, Hetnarski and Wilkinson, unpublished) on the purified, proteo-lytically solubilized flavoprotein (NADPH cytochrome _c_ reductase) from armyworm (_Spodoptera eridania_) midgut microsomes, have shown it to have catalytic and structural characteristics almost identical to the rat liver enzyme right down to the level of amino acid composition. The two proteins are immunochemically distinct, however, suggesting some degree of structural difference. Although progress in the solubilization and purification of the cytochrome P-450s from a non-mammalian species has not yet progressed sufficiently to allow meaningful comparisons, it is likely that a strong conservatism of active site structure will eventually emerge[48], and that the structural differences that do exist will be found largely in the remainder of the protein. Consequently, although we can probably expect to find a large number of structurally diverse "cytochrome P-450 families" in different organisms (already multiple forms of cytochrome P-450 have been reported in various insect tissues[49] and in fish[30]) it is unlikely that these differences will be associated with significant qualitative variations in their combined catalytic function.

In considering the biological function of the animal microsomal cytochrome P-450-mediated oxidase system it becomes apparent that it is beautifully adapted for its role as a biochemical clearing-house for xenobiotics. Let's briefly review some of its characteristics in this respect.

1. As we have discussed earlier the system is able to accept any of a large number of lipophilic foreign compounds; i.e., it shows a remarkable degree of nonspecificity.

2. A brief look at the distribution of oxidase activity in the organs of different animals reveals that the enzymes are located primarily in tissues associated with the major portals of entry of xenobiotics into the body[3,32]. Thus in mammals they are found in the lung, skin and intestine[18] and it is of interest to note that the liver, the major site of microsomal oxidation in mammals, itself is derived embryologically from the intestine; a similar pattern of strategic location is observed in fish where oxidase activity occurs mainly in liver, kidney and gill[30]. In insect species studied, oxidase activity is usually found in either the gut or in the fat body[32] (occasionally the Malpighian tubules), tissues that presumably represent the first lines of defense against naturally occurring foreign compounds entering the body in the diet or by cuticular penetration. The digestive tract is also the major tissue involved in microsomal oxidation in the earthworm[37] and presumably other annelids. In summary, therefore, the oxidase system appears to be located in those tissues where it is likely to function to maximum advantage against foreign compounds entering the body.

3. Through its ability to be induced by a wide variety of foreign compounds the oxidase system is well prepared to respond rapidly to periods of unusually severe environmental (chemical) stress, and in some situations this may prove sufficient to ensure the immediate survival of the animal against xenobiotic assault. The rapidity with which enzyme induction can occur is not always obvious in mammals but becomes much clearer in other species. Thus our studies with southern armyworm larvae have shown a dramatic 4-fold increase in gut mixed-function oxidase activity within the first 5 hours of dietary exposure to pentamethylbenzene[50] and a significant increase in activity has been observed only 30

minutes after ingestion of small doses of the natural products α-pinene and sinigrin[51]. As we have discussed earlier, induction with different compounds does not cause a simultaneous increase in all types of cytochrome P-450 but in many cases results in an increase in a specific type of the cytochrome most appropriate for the animal's immediate needs. The full extent of this specificity remains to be established. The remarkable flexibility of the oxidase system is further emphasized by the fact that once the foreign compound inducer is removed from the tissues enzyme activity rapidly returns to previous levels, a factor which minimizes the energy load imposed by increased protein synthesis.

4. The strict conservatism of animals with regard to energy expenditure on the mixed-function oxidases is further shown by the fact that the enzymes are synthesized and maintained only during those periods when they are required. It has long been recognized that fetal and neonate mammals have low titers of oxidase activity which steadily develop to attain maximum levels only in adults. It could be argued that in this case, the fetus relies on the maternal oxidases for protection against foreign compounds. But again we have to go to the results of comparative studies to fully appreciate what controls exist -- particularly to insects where development is characterized by sharply defined periods of feeding and inactivity. In considering insect species it is interesting to note that mixed-function oxidase activity is found only in those stages actively engaged in feeding[32]. This is particularly clear in lepidopterous larvae such as the southern armyworm, where within a few hours of finishing feeding in preparation for pupation, oxidase activity in the gut virtually disappears[52]. It is further shown in the lack of oxidase activity during larval and nymphal molts of various species and by the general absence of activity in pupae and in some adult insects which do not feed[32]. This evidence strongly suggests that the microsomal oxidases have indeed evolved to protect animals from naturally occurring foreign compounds and that control mechanisms have been developed whereby enzyme activity is synchronized with periods of maximum xenobiotic exposure.

In considering the cytochrome P-450-mediated mixed-function oxidases of plants, our original arguments regarding their function in animals (i.e. to convert lipophilic xenobiotics into a more excretable form) is no longer valid. Obviously plants do not excrete foreign compounds like mammals. However, plants are themselves the primary sources of the many naturally occurring lipophilic foreign compounds (alkaloids, terpenes and other allelochemicals) against which animals, especially herbivores, need protection[22,53]. Plants, therefore, have developed the ability to synthesize these same foreign compounds in the course of their evolutionary struggles against herbivorous enemies and it seems reasonable to suppose that many of the enzymatic steps necessary for the biosynthesis of these compounds might be similar to those required for their catabolism. In addition, it is probable that mixed-function oxidases may be involved in the biosynthesis of the plant growth hormone, gibberellin[54]. Little is known concerning the substrate specificity of these enzymes in higher plants although several rather non-specific xenobiotic oxidations (e.g. aldrin epoxidation) have been reported[41,42]. Like the oxidases from animal sources, those from plants are microsomal enzymes; although few detailed studies have been reported, they appear to require NADPH and O_2 and are associated with cytochrome P-450 and a flavin-dependent reductase. This is also true of the oxidases which have been reported from some of the lower yeasts and fungi although here they seem to have developed to enable these organisms to grow on a variety of non-physiological carbon sources. In a functional sense, therefore, they tend to show a closer resemblance to the bacterial oxidases than to those of higher plants.

Since most of the basic biochemical pathways were developed by bacteria at an early stage of evolution, the cytochrome P-450 mixed-function oxidases in prokaryotes are particularly interesting. Like those in the yeasts and fungi the cytochrome P-450-dependent oxidases in aerobic bacteria catalyze the initial oxidations of a variety of lipophilic hydrocarbons into phenols and alcohols and set the stage for a variety of other reactions which result ultimately in the production of normal intermediary metabolites which can be completely oxidized in respiration[46]. In this way aerobic bacteria are able to convert petroleum into a fully utilizable source of energy.

Aerobic bacteria are able to catalyze mixed-function oxidations of several types and employ a variety of mechanisms involving flavoproteins and iron-sulfur proteins[46]. Mention will be made here only of those mediated by cytochrome P-450. Although it is likely that many of the oxidations carried out by bacteria will be shown to involve cytochrome P-450, so far only two have been studied in detail; these are the conversion of n-octane to n-octanol in Corynebacterium sp.[55] and the oxidation of D-camphor to its 5-exo-alcohol in Pseudomonas putida[47]. The latter reaction which is the initial step in the conversion of D-camphor to acetate and iso-butyrate has received maximum attention. NADH is the electron donor and reducing equivalents are transported to the cytochrome P-450 via a flavoprotein (NADH-putidaredoxin reductase) and an iron-sulfur protein, putidaredoxin (Figure 4). Since all components of the system are soluble proteins they have been studied intensively in a highly purified state and the results have contributed very substantially to our present understanding of the mechanism of mixed-function oxidations involving cytochrome P-450. The hydroxylating activity of P. putida is quite specific for a limited range of camphor

262

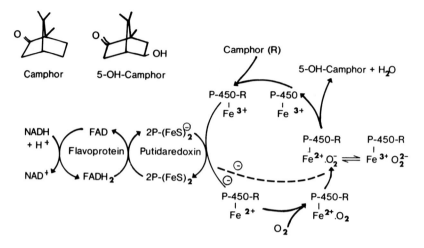

Fig. 4. Electron transport pathway in <u>Pseudomonas</u> <u>putida</u>.

derivatives and occurs only when the bacteria are grown on media enriched by camphor-related compounds. It is, therefore, inducible as is the system in <u>Corynebacterium</u> sp.

   Despite their distant evolutionary relationship, the bacterial hydroxylases bear a striking resemblance to the steroid hydroxylating enzymes of mammalian adrenal mitochondria; both employ an electron transport pathway involving a flavoprotein, iron-sulfur protein (putidaredoxin and adrenodoxin) and cyto-chrome P-450 and both are quite specific for their respective substrates. Indeed the only real differences are that the bacterial systems are soluble and require NADH whereas those in the adrenals are membrane bound and rely on NADPH. The similarities become even more apparent when the characteristics of some of the purified components are compared. Thus both putidaredoxin and adrenodoxin have similar molecular weights (12,500 and 13,100 respectively), similar active centers containing two atoms each of iron and labile sulfide and a similar amino acid composition[56]. Similarities have also been noted between the correspond-ing flavoproteins and cytochrome P-450s.

   In summary, therefore, we find cytochrome P-450 participating in several types of mixed-function oxidation reactions ranging from the highly specific reactions in aerobic bacteria to the highly non-specific microsomal reactions involved in xenobiotic metabolism. It is of interest to note that, wherever specificity is observed (i.e. in the bacterial and adrenal mitochondrial systems), the reactions involve an iron-sulfur protein. This suggests that the latter may play an important role in determining specificity, and in this respect it may be relevant that in the reconstituted camphor hydroxylating system, adrenodoxin cannot be substituted for putidaredoxin.

THE EVOLUTION OF CYTOCHROME P-450 MEDIATED OXIDASES

It seems clear from the current ubiquitous distribution of cytochrome P-450 in both eukaryotes and aerobic prokaryotes that the evolutionary origins of the enzyme system go back to the dim and distant era when life was just developing on planet earth. The events which took place during this period are, of course, unclear and any discussion concerning them is highly speculative. However, let's begin by outlining a few of the major events which are known to have occurred during this momentous period of our history (Figure 5).

Until relatively recent times the fossil record could be traced back with any degree of certainty only to the beginning of the Cambrian period about 600 million years ago. This represented a puzzling discontinuity in geologic history since the fossil record of the Cambrian is rich in many forms of life (worms, molluscs and arthropods) found today and earlier sedimentary rocks provided little or no evidence of their immediate ancestors. More recent microscopic examination of Precambrian deposits has now clearly established the presence of a variety of micro-fossils and has extended the fossil record back to around 3.2 billion years. The origin of life is considered to have occurred somewhere around 3.5 billion years ago, only about 1 billion years after the earth was formed. Since we know that during the very early period of earth's history conditions were anoxic and since we know that by the start of the Cambrian period a large number of well-developed multicellular eukaryotes were thriving in an atmosphere not dissimilar to the one we know today, two major events must

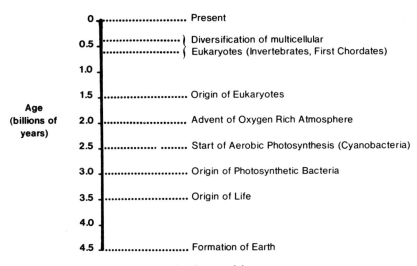

Fig. 5. Major events in evolutionary history.

have occurred during the Precambrian period. One of these was the formation of
an oxygen atmosphere (around 2 billion years ago) and the other was the emergence
of the eukaryotic cell (around 1.5 billion years ago).

The very earliest forms of life were almost certainly heterotrophic organisms
which obtained their nutrients (amino acids, carbohydrates and other organics)
from the abundant "abiotic soup" of the primordial earth[57, 58]. They were anaerobic and their survival depended on few, if any, complex biochemical transformations. As the supply of preformed, readily-utilizable abiotic nutrients steadily
declined, it is postulated that there was increasing selection in favor of organisms capable of obtaining their nutrients from alternative compounds, a process
which led to the development of the anaerobic fermentative bacteria and which
was responsible for the formation of the first multistep synthetic pathways. It
is likely that many of the basic anaerobic biochemical pathways originated in
these organisms and that they possessed simple electron transport pathways involving flavoproteins and iron-sulfur proteins. They were, however, unable to
synthesize the tetrapyrrole nucleus and consequently were devoid of cytochromes
and chlorophylls[57,58]. Life could not depend for long, however, on a ready
supply of abiotic material and it is perhaps not surprising that the next organisms to make their appearance were the photosynthetic bacteria capable of utilizing light energy as a source of ATP. The photosynthesis carried out by these
organisms was quite different from that of the higher plants of today since
instead of water they employed H_2S as a source of reducing power for converting
CO_2 to glucose. The reaction proceeded anaerobically and indeed was inhibited
by traces of oxygen. These organisms may have been the first to synthesize the

$$12H_2S + 6CO_2 \xrightarrow{hv} \text{Glucose} + 12S + 6H_2O$$

tetrapyrrole structure and to employ it in the form of bacterial chlorophyll and
cytochromes[58]. They were probably also the organisms which 2 billion years ago
gave rise to the early cyanobacteria which were the first organisms to effect aerobic photosynthesis using water instead of H_2S and more importantly liberating
O_2 as a by-product of the reaction. The first appearance of oxygen in the

$$12H_2O + 6CO_2 \xrightarrow{hv} \text{Glucose} + 6O_2 + 6H_2O$$

atmosphere represented a dramatic change in the environment. Many anaerobes
either became extinct or were forced to adapt to anerobic habitats, whilst others
began to develop alternative aerobic pathways for respiration and biosynthesis.
These were the so-called facultative aerobes, which could switch from aerobic to
anaerobic pathways readily, and were thus in tune with the fluctauting environmental levels of oxygen. The appearance of oxygen provided organisms with a

much more efficient means of respiration than had hitherto been available and most facultative aerobes made use of aerobic respiration whenever possible; it also made possible the development of a wide variety of other metabolic reactions involving oxygen and it is possible that mixed-function oxidation via cytochrome P-450 was first developed by these organisms.

As Mason[48] pointed out, however, by the time oxygen first appeared many enzyme proteins were already under well-developed genetic control and it is probable that the first oxidases were modifications of existing proteins rather than totally novel macromolecules. It is unlikely, therefore, that cytochrome P-450 suddenly appeared and assumed its role in mixed-function oxidation. One suggestion of a possible earlier role of cytochrome P-450 is that it may have been involved in oxygen detoxication[59]. Cytochrome P-450 is known to reduce oxygen to hydrogen peroxide and its low redox potential (-410mv) would have allowed it to operate efficiently at very low oxygen levels either before the development of superoxide dismutase and catalase or in conjunction with them. Another possible reductive role is suggested by the presence of cytochrome P-450 in the nitrogen-fixing bacteroid Rhizobium japonicum[60] and, indeed, under anaerobic conditions, hepatic cytochrome P-450 can catalyze several reductive reactions (e.g. nitro-reductase, azoreductase).

Whatever the very early origins of cytochrome P-450 it was certainly well-developed as an oxidase in the aerobic bacteria and allowed them to thrive on a variety of new carbon sources such as petroleum hydrocarbons which were undoubtedly prevalent in the Precambrian environment. Indeed, the basic problem faced by many of these bacteria -- how to utilize many of these apolar, lipophilic hydrocarbons for respiratory purposes -- is not dissimilar to the problems faced by contemporary animals -- how to remove such compounds from their tissues. In light of the fact that mixed-function oxidation remains the only known biochemical mechanism for activation of non-activated carbon-hydrogen bonds, the development of a cytochrome P-450 system for this purpose seems in retrospect to be a logical (perhaps inevitable) evolutionary step.

Precisely how our story progresses through the next momentous event in evolutionary history, the appearance of the eukaryotic cell, and continues through the subsequent development of multicellular plants and animals remains obscure. One can argue plausibly that the specific cytochrome P-450-mediated oxidases in the mitochondria of mammalian endocrine tissues are directly descended from those of the prokaryotes. This is consistent with the widely held view that mitochondria originated as symbiotic prokaryotic inclusions in early eukaryotes[61] and as we have discussed, there are remarkable similarities between the two enzyme systems. But the origins of the mixed-function oxidases found in the endoplasmic reticulum of various plant and animal tissues and the development of their roles in biosynthesis and xenobiotic metabolism are more difficult to explain. At some point in evolution the soluble prokaryotic oxidases became associated with the phospholipids of the eukaryotic endoplasmic reticulum and it appears that this, combined with loss of the iron-sulfur protein component and the development of multiple forms of cytochrome P-450, have been responsible for a general broadening of substrate specificity and a marked enhancement in functional flexibility.

It appears, therefore, that cytochrome P-450 and its associated electron transport components have ancient prokaryotic origins and that following the emergence of eukaryotes, the oxidase system has developed along two separate evolutionary lines. One of these has retained its specificity for important biosynthetic processes, whilst the other has been adapted to serve an important role in xenobiotic defense. It is the latter that may well prove to be our saviour in an increasingly polluted environment.

REFERENCES

1. Maugh, T. H., II (1978) Science, 199, 162.

2. Hutson, D. H. (1977) in Foreign Compound Metabolism in Mammals (Hathway, D.E., Ed.), Vol. 4, The Chemical Society, London, pp. 259-346.

3. Nakatsugawa T. and Morelli, A. (1976) in Insecticide Biochemistry and Physiology (Wilkinson, C. F., Ed.), Plenum, N.Y., pp. 61-104.

4. Ullrich, V., Roots, I., Hildebrandt, A., Estabrook, R. W. and Conney, A. H. (Eds.) (1977) Microsomes and Drug Oxidations, Pergamon, N. Y. pp. 1-768.

5. Estabrook, R. W., Gillette, J. R. and Leibman, K. C. (Eds.) (1973) Microsomes and Drug Oxidations, Williams and Wilkins, Baltimore, Md., pp. 1-486.

6. Testa, B. and Jenner, P. (1976) Drug Metabolism: Chemical and Biochemical Aspects. Dekker, N.Y., pp. 1-500.

7. LaDu, B. N., Mandel, H. G. and Way, E. L. (Eds.) (1971) Fundamentals of Drug Metabolism and Drug Disposition, Williams and Wilkins, Baltimore, Md., pp. 1-615.

8. Jerina, D. M. (Ed.) (1977) Drug Metabolism Concepts, A. C. S. Symposium Series 44, American Chemical Society, Washington, D. C., pp. 1 - 196.

9. Jollow, D. J., Kocsis, J. J., Snyder, R. and Vainio, H. (Eds.) (1977) Biological Reactive Intermediates, Plenum, N. Y., pp. 1-514.

10. Lu, A. Y. H., Ryan, D., Kawalek, J., Thomas, P., West, S. B., Huang, M. T. and Levin, W. (1976). Biochem. Soc. (London) Trans., 4, 169-172.

11. Coon, M. J., Vermilion, J. L., Vatsis, K. P., French, J. S., Dean, W. L. and Haugen, D. A. in ref. 8, pp. 46-71.

12. Conney, A. H. (1967) Pharmacol Rev., 19, 317-366.

13. Conney, A. H. (1972) in ref. 7 pp. 253-273.

14. Remmer, H. (1972) Eur. J. Clin. Pharmacol., 5, 116-136.

15. Lu, A. Y. H. and Levin, W. (1974) Biochim. Biophys. Acta, 344, 205-240.

16. Lu, A. Y. H., Kuntzman, R., West, S., Jacobson, M. and Conney, A. H. (1972) J. Biol. Chem. 247, 1727-1734.

17. Kawalek, J. C. and Lu, A. Y. H. (1975) Mol. Pharmacol., 11, 201-210.

18. Bend, J. R. and Hook, G. E. R. (1977) in Handbook of Physiology, Section 9, American Physiological Society, Washington, D. C., pp. 419-440.

19. Ullrich, V. and Duppel, W. (1975) in The Enzymes, Vol. 12, pp. 253-297.

20. Sih, C. J. and Whitlock, H. W. Jr. (1968) Ann. Rev. Biochem., 37, 661-694.

21. Wickramasinghe, R. H. (1975) Enzyme, 19, 348-376.

22. Brattsten, L. B. (1979) in Herbivores: Their interactions with Secondary Plant Metabolites (Rosenthal, G. A., Janzen, D. H., Eds.) Academic, N. Y. In Press.

23. Khan, M. A. Q. and Bederka, J. P., Jr. (Eds.) (1974) Survival in Toxic Environments, Academic Press, N. Y., pp. 1-553.

24. Paulson, G. D., Frear, D. S. and Marks, E. P. (Eds.) (1979) Xenobiotic Metabolism: In Vitro Methods, ACS Symposium Series No. 97, American Chemical Society, Washington, D. C.

25. Machinist, J. M., Dehner, E. W. and Ziegler, D. M. (1968) Arch. Biochem. Biophys., 125, 854-864.

26. Pan, H. P., Hook, G. E. R. and Fouts, J. R. (1975) Xenobiotica, 5, 17-24.

27. Pan, H. P., Fouts, J. R. and Devereux, T. R. (1975) Life Sci., 17, 819-826.

28. Garfinkel, D. (1963) Comp. Biochem. Physiol., 8, 367-379.

29. Creaven, P. J., Davies, W. H. and Williams, R. T. (1967) Life Sci., 6, 105-111.

30. Bend, J. R. and James, M. O. (1978) in Biochemical and Biophysical Perspectives in Marine Biology. (Malins, D. C. and Sargent, J. R., Eds.), Vol. 4. Academic Press, N. Y. pp. 125-188.

31. Bend, J. R., James, M. O. and Dansette, P. M. (1977) Ann. N. Y. Acad. Sci., 298, 505-521.

32. Wilkinson, C. F. and Brattsten, L. B. (1972) Drug Metab. Revs., 1, 153-228.

33. Neuhauser, E. and Hartenstein, R. (1976) Comp. Biochem. Physiol., 53C, 37-39.

34. Malins, D. C. (1977) Ann. N. Y. Acad. Sci., 298, 482-496.

35. Corner, E. D. S., Harris, R. P., Kilvington, C. C. and O'Hara, S. C. M. (1976) J. Marine Biol. Assoc., U. K., 56, 121-133.

36. Wilkinson, C. F. (1979) in ref. 24, pp. 249-284.

37. Nelson, P. A., Stewart, R. R., Morelli, M. A. and Nakatsugawa, T. (1976) Pestic. Biochem. Physiol., 6, 243-253.

38. Willis, D. E. and Addison, R. F. (1974) Comp. Gen. Pharmacol., 5, 77-81.

39. Markham, A., Hartman, G. C. and Parke, D. V. (1972) Biochem. J., 30, 90 p.

40. Meehan, T. D. and Coscia, C. J. (1973) Biochem. Biophs. Res. Comm., 53, 1043-1048.

41. Mehendale, H. M. Skrentny, R. F. and Dorough, H. W. (1972) J. Agric. Food Chem., 20, 398-402.

42. Earl, J. W. and Kennedy, I. R. (1973) Aust. J. Biol. Sci., 26, 341-347.

43. Rich, P. R. and Bendall, D. S. (1975) Eur. J. Biochem., 55, 333-341.

44. Duppel, W., Lebeault, J. M. and Coon, M. J. (1973) Eur. J. Biochem., 36, 583-592.

45. Ambike, S. H. and Baxter, R. M. (1970) Phytochemistry, 9, 1959-1962.

46. National Academy of Sciences (1972) Degradation of Synthetic Organic Molecules in the Biosphere, Washington, D.C., pp. 1-146.

47. Gunsalus, I. C. (1972) in ref. 46, pp. 137-146.

48. Mason, H. S. (1968) in Homologous Enzymes and Biochemical Evolution (Thoai, N. V. and Roche, J., Eds.), Gordan and Breach, N.Y., pp. 69-91.

49. Agosin, M. (1976) Mol. Cell. Biochem., 12, 33-44.

50. Brattsten, L. B. and Wilkinson, C. F. (1973) Pestic. Biochem. Physiol., 3, 393-407.

51. Brattsten, L. B., Wilkinson, C. F. and Eisner, T. (1977) Science, 196, 1349-1352.

52. Krieger, R. I. and Wilkinson, C. F. (1969) Biochem. Pharmac., 18, 1403-1415.

53. Brattsten, L. B. (1979) Drug Metab. Revs., in press.

54. Murphy, P. J. and West, C. A. (1969) Arch. Biochem., Biophys., 133, 395-400.

55. Cardini, G. and Jurtshuk, P. (1970) J. Biol. Chem., 245, 2789-2796.

56. Tsai, R. L., Gunsalus, I. C. and Dus, K. (1971) Biochem. Biophys. Res. Comm., 45, 1300-1306.

57. Schopf, J. W. (1978) Scientific American, 239(3), 111-139.

58. Lascelles, J. (1964) in Oxygen in the Animal Organism, IUB Symposium Series, Vol. 31, Macmillan, London, pp. 657-669.

59. Wickramasinghe, R. H. and Villee, C. A. (1975) Nature, 256, 509-511.

60. Appleby, C. A. (1969) Biochim. Biophys. Acta, 172, 71-87.

61. Margulis, L. (1970) Origin of Eukaryotic Cells, Yale University Press, New Haven.

TOXICOLOGY AS A PREDICTIVE SCIENCE - THE FUTURE

Chairman: Stata Norton

TOXICOLOGY AS A PREDICTIVE SCIENCE: INTRODUCTION

STATA NORTON

Department of Pharmacology, University of Kansas Medical Center, Rainbow Boulevard at 39th, Kansas City, Kansas 66103

Recent events have caused many toxicologists, particularly those in government and industry, to focus on the problems associated with prediction from present data on a toxic agent to future risk or benefit to man.   The role of prediction in science, however, is not new.   The ability to predict is in fact a tenet of the scientific method, an established way of testing a scientific hypothesis or generalization.   The new role for prediction in toxicology is the estimation of the probable occurrence of an event from biological data which have a known or assumed variability.   Often extrapolation of risk must be made from data in one animal species to outcome in another species.

One result of the process of using toxicologic data for prediction has been an increased awareness among toxicologists of the need for validation of their test methods.   If an effect is obtained from exposure of an animal to a toxic agent, is it reproducible and what is the likelihood that it will occur at another dose?   Attempts to answer these questions in a scientific way have resulted in new statistical concepts for prediction from animal data. These are discussed in the paper by Drs. Van Ryzin and Rai.

An excellent example of the need in prediction for adequate data which have been obtained from valid tests and the use to which these data can be put is given by Drs. Fry, Storer and Ullrich in their paper on radiation-induced carcinogenesis.   As Fry and his co-workers point out, the more we know about the effects of radiation, the more we realize what we need to know.   "No carcinogenic agent has been studied in both man and experimental animals with such accurate dosimetry as can be made with radiation, and perhaps no carcinogenic agent has revealed the complexities of cancer induction and expression more explicitly than radiation."[1]

As mentioned above, findings of general scientific applicability have resulted from recent attempts to answer questions of the validity of tests and predictability of risk. However, in the process of prediction one more question which must be answered is how to estimate the likelihood of an effect in one species from data obtained in another species.

---

[1]Fry, R. J. M. and J. B. Storer, Abstract for this Symposium.

This question can best be answered by understanding mechanisms. In the final paper of this session, Dr. Aldridge addresses this problem and illustrates the definitive contribution of knowledge of mechanisms in toxicology to decisions of risk to man from toxic agents.

© 1980 Elsevier/North-Holland Biomedical Press
The Scientific Basis of Toxicity Assessment
H. Witschi, editor.

THE USE OF QUANTAL RESPONSE DATA TO MAKE PREDICTIONS

JOHN VAN RYZIN and KAMTA RAI
The Rand Corporation, Santa Monica, California and California State Polytechnic
University, Pomona, California

INTRODUCTION

This paper discusses the use of quantal response toxicity data from animal
tests to make predictions concerning toxic responses in man. By quantal response data, we mean response rates for a specified toxic endpoint (death,
tumor, etc.) in an animal toxicity test. Such data is usually gathered at a
variety of dose levels which are much higher than the exposure levels of man.
Using such data to predict the probability of a toxic response in man at a low-
dose environmental exposure level becomes an exceedingly difficult problem.
Yet, with the advent of more precise detection methods (now in the ppm. range),
with the need for regulation under the Toxic Substances Control Act of 1976,
and the increasing realization of the presence of such toxic substances in the
environment, it becomes necessary to make such predictions. With the aid of
the concept of a dose-response curve such predictions are possible. Such predictions are fraught with uncertainties. The two main variables are: (1) the
extrapolation of high-dose exposure levels in animals to low-dose levels consistent with environmental exposure levels, and (2) the conversion from the
animal test species prediction to man. The first of these problems is primarily statistical, but must include biological mathematical modeling and biological relevance. The second problem is primarily biological and we refer to discussions in the DHEW report of Hoel et al.[1] and the Report of the Scientific
Committee of the Food Safety Council[2] and references therein for further information. In this paper we concentrate on the first of these problems: low-dose
prediction or extrapolation in the animal.

We first present a brief review of dose-response models. Second, we discuss
the statistical methodology of low-dose prediction or extrapolation. Next, we
apply this methodology to three sets of data to illustrate certain important
points in prediction. The vinyl chloride example shows the importance of using
the *effective* dose rather than the *administered* dose. The question of linearity
versus non-linearity at low doses is discussed in relation to the example of
ethylene thiourea. This is of crucial concern for low-dose prediction. In this
context, we discuss three proposed stochastic biological models: the one-hit
model, the multi-hit model and the multi-stage model. Next, we present a

modification of the multi-hit model for accommodation of possible low-dose linearity. Following this, we discuss the use of dose-response models for non-carcinogenic (and reversible) low-dose prediction as opposed to the commonly used toxicological procedure of using a no observed effect level (NOEL). We conclude the paper with some observations about low-dose prediction and future directions of research.

DOSE-RESPONSE MODELS

The notion of dose-response model is a familiar concept in toxicology. It forms the basis for the theory of probit analysis (see e.g., Finney[3]).

Consider an animal on test for a fixed time period in which the outcome of interest is some toxic event (e.g., death, tumor, paralysis). The probability, P, of an animal having such a response is taken to be a function f, $P = f(d)$, of the administered dose, d, of the substance under test. With time fixed we are not considering models designed to look at time to the toxic effect. Four of the models proposed in the literature, and which we use later in the paper, are given in Table 1 below. For a discussion of other models such as the logistic model, the extreme value model, and the Weibull model, see Chand and Hoel[4], Rai and Van Ryzin[5] and the Food Safety Council Report[2] and references therein.

TABLE 1

MATHEMATICAL DOSE-RESPONSE MODELS

Models	P(d)	Parameter Values	Equation Number
Probit[3]	$\Phi(\alpha+\beta\log d)$, $$\Phi(t) = \int_{-\infty}^{t} (2\pi)^{-1/2} e^{-u^2/2}\, du$$	$-\infty < \alpha < \infty$ $\beta > 0$	(1)
One-hit[1]	$1 - e^{-\beta d}$	$\beta > 0$	(2)
Multi-hit[2,5,6]	$$\int_0^{\beta d} (u^{k-1}e^{-u}/\Gamma(k))\,du,$$ $$\Gamma(k) = \int_0^{\infty} u^{k-1}e^{-u}\,du$$	$k > 0$ $\beta > 0$	(3)
Multi-stage[7,8,9]	$1 - e^{-\sum_{i=1}^{k} \alpha_i d^i}$	k a positive integer $\alpha_i \geq 0$	(4)

For the detailed motivation behind the various models see the references cited. For the models in Table 1, we give the following brief descriptions.

The probit model is based on the notion of a tolerance distribution for the population of animals under study. If an animal's tolerance is exceeded by the toxic dose, then a toxic response occurs. In the probit model, the tolerance is assumed to have a log normal distribution.[3,5]

The other three models in Table 1 are *stochastic biological models.*[5] For the one-hit model, the toxic response is envisioned as the result of one or more hits to the target organ which results in a toxic response, where the number of hits is a homogeneous Poisson process in dose with intensity parameter β. Such a model was recommended in the BEIR report[10] and a DHEW subcommittee report.[1] This model is often referred to as the linear model because in the low-dose range P(d) is approximately equal to βd, a straight line through the origin.

The multi-hit model is a generalization of the one-hit model. If the parameter k is an integer, then the toxic response is envisioned as the result of k or more hits to the target which results in a toxic response, where again the number of hits is a homogeneous Poisson process in dose with intensity parameter β. A second interpretation for this model with non-integer k is that the animal population under study has a gamma tolerance distribution with scale parameter β and shape parameter k. Statistical procedures for this model are given by Rai and Van Ryzin.[5,6] For a biological basis for this model see Cornfield,[11] Nordling[12] and Marshall and Groer.[13]

The multi-stage model was first proposed by Armitage and Doll[8] for carcinogenic toxicity and has been generalized by Crump et al.[7,9] This model has recently been extensively used by the National Academy of Science in its report on Drinking Water and Health.[14]

When k = 1 in the multi-hit or multi-stage model, these models reduce to the one-hit model.

Incorporation of background response

For the models of Table 1, the spontaneous or background response rate is assumed to be zero, i.e., P(0) = 0. To incorporate non-zero background response $p \geq 0$ in these models we use Abbot's correction.[15] The extended model with background, denoted by P*(d), becomes:

$$P^*(d) = p + (1-p)P(d), \tag{5}$$

where P(d) is as in Table 1.

A quantity of particular interest, especially from the viewpoint of regulation, is a quantity called the *added risk over background* (AROB) due to the
added dose d, defined by

$$P(d) = \frac{P^*(d)-p}{1-p}. \tag{6}$$

Note that if there is no background response (p=0), $P^*(d) = P(d)$. The AROB is
of particular interest regulation-wise since it measures the added probability
of toxic response due to the added dose d.

For some preassigned small risk level P_0, e.g., 10^{-6}, of acceptable risk, if
one solves the equation $P(d^0) = P_0$ for d^0 one obtains a dose level d^0 called
the *virtual safe dose* (VSD), a term due to Mantel and Bryan.[16] Note that d^0 is
the dose level whose expected number of additional toxic responses over background is $NP(d^0)$ in a population of N animals on test. For example, if $P_0 =$
10^{-6} represents the lifetime risk of, say, bladder cancer due to the added
daily saccharin dose in mg./kg./body weight, then the solution d^0 would be that
dose level leading to approximately three additional bladder cancers in the U.S.
per year. This calculation assumes a U.S. population of 210 million people
with an average lifetime of 70 years leading to N = 210/70 = 3 million people
at risk per year, i.e., $NP_0 = (3,000,000) \times 10^{-6} = 3$. Obviously, this calculation is over-simplified since it ignores varying saccharin consumption, sex,
etc. More realistic assessment requires looking at selected subgroups of the
population. However, the above calculation gives some feel for a risk of 10^{-6}
in terms of the U.S. population.

We now turn to the problem of low-dose prediction using dose-response models
as given in Table 1.

LOW-DOSE PREDICTION (EXTRAPOLATION)

Once the mathematical form of the dose-response curve is assumed, the next
problem is that of low-dose prediction based on the observed response data. Table
2 shows the format of the available data from a typical animal toxicity test.
The test is carried out at, usually, a control group dose level $d_0 = 0$ and m
increasing dose levels $0 < d_1 < d_2 < \ldots < d_m$.

If the animal responses (the x_i's) are occurring as statistically independent
realizations (a sample) of dichotomous response variables, then the probability associated with the experimental outcome of Table 2 is

$$\Pi_{i=0}^{m} \binom{n_i}{x_i} [P^*(d_i)]^{x_i} [1-P^*(d_i)]^{n_i-x_i}, \tag{7}$$

where $P^*(d)$ is given by equation (5), $\binom{n}{x}$ is the usual combinatorial number of x objects chosen from n indistinguishable objects, and $\prod_{i=0}^{m}$ indicates an (m+1) fold product.

TABLE 2

ANIMAL TOXICITY TEST DATA

Dose Level (d)[a]	No. of Animals Tested (n)	No. of Responders (x)
$d_0 = 0$	n_0	x_0
d_1	n_1	x_1
.	.	.
.	.	.
.	.	.
d_m	n_m	x_m

[a] $0 = d_0 < d_1 < \ldots < d_m$, $d_0 = 0$ is the control dose.

Equation (7) represents the likelihood function for the observed sample and as such can be used to estimate the parameters of the model assumed.

Estimation procedures for the models

The estimation of the parameters p, α and β for the probit model are discussed in Finney.[3] The one-hit model in its linear form has simple estimates given by Hoel et al.,[1] while the maximum likelihood estimates are obtainable from the computer program called GLOBAL of Crump et al.[9] for the multi-stage model by taking k = 1. For the multi-hit model, the maximum likelihood estimates of p, k and β are given by Rai and Van Ryzin[5,6] and the computer program is obtainable from the authors. Maximum likelihood estimates for the multi-stage model with an unknown (or fixed) number k are given by Guess and Crump[17] and are obtainable in the GLOBAL computer program of Crump et al.[9]

Having estimated the parameters of the model one can substitute the estimated values into the added risk over background function, P(d), to obtain, $\hat{P}(d)$ an *estimated added risk over background.*[*] Solving the equation $\hat{P}(d) = P_0$ for d yields a $\hat{d}^0$, which is the *estimated virtual safe dose* at the acceptable risk level P_0.

[*]Crump et al.[9] estimate $P^*(d) - p$ instead of P(d). To obtain the estimate $\hat{P}(d)$ this requires dividing their estimate by $1-\hat{p}$, which is usually very close to unity.

Confidence limits on VSD

Based on appropriate statistical arguments one can find for the parametric models in Table 1 an *estimated upper curve* for P(d) given by $\hat{P}^u(d)$. This curve is such that the probability that $P(d) \leq \hat{P}^u(d)$ for all d holds (or, at least holds approximately in a suitable large sample sense) is some preassigned confidence level $\gamma, 0 < \gamma < 1$. Then solving the equation $\hat{P}^u(d) = P_0$, one obtains a one-sided $100(1-\gamma)\%$ lower confidence limit $\hat{d}_L^0$ satisfying $\hat{P}^u(\hat{d}_L^0) = P_0$ and such that the probability that $\hat{d}_L^0 < d^0$ holds is approximately $1 - \gamma$. If $\gamma = .05$, one would obtain a one-sided 95% lower confidence limit on d^0, the virtual safe dose. Usually, one is interested in lower limits on VSD since such a resulting dose level will be below the true VSD $100(1-\gamma)\%$ of the time. This provides a conservative estimate of VSD if the model is correct. We shall discuss the use of lower confidence limit estimates for the various models when the examples are presented later in the paper.

The construction of the above estimates of the VSD and their corresponding lower limits for the various models are described in detail in the papers cited in the section on estimation procedures for the models.

APPLICATION TO DATA: EXAMPLE--VINYL CHLORIDE

In this section we do two things: (1) illustrate the methods for the models of Table 1 by applying the methods to the vinyl chloride data of Maltoni[18] on hepatic angiosarcoma with dose levels as adjusted for metabolic activation as given by Gehring et al.;[19] and (2) apply three of the four models (probit omitted) to the unadjusted data to illustrate the importance of using the effective dose to the target organ rather than the administered dose when biologically reasonable. The second application also illustrates the important role of metabolism in low-dose extrapolation.

Application of models to metabolized doses

Table 3 below presents the dose and toxicity data for the vinyl chloride experiment of Maltoni.[18] The original dose levels in column one are in ppm. of vinyl chloride inhaled by Sprague-Dawley rats for 4 hr./day, 5 days/wk. for 12 months. The toxic response of interest is hepatic angiosarcoma at the end of the experiment (135 weeks). The second column represents the dose levels in μg, metabolized/4 hr. as determined by Gehring et al.[19] The estimated conversion equation of dose d = ppm. exposed to d' = μg. metabolized/4 hr. exposed is given by

$$d' = \frac{(5706)(2.56)d}{860 + (2.56)d} \qquad (8)$$

For details see Gehring et al.[19]

TABLE 3

TOXIC RESPONSE DATA FOR VINYL CHLORIDE

Dose (ppm.)	Dose (µg. met./4 hrs.)	No. of animals tested	No. of responders
0	0	58	0
50	739	59	1
250	2,435	59	4
500	3,413	59	7
2,500	5,030	59	13
6,000	5,403	60	13
10,000	5,521	61	9

Using the metabolized dose levels, the four models of Table 1 yield the following results using all seven dose levels.

TABLE 4

ESTIMATED VSD (AND CONF. LIMITS) FOR VINYL CHLORIDE
VSD and 95% lower conf. limit in parentheses based on metabolized dose levels

Model	Risk level $P_0 = 10^{-4}$ µg./4 hrs.	ppm.	Risk level $P_0 = 10^{-6}$ µg./4 hrs.	ppm.
Probit[a]	76.3(.51)	4.6 (.03)	---	---
One-hit[b]	2.6(2.1)	.15(.12)	.026(.021)	.0015(.0012)
Multi-hit[c]	15.8(3.9)	.93(.23)	.507(.095)	.030 (.006)
Multi-stage[d]	4.1(1.8)	.24(.11)	.041(.018)	.002 (.001)

[a]Taken from Gehring et al.[19]
[b]Maximum likelihood estimates for p and β are $\hat{p} = 0$, $\hat{\beta}$ = .0000381.
[c]Maximum likelihood estimates for p, β and k are $\hat{p} = 0$, $\hat{\beta}$ = .0000739 and $\hat{k}$ = 1.34.
[d]GLOBAL program of Crump et al.[9] indicates a two-stage model with maximum likelihood estimates for p, α_1 and α_2 are $\hat{p} = 0$, $\hat{\alpha}_1$ = .000241 and $\hat{\alpha}_2$ = 3.077 x 10^{-8}.

Observe that the models differ in VSD by about a factor of 30 from largest
to smallest. The current standard set by the Department of Labor is one ppm.
average for 8 hrs. per day (see e.g., DHEW report [20]) appears to be well-
warranted to protect workers from an added risk of one in 10,000 from hepatic
angiosarcoma due to vinyl chloride if one assumes a 4 hr. daily exposure in
the rat as the equivalent of an 8 hr. daily exposure in man. If lower than
95% confidence limits are used, the standard indicated would be .1 to .2 ppm.
Thus, the estimates in this case, although they do not give an exact prediction of added risk and are quite variable, do provide some guideline for
regulation.

Use of administered dose versus effective dose

The example of vinyl chloride in this section illustrates vividly the need
for using the effective dose (here, the metabolized dose) rather than the
administered dose in doing predictions. By effective dose level we mean the
dose available to effect biologically the target organ. As demonstrated by
Gehring et al.[19] and their cited references, there is considerable evidence
that metabolic activation of vinyl chloride is required to transform it into a
bioactivated effective metabolic dose.

In Table 5, we present the low-dose predictions (with 95% lower limits) of
VSD using the three stochastic biological models using respectively 4, 5, 6,
and 7 of the dose levels of the data.

Examining Table 5, it is evident the models are more self-consistent over
varying dose levels included and more cross-consistent over models when applied
to the effective (metabolized) doses than when used on the administered doses.
Furthermore, if one uses administered doses there are vast differences between
the predictions using the multi-stage model (one-hit, here) and the multi-hit
model. The reason for this discrepancy is that both models try desperately to
"fit" the data at the higher dose levels whose observed response rates of 13/60
= .217 at 6,000 ppm. and 9/61 = .0148 at 10,000 ppm. are actually smaller than
the observed response rate of 13/59 = .222 at 2,500 ppm. Such reversals for
distantly placed dose levels are contrary to the model since P(d) is supposed
to be an increasing function of dose. Thus, in attempting to fit the data the
models are forced to make estimates of the parameters which are quite inaccurate.
This has a profound effect on the low-dose behavior of the predictions. For the
multi-hit model this forces $\hat{k}$ to be less than 1 and decreasing with more dose
levels included yielding increasingly concave upward dose-response curves near
the origin. This leads to extremely small predictions of VSD. See Rai and
Van Ryzin[5] for further discussion. For the one-hit (multi-stage) model the

TABLE 5

VSD FOR VINYL CHLORIDE FOR STOCHASTIC BIOLOGICAL MODELS

The number of dose levels used in each case starts from 0 dose level on up.
95% confidence limits are in parentheses.

Model	No. of dose levels	VSD at 10^{-4}	VSD at 10^{-6}	Remarks
One-hit[a]	4	.37(.25)	.0037(.0025)	$\hat{\beta}$=.00027
(administered	5	.84(.59)	.0084(.0059)	$\hat{\beta}$=.00012
dose level)	6	2.0 (1.5)	.0200(.0150)	$\hat{\beta}$=.000052
	7	5.0 (3.3)	.0500(.0330)	$\hat{\beta}$=.000023
One-hit[b]	4	.18(.12)	.0018(.0012	---[b]
(effective	5	.15(.11)	.0015(.0011)	---[b]
dose-level)	6	.14(.11)	.0014(.0011)	---[b]
	7	.15(.12)	.0015(.0012)	---[b]
Multi-hit	4	.12(.02)	$5 \times 10^{-4} (8 \times 10^{-5})$	$\hat{k}$=.89
(administered	5	$2 \times 10^{-3} (7 \times 10^{-4})$	$5 \times 10^{-7} (2 \times 10^{-7})$	$\hat{k}$=.55
dose level)	6	$3 \times 10^{-5} (9 \times 10^{-7})$	$4 \times 10^{-10} (1 \times 10^{-10})$	$\hat{k}$=.41
	7[c]	VSD<10^{-7}	VSD<10^{-12}	N.A.
Multi-hit[b]	4	.99(.18)	.03(.004)	$\hat{k}$=1.35
(effective	5	2.1 (.63)	.12(.03)	$\hat{k}$=1.62
dose level)	6	1.9 (.57)	.09(.02)	$\hat{k}$=1.57
	7	.93(.23)	.03(.006)	$\hat{k}$=1.34
Multi-stage[b]	4	.33(.10)	.0033(.0010)	2 stage[d]
(effective	5	.28(.07)	.0028(.0007)	3 stage[d]
dose level)	6	.34(.08)	.0034(.0008)	3 stage[d]
	7	.24(.11)	.0024(.0011)	2 stage[d]

[a]The multi-stage model reduces to the one-hit model in all cases for the administered dose level since GLOBAL indicates k = 1 stage.

[b]Predicted low-dose levels for this table have been converted to ppm. equivalents using equation (8). $\hat{\beta}$ is not available due to conversions.

[c]Computer program terminated due to lack of time.

[d]Number of stages as determined by GLOBAL.

effect is the exact opposite. The "best" estimate of the slope parameter $\hat{\beta}$ decreases from $\hat{\beta}$ = .00027 to $\hat{\beta}$ = .000023 since model is trying to compensate for the flattening of the response rates at the higher dose levels unadjusted for

metabolic activation. Since in the linear (one-hit) model the low-dose predictions are linear in d with slope $\hat{\beta}$, a smaller $\hat{\beta}$ yields larger safe dose levels
for a fixed P_0. This trend is clearly visible in Table 4. The discrepancy
between the models becomes quite dramatic at $P_0 = 10^{-6}$ for 6 and 7 dose levels
where the discrepancy is more the 7 orders of magnitude.

Some conclusions we feel warranted from this example are:

(1) Use effective dose levels in making low-dose predictions whenever
possible. Metabolism will play an important role with many other chemicals
beside vinyl chloride which need metabolic activation to become toxic.

(2) High doses in the experiment leading to reversals in the observed response rates and not adjustable as in (1) should be omitted based on some
goodness-of-fit criteria before a parametric model is fit and low-dose predictions are attempted. For an interesting further discussion see Brown.[21]

(3) More than one model should be used to make predictions. The understanding of discrepancies between models can be enlightening.

(4) The future understanding of metabolism and detoxification mechanisms,
including DNA repair, should help in getting biologically relevant effective
doses for better use of dose-response low-dose predictions.

LOW-DOSE LINEARITY VERSUS NON-LINEARITY

Many researchers feel that low-dose predictions for irreversible, delayed
toxic effects, such as carcinogenesis, should be done almost always by the one-
hit model. See, for example, the DHEW subcommittee report[1] and Peto[22] who
advocates this as a dogma. However, to always expect low-dose linearity seems
implausible to us. Non-linearity leading to concave dose-response curves can
be the result of metabolism, see, for example, Cornfield et al.,[23] Gehring and
Blau,[24] and Chapter 7 of the Food Safety Council Report.[2] Furthermore, the
possibility of repair mechanisms at low-dose levels, including DNA repair, may
well account for low-dose non-linearities in dose-response curves.

As we see it, the real question is when does one have enough evidence,
biologically or from data, to justify non-linearity at low doses. As shown in
a recent paper by Van Ryzin et al.,[25] the one-hit model gave an unacceptable fit
for four out of ten sets of carcinogenic response data, while the multi-stage
and multi-hit models gave acceptable fits in nine and ten cases respectively.
Both of these models do exhibit non-linearity of the added risk over background
model. The multi-stage model of equation (4) is non-linear if $\alpha_1 = 0$ and the
multi-hit model of equation (5) is non-linear if $k < 1$ or $k > 1$. Thus, the use
of a model for prediction allowing non-linearity seems warranted. To illustrate
this phenomena we give the following example.

An example of low-dose non-linearity

The set of data given in Table 6 is for rats exposed to ethylene thiourea and the response is thyroid carcinoma taken from Graham et al.[26]

TABLE 6

TOXIC RESPONSE DATA FOR ETHYLENE THIOUREA

Dose level (ppm.)	No. of animals tested	No. of responses
0	72	2
5	75	2
25	73	1
125	73	2
250	69	16
500	70	62

These data were applied to the three stochastic biological models of Table 1. Table 7 gives the VSD and the lower 95% confidence limits for each of the models.

Note that the multi-hit and multi-stage models show relatively close agreement for the predicted VSD at both risk levels, being within one order of magnitude in each case. However, the estimate of VSD from the one-hit model is approximately 1/1000th (1/60,600th) that of the multi-hit model and 1/400th (1/8050th) that of the multi-stage model at risk levels of 10^{-4} (10^{-6}), respectively. This is because the multi-hit and multi-stage best fitted models are both non-linear at low-dose, while the one-hit model forces linearity. Hence, the use of the one-hit or linear model is very conservative in the prediction of safe doses; unnecessarily, we feel, considering the non-linearity exhibited in the observed dose-response curve.

Comparing the 95% lower confidence limits, the multi-hit and multi-stage differ widely. This is because although the best fit to the multi-stage model is non-linear at low-dose, the estimated upper confidence curve allows a linear term which dominates in constructing the low-dose predictions. Although this may be useful from a regulatory point of view, where conservatism may be demanded, it is less useful as a scientific estimate of the low-dose risk.

The reason no such phenomenon occurs with the lower confidence limits in the multi-hit model is partly due to the method of their construction in Rai and

TABLE 7

VSD FOR ETHYLENE THIOUREA FOR THREE MODELS

95% confidence limit estimates are in parentheses.

Model	Maximum likelihood estimates of parameters	VSD at 10^{-4}	VSD at 10^{-6}
One-hit[a]	$\hat{p} = .012$, $\hat{\beta} = .0018$	.055(.046)	.00055(.00046)
Multi-hit	$\hat{p} = .022$, $\hat{\beta} = .0235$ $\hat{k} = 8.23$	62.8 (49.0)	33.4 (25.3)
Multi-stage	4 stages with $\hat{p} = .027$, $\hat{\alpha}_1 = \hat{\alpha}_2 = 0$ $\hat{\alpha}_3 = 1.1 \times 10^{-8}$ $\hat{\alpha}_4 = 1.28 \times 10^{-11}$	20.4 (.15)	4.4 (.0012)

[a]The one hit model is rejected by a chi-squared one-hit model goodness-of-fit test at significance level < .01.

Van Ryzin[5] based on large sample approximations and partly in the non-linearity for $k > 1$. To modify, in a conservative direction, the first of these, namely the method of constructing confidence intervals, we propose an alternative more conservative method in the next section.

However, before closing this section we raise the specter of possible non-linearities in the low-dose range which would include concave dose-response curves--the hyper-linear case. Such a curve is given by the multi-hit model whenever $0 < k < 1$. In such a case the added risk over background is approximately cd^k, $c > 0$ (see Rai and Van Ryzin[5]) leading to a curve rising faster than linear in the low-dose range. The vinyl chloride data of Tables 4 and 5 exhibited this behavior for the administered doses, but not the metabolized doses. Whether such behavior is justified biologically (it disappeared when applied to the proper metabolized doses) seems questionable. However, if there are highly toxic chemicals at low-dose which later saturate the system to some level of toxicity such could be the case. From a tolerance distribution view, the gamma density with $k < 1$ is possible. Such a population of tolerances would have a density function tending to $+\infty$ as the tolerance level approaches zero; steeper than the exponential when $k = 1$. Such a density would indicate a high frequency of very susceptible animals to the toxic response. Neither the one-hit nor multi-stage model allows hyper-linearity.

MODIFICATION OF THE MULTI-HIT MODEL CONFIDENCE LIMITS

The multi-hit model lower confidence limits as given by Rai and Van Ryzin[5] are based on standard large sample approximations (Taylor expansions). Such confidence limits are not very sensitive to changes in k while the model itself is. To remedy this consider the added risk over background function

$$P(d) = P(d;\beta,k) = \int_0^{\beta d} \frac{u^{k-1} e^{-u}}{\Gamma(k)} \, du.$$

as a function of β and k. It can be shown mathematically, for $k \geq 1$, that $P(d; \beta,k)$ is strictly decreasing in k. Also it is strictly increasing in β for all k. We omit the details of proof here. This observation immediately suggests the following method of low-dose extrapolation.

Method

1.) Find an upper $100(1-\gamma)\%$ confidence limit for β, denoted by $\beta_u(\gamma)$. Since $\hat{\beta}$ is asymptotically normal (see Rai and Van Ryzin[5]), this implies taking $\beta_u(\gamma) = \hat{\beta} + Z_\gamma \hat{\sigma}(\hat{\beta})$, where Z_γ is the $(1-\gamma)^{th}$ percentile of the standard normal distribution and $\hat{\sigma}(\hat{\beta})$ is the estimated standard error of $\hat{\beta}$.[5]

2.)' Find a lower $100(1-\gamma)\%$ confidence limit for k, denoted by $k_L(\gamma)$. Again, this is given approximately by $k_L(\gamma) = \hat{k} - Z_\gamma \hat{\sigma}(\hat{k})$ by the large sample theory in Rai and Van Ryzin,[5] where $\hat{\sigma}(\hat{k})$ is the estimated standard error of $\hat{k}$.[5]

3.) Use $P(d;\beta_u(\gamma),k_L(\gamma))$ as an upper limit on $P(d;\beta,k)$. This is an upper limit with probability at least $(1-\gamma)$ by the above montonicity property and the fact that both of the events $\beta \leq \beta_u(\gamma)$ and $k \geq k_L(\gamma)$ has probability larger than $(1-\gamma)$, the probability of each of the events.

4) Solve the equation $P(d^*;\beta_u(\gamma),k_L(\gamma)) = P_0$ to obtain d^* as a stringent lower confidence limit on VSD, since clearly $d^* \leq d^0$ with probability at least $(1-\gamma)$.

We illustrate this procedure for the ethylene thiourea data of Tables 5 and 6. For this data, $\hat{\sigma}(\hat{\beta}) = .0061$ and $\hat{\sigma}(\hat{k}) = 2.09$. Thus to obtain a 95% lower confidence limit, we take $\gamma = .05$, $Z_{.05} = 1.645$ and obtain

$$\beta_u(.05) = .0235 + (1.645)(.0061) = .0335$$

and

$$k_L(.05) = 8.23 - (1.645)(2.09) = 4.79,$$

where $\hat{\beta} = .0235$ and $\hat{k} = 8.23$ from Table 6. The results using this procedure are illustrated in Table 8. A computer program for these computations is available from the authors.

286

TABLE 8

RESULTS OF METHOD FOR ETHYLENE THIOUREA

Risk Level	Maximum likelihood estimate of VSD	Lower 95% conf. limit on VSD (standard)	Lower 95% conf. limit on VSD (conservative)
10^{-4}	62.8	50.1	11.9
10^{-6}	33.3	25.8	4.6
10^{-8}	18.4	13.9	1.6

In practice if $k_L(\gamma) \leq 1$, we recommend use of the one-hit model and if $k_L(\gamma) > 1$ use the above conservative method, if one wants a conservative confidence limit predictor. However, for scientific understanding as opposed to regulation, we feel that the maximum likelihood prediction of VSD is preferable.

CARCINOGENIC VERSUS NON-CARCINOGENIC TOXICITY

The argument has been put forward that the one-hit and multi-stage model with lower confidence limits (thus essentially a linear model) are most appropriate for carcinogenic (and other, irreversible) toxic effects, since these models explain the biology better. See Hoel et al.,[1] Peto[22] and Crump et al.[7] This is not evident to us and has been disputed in the literature by Mantel,[27] Cornfield[28] and Cornfield et al.[23] In view of the example of ethylene thiourea and other examples in the Food Safety Council Report,[2] we feel the use of the multihit (and other models) allowing for low-dose non-linearity makes eminent sense for carcinogenic data, as in the case of ethylene thiourea.

Let us now consider the use of dose-response models for non-carcinogenic toxicity. The common toxicological procedure for such data is to establish a *no observed effect level* (NOEL). By a NOEL is meant the determination of the highest dose level at which there is no statistically significant toxic effect over background and then dividing this dose by an arbitrary factor (10, 100, or 1,000) based on severity of the toxic effect. This procedure is undesirable because:

1) It has no biological basis
2) It is quite arbitrary
3) It uses no systematic dose-response information from all dose levels simultaneously
4) It is insensitive to sample size. Small experiments are rewarded for

not detecting differences. This is contrary to good dose-response methods which improve their estimates with increasing sample size.
The use of NOELs has been critized by a DHEW subcommittee report.[1]

The use of dose-response curves to predict low-dose toxicity should be encouraged. Such an approach has recently been recommended by the Scientific
Committee of the Food Safety Council.[2]

To illustrate the use of models for non-carcinogenic data, we now apply the
three stochastic biological models to the data of Table 9 for botulinum (type A)
toxicity data furnished by E.M. Foster of the Food Research Institute, University of Wisconsin-Madison to the Food Safety Council. The animals on test for
this data are mice weighing between 17-20 grams, the toxic response is death
due to botulism within 24 hours and the dose units are nanograms. The results
for the three models are given in Table 10.

TABLE 9

BOTULINUM TOXICITY DATA

Dose (ng.)	No. of animals tested	No. of responses
.010	30	0
.015	30	0
.020	30	0
.024	30	0
.027	30	0
.030	30	4
.034	30	11
.037	30	10
.040	30	16
.045	30	26
.050	30	26

For these data the dose-response curve is extremely steep. This is captured
by both the multi-hit ($\hat{k}$ large) and multi-stage (first five $\hat{\alpha}_i$'s are zero) and
in their respective VSD predictions. However, the linear model totally misses
this steepness resulting in ridiculously small VSD predictions. Thus, the multi-
stage and multi-hit models are flexible enough to detect non-linearity for steep
dose response curves. This example of use of dose response models for non-
carcinogenic data illustrates their usefulness for such data. For further

applications to such data see Rai and Van Ryzin.[5] For a further discussion of the use of dose-response models for non-carcinogenic risk assessment see Cornfield, p. 696.[28]

TABLE 10

VSD PREDICTIONS FOR BOTULINUM

95% confidence limits in parentheses

Model	Parameter estimates	Estimate of VSD at risk level 10^{-4}	10^{-6}
One-hit[a]	$\hat{p} = 0$ $\hat{\beta} = 11.92$	8.4×10^{-6} (5.7×10^{-6})	8.4×10^{-8} (5.7×10^{-8})
Multi-hit	$\hat{p} = 0$ $\hat{\beta} = 700.8$ $\hat{k} = 27.5$	.017 (.016) $(.007)^{b}$	.013 (.012) $(.005)^{b}$
Multi-stage	6 stage $\hat{p} = 0$ $\hat{\alpha}_1 = \hat{\alpha}_2 = \hat{\alpha}_3 = \hat{\alpha}_4 = \hat{\alpha}_5 = 0$ $\hat{\alpha}_6 = 1.77 \times 10^{10}$	.0091 (8.8×10^{-7})	.0042 (5.3×10^{-9})

[a]The one-hit model is rejected by a chi-squared goodness-of-fit test at significance level < .001.
[b]Lower 95% conservative confidence limit of previous section.

SUMMARY

We have tried to illustrate the use of some dose-response models for low-dose prediction. Our conclusions are:

(1) For scientific purpose, a variety of models, especially those allowing non-linear behavior should be used. Indeed, more should be developed by alternative methods of stochastic biological modeling as biological understanding improves.

(2) Metabolic activation of toxic substances may be crucial in the modeling and application of dose-response curves to low-dose prediction.

(3) Currently, the multi-hit and multi-stage appear to be highly useful and flexible models.

(4) The problem of transforming the low-dose animal predictions to man is a biological question whose answer may well depend on the species involved and

mechanism of the toxic substance.

(5) Effective biological doses should always replace administered doses in such predictions when the biology is well enough understood.

(6) With the present lack of knowledge many models should be tried.

(7) Dose-response predictions should replace NOELs whenever possible.

(8) For regulatory purposes conservative procedures are more warranted than for scientific purposes. This distinction should be paramount in applying these models.

(9) More realistic models are greatly needed in view of the tough environmental decisions facing man.

ACKNOWLEDGEMENTS

Research was supported by Grant No. 1-RO-1-GM23129, National Institute of General Medical Sciences, DHEW and pursuant to a grant to Rand from the U.S. Department of Health, Education and Welfare.

We wish to thank Ms. Patti Masthay, The Rand Corp., for certain computations in this paper and for implementing the GLOBAL program at Rand.

REFERENCES

1. Hoel, D.G., Gaylor, D.G., Kirschstein, R.L., Saffiotti, U., and Schneiderman, M.A. (1975) Jour. Toxicol. Env. Health, 1, 133-151.

2. The Scientific Committee, Food Safety Council (1978) Fd. and Cosmet. Toxicol., 16, Supp. 2, pp. 1-136.

3. Finney, D.J. (1952) Statistical methods in biological assay, Hafner Publishing Co., New York.

4. Chand, N. and Hoel, D.G. (1974) Reliability and Biometry: Statistical Analysis of Lifelength, SIAM Press, Phil., PA

5. Rai, K. and Van Ryzin, J. (1979) Energy and Health, SIAM Press, Phil., PA

6. Rai, K. and Van Ryzin, J. (1979) Rand publication, P-6305, Santa Monica, CA, submitted for publication.

7. Crump, K.S., Hoel, D.G., Langley, C.H. and Peto, R. (1976) Cancer Research, 36, 2973-2979.

8. Armitage, P. and Doll, R. (1961) Proc. of Fourth Berkeley Symp. on Stat. and Prob., 4, 19-38.

9. Crump, K.S., Guess, H.A., and Deal, K.L. (1977) Biometrics, 33, 437-451.

10. National Academy of Sciences, National Research Council (1972) Report of the advisory committee of the biological effects of ionizing radiation Govt. Printing Office Publ. No. 0-489-797, Washington, D.C.

11. Cornfield, J. (1954) Statistics and Mathematics in Biology, Iowa State Univ. Press, Ames, 123.

12. Nordling, C.O. (1953) Br. J. Cancer, 7, 68-72.

13. Marshall, J.H. and Groer, P.G. (1977) Radiation Research, 71, 149-192.

14. National Academy of Sciences, (1977) Drinking water and health, Washington, D.C.

15. Abbott, W.S. (1925) J. Econ. Entom., 18, 265-267.

16. Mantel, N. and Bryan, W.R. (1961) J. Natl. Cancer Inst., 27, 455-470.

17. Guess, H.A. and Crump, K.S. (1978), Ann. Stat., 6, 101-111.

18. Maltoni, C. (1975) Ambio, 4(1), 18-23.

19. Gehring, P.J., Watanabe, P.G., and Park, C.N. (1978) Toxicol. Appl. Pharmacol. 44, 581-591.

20. Department of Health, Education and Welfare (1978) Vinyl Chloride DHEW Publ. No., (NIH) 78-1599, pp. 1-91.

21. Brown, C.C. (1978) J. Natl. Cancer Inst., 60(1), 101-108.

22. Peto, R. (1978) Environ. Health Persp., 22, 155-159.

23. Cornfield, J., Carlborg, F. and Van Ryzin, J. (1978) Proc. First Intl. Cong. Toxicol., Plaa and Duncan (Ed.), Academic Press, 143-164.

24. Gehring, P.J. and Blau, G.E. (1977) J. Environ. Pathol. Toxicol, 1, 163-179.

25. Van Ryzin, J., Rai, K. and Cornfield, J. (1979) Submitted for publication.

26. Graham, S.L., Davis, K.S., Hansen, W.H., Graham, C.H. (1975) Fd. Cosmet. Toxicol., 13, 493-499.

27. Mantel, N. (1978) Cancer Research, 38, 1835-1838.

28. Cornfield, J. (1977) Science, 198, 693-699.

© 1980 Elsevier/North-Holland Biomedical Press
The Scientific Basis of Toxicity Assessment
H. Witschi, editor.

RADIATION TOXICOLOGY: CARCINOGENESIS[*]

R. J. M. FRY, J. B. STORER AND R. L. ULLRICH

Biology Division, Oak Ridge National Laboratory, Oak Ridge, Tennessee 37830

INTRODUCTION

The study of radiation toxicology is about as old as the proverbial life span of man. Despite intensive research and the development of a remarkable body of information about the effects of radiation of different qualities, there is still no absolute agreement on how radiation kills cells or induces tumors. Not only is there a practical need for an understanding of various radiation effects but there is still the excitement of investigating the mechanisms by which deposition of energy results in major biological effects.

Radiations of different wavelengths vary in their biological effects (Table 1). Radiations with wavelengths greater than 320 nm are considered noncarcinogenic but very few systematic late effects studies have been carried out with the longer wavelengths. With raditions such as infrared and radio-waves, thermal damage is the common feature. There are no data on the carcinogenic effects of hyperthermia in animals, and heat does not transform cells[1]. The relative amounts of the different types of radiation-induced macromolecular damage vary considerably for the spectrum of radiations that are carcinogenic. It is clear that the more densely ionizing radiations (probably up to about 100 kev/μ) are more effective than the sparsely ionizing for several biological endpoints including tumorigenesis. But there is yet no evidence that a DNA lesion common to the various radiation qualities is involved in carcinogenesis. In the case of ultraviolet radiation there seems to be a correlation between the wavelengths that interact with DNA and those that result in skin cancer. The spatial and temporal characteristics of the deposition of energy of radiation of different qualities provide a potentially powerful probe for investigating the mechanisms of malignant transformation.

---

[*]Research sponsored by the Office of Health and Environmental Research, U.S. Department of Energy, under contract W-7405-eng-26 with the Union Carbide Corporation. Some of the research reported in this paper was carried out by R. J. M. Fry and colleagues at the Division of Biological and Medical Research, Argonne National Laboratory, Argonne, Illinois, under contract W-31-109-eng-38.

TABLE I

Type of Radiation	Source		Wavelength NM	Molecular Lesions	Adverse Biological Effects
	Natural	Other			
Gamma	Radioactive minerals	Medical	1×10^{-4} 1.4×10^{-1}	Single strand breaks Double strand breaks Base Damage	Cell killing Mutagenesis Teratogenesis Carcinogenesis
X-rays	Sun	Medical	$5 \times 10^{-4} - 20$		Cell killing Carcinogenesis
Ultraviolet	Sun		$40 - 390$	Pyrimidine dimers Base damage Thymine photoproducts DNA-protein crosslinks	320 nm considered noncarcinogenic
Visible	Sun		$390 - 780$		
Infrared	Sun		$780-4 \times 10^{5}$	Thermal damage	Cell killing
Radio waves	Sun	Radar TV Radio	$10^{5}-3 \times 10^{13}$	Thermal damage	Cell killing Deafness ?
Power A.C.		Electric Power lines	10^{5}	?	?

Radiation, unlike some of the chemicals about which there is concern today, has been present through man's evolution. The heat from the radioactive elements in the earth's crust has helped shape its surface. We know less about the way in which radiation has influenced the design of man although it seems reasonable to believe exposure to both ionizing and nonionizing radiation has influenced the development of systems capable of repairing damage to DNA and recovery from both the consequences of DNA damage and also from lesions in molecules and structures not associated with DNA. Although a small fraction of the incidence of cancer is attributed, by some, to environmental radiation it is not known with certainty whether or not this level of radiation does cause cancer.

The natural radiation background varies, depending on geographical location, by as much as a factor of 20^2. Unfortunately, there are no adequate studies of the human populations such as those on the Kerala coast in India that are exposed to about 2 rem/yr background radiation or those in Brazil exposed to high background radiation from the monozite sand. It would be very valuable to compare the effects of background irradiation in these populations and those exposed to less than 100 mrem/yr. Despite the profound difficulties in such an epidemiological approach Frigerio and Stone[3] considered it so attractive that they examined cancer rates in relation to the varying levels of background radiation within the U.S. Although the results suggested a negative correlation between radiation levels and cancer mortality the problems of lack of uniformity of medical treatment, the recording of cancer mortality, and the fact that the range in the background levels is small, compromise any conclusions.

In the case of ultraviolet radiation (UVR) a distinct association has been established between the environmental level of the radiation at different latitudes and the incidence of skin cancer[4,5].

Time and Radiation. Time after irradiation is important for the expression of the biological effects and the interval, or latent period, between the exposure and the development of tumors is long. Time-dose relationships, such as dose-rate and fractionation have a profound influence on the effect of irradiation.

Latent Period. The amount of time necessary for the expression of different types of radiation-induced lesions varies with the nature of the lesion and is also influenced by the total dose of radiation. Some effects, such as cancer, are expressed months or years after exposure and this is one of the diffi- culties in epidemiological studies of cancer. Obviously, exposure to many other factors in the interval between radiation exposure and tumor appearance complicates the studies. Similarly in animal experiments competing risks from diseases other than that under study confound the analyses. It is established that radiation can act as a complete carcinogen, as an initiator, and also interacts as a co-carcinogen. But the role of irradiation, particularly low dose protracted irradiation, in enhancing or promoting the expression of tumors induced by various other agents is not understood. The importance of such interaction is shown by the finding that uranium miners who smoke had 10 times the excess of lung cancers than miners who did not smoke[6].

In the case of UVR, Blum suggested that the effect of many of the later fractions in the multifraction regimes necessary for carcinogenesis was on the expression of the initiation events[7]. This idea has been confirmed. When the promoter phorbol ester is used after a regime of UVR a comparable incidence of tumors is produced with fewer fractions of UVR[8]. In the case of protracted or fractionated exposures of ionizing radiation there has been very little work that allows a separate examination of the effect on initiation and an expression of the initial lesions.

Experimentally, the term "latent period" has various meanings depending on the organ, the endpoint, and the methods of detection of the selected endpoint. For example, the latent period for skin tumor development may be from the time of exposure to the appearance of the first tumor of a size that can be recognized. As very small tumors can be recognized in the skin the estimate of time of appearance may not be much greater than the time for the necessary cell divisions for the growth to a size that can be seen by the eye, and any time that may exist between the exposure and the onset of tumor growth. The latent period, for lung tumors, if based on the time from the exposure to time of death due to the tumor, will depend very much on the degree of malignancy and site of the tumor. Admittedly, most of the natural history of a tumor is over by the time it is detected. Despite the lack of understanding of the biology of the latent period, Blum[7], Druckery[9], and more recently Albert and Altshuler[10] have found that the time of tumor appearance has a log normal distribution that is dependent on dose rate and that the dose rate multiplied by a power of the median time to appearance is a constant. It has been accepted by some authors that higher doses result in earlier appearance of tumors than with lower doses[11,12]. Unfortunately, there is no body of data that shows unequivocally the time of appearance to be dependent on dose and independent of the change in incidence that accompanies higher doses of the carcinogenic agents.

The distinction between advancement of the time of appearance of naturally

occurring tumors and the induction of tumors is not a trivial matter and is
fundamental to the understanding of mechanisms and susceptibility to cancer
induction. There are a number of tumors which occur with a high natural
incidence in rodents; in some strains the incidence may reach nearly 100%, for
example, liver tumors in C3H mice, and mammary tumors in Sprague Dawley rats.
Presumably the observed radiation effect in such cases can only be related to
the time of appearance. In Figure 1 the dose-dependent change in time at
death from lung tumors after exposure to fission neutrons is shown. In this
hybrid mouse no dose-dependency for the number of mice dying from lung tumors
was found but only a change in time of death after exposure[13].

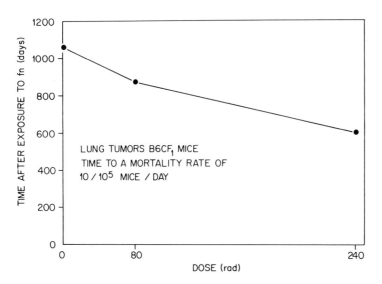

Fig. 1. Time to a selected mortality rate due to lung tumors in female B6CF[1]
/Anl mice as a function of dose of Janus fission neutrons.

    The marked difference in time to appearance of tumors in various species
is one of the facets that must be understood if extrapolations across species
are to be made: The equally marked difference in life span between species
has encouraged interest in the idea that the temporal pattern of tumor response
is dependent on life span[14,15]. The idea of finding a correction factor for
life span differences that allows meaningful comparisons or even extrapolations
for tumor rates across species is attractive but perhaps too optimistic.
    Dose-Response Relationships. The data for radiation-induced cancer in humans
are still insufficient to determine the shape of the dose response curves.
Furthermore, human studies have shed little or no light on the mechanisms of

tumorigenesis. Studies in radiation carcinogenesis in experimental animals are useful for the investigation of mechanisms, for the determination of time-dose relationships, such as the effect of dose rate and fractionation, and to obtain dose response curves at least of sufficient quality to test models.

The simplest models suggested for the dose response curves for high linear energy transfer (LET) radiation, such as neutrons, and low-LET radiation such as gamma radiation are linear and curvilinear respectively (Fig. 2). Nowadays

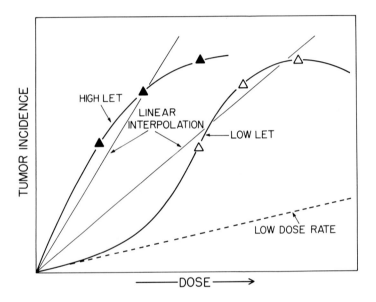

Fig. 2. Schematic dose response curves for tumor incidence after exposure to high and low LET radiation with linear interpolations through selected points of the curves.

the equations that describe the curves usually have some correction for cell killing. It is not surprising that these models, if it is appropriate to call them that, are too simple. First of all it is clear that the mechanism of tumorigenesis, though not necessarily induction, involves different factors. For example, the mechanisms involved in the production of hormonal dependent tumors must surely be different from the production of a sarcoma. So there is no a priori reason that one model will be suitable for more than one or a small number of tumor types. In tumor dose-response curves tumor incidence is often plotted as a function of dose but the occurrence of a tumor involves not only the malignant transformation of a cell but also the factors that influence the subsequent expression (and repression). The models for dose response curves

are really based on the dose response of initial events or transformation and
not sufficient for what many workers believe to be a multistage process.

An example of the influence of hormones on radiation-induced cancer is
shown in Fig. 3. Pituitaries were grafted into the spleens of mice to increase

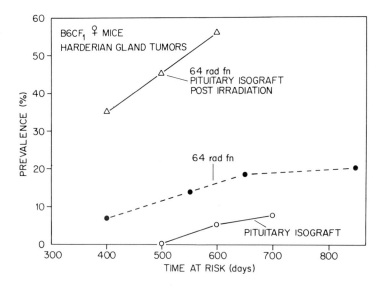

Fig. 3.   The prevalence of Harderian gland tumors in female B6CF$_1$/Anl after
pituitary isograft only o——o after a single exposure to 64 rad fn only ●---●
and to 64 rad fn followed by pituitary isograft on the same day Δ——Δ.

the level of prolactin. This treatment advanced the time of appearance of the
small number of naturally occurring Harderian gland tumors (data not shown in
Fig. 3) without any significant increase in the incidence. When pituitaries
were grafted into mice after they had been irradiated there was marked increase
in the tumor prevalence compared to mice exposed only to radiation. For
Harderian gland tumors the increased prolactin level appears to act as a promoter.

The effect of the pituitary isografts on mammary tumors was quite different.
The cumulative natural incidence of mammary tumors in B6CF$_1$ mice is about 1%.
The increased prolactin levels from the pituitary isograft resulted in an incidence of 43% of mammary tumors. If we assume that the raised prolactin levels
maximize the expression of the radiation-induced transformation in both the
mammary and Harderian glands then the excess tumors in mice exposed to radiation
compared to the tumor incidence in mice with pituitary isografts and irradiation

should be a measure of the radiation induced initial events. It was found that the effect of both gamma and neutron irradiation on the incidence of mammary tumors was very small compared to the effect of altering the prolactin level. Furthermore the effect on tumorigenesis of the combined hormone and radiation treatment that could be attributed to the radiation was much less in the mammary gland than with the Harderian gland.

The results shown in Fig. 4 (unpublished data, Fry, R. J. M., Grube, D. and

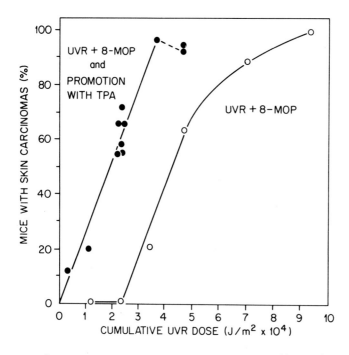

Fig. 4. The percent of mice with squamous cell carcinomas as a function of total dose of 320-400 nm UVR given in various numbers of fractions plus 8-methoxy-psoralen o——o and similar exposures but followed at the end of the fractionation regime by treatment with 5 µg of TPA 3/week.

Ley, R. D.) provide a good example how the expression of the initial tumor induction events influence the shape of the dose response curve. The curve on the right representing the incidence of skin cancer as a function of total dose of UVR in mice photosensitized with 8-methoxypsoralen (8-MOP) appears sigmoid in shape and shows a threshold. When the total doses were reduced by decreasing the number of fractions but the exposures to UVR + 8-MOP regimes were followed by promotion by 12-0-tetradecanoyl phorbol-13-acetate (TPA) the

shape of the dose response curve appears to be more linear and without a threshold. These results suggest: (1) that with the UV radiation some of the transformed cells did not express their tumor potential, and (2) accurate dose
response relationships for the induction or initial events of transformation
are not necessarily represented by the incidence of cancer as a function of
dose.

For other tissues and organs, we need similar techniques that will allow
us to dissect out the radiation-induced initial events from the influence of
endogenous and exogenous factors that influence the final tumor incidence.

The Influence of Experimental Results on Human Risk Estimates. The use of
linear interpolation from higher dose levels for estimating the human risk of
cancer has been accepted as a conservative approach for handling the data for
low-LET radiation and a reasonable method for high-LET radiation. Recently,
it has been suggested that even in the case of low-LET radiation that interpolation could underestimate the effects[16]. The available experimental data
do not support such a suggestion.

In an attempt to illustrate some aspects of this question we have made a
comparison of linear fits of the data for dose responses from a number of
different tumor types obtained after exposure to radiation at (a) high dose
rate (above 7 rad/min) and (b) low dose rate (below 0.06 rad/min)[17-20]. The
results are shown in Fig. 5. The solid lines indicate the range of slopes
obtained from linear fits to the data for the responses of the selected tumors
after exposure to radiation at a high dose rate. The slopes of the linear
fits of the data for the responses of the same tumor types after exposure to
low dose-rate irradiation are shown individually. It can be seen that all of
the responses to irradiation at low dose rates are less than the range of
responses to irradiation at high dose rates. The relative range of dose
levels is indicated for the different tumor types. For example, the zero
slope for thymic lymphoma is for the data up to 100 rad. It is clear that the
effect of lowering the dose rate is tissue dependent and varies considerably.
The results for myeloid leukemia after low dose irradiation are of particular
interest. The experiments of Upton et al., and Ullrich and Storer were carried
out on the same strain of mouse (RFM) but in the case of Ullrich and Storer's
experiment the mice were maintained in a specific-pathogen-free facility.
The explanation for the difference in the results from these studies is not
known but perhaps the different microbial environment results in a difference
in the number of myeloid stem cells at risk. What is clear is that simple
interpretations of dose response curves based purely on biophysical aspects are
unwise. It can be seen from Fig. 2 that in the case of low-LET radiation that

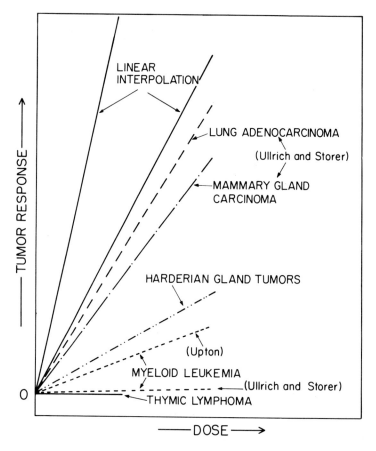

Fig. 5. Plot of the slopes of tumor incidence as a function of dose derived from linear interpolation of data assuming no threshold for exposures to high dose rate irradiation solid lines and for the same

linear interpolation will overestimate risks for tumors with a curvilinear dose-response. But without a precise knowledge of the dose response relationships for different types of radiation-induced cancer there was no choice for the advisory bodies concerned with radiation protection; they had to recommend the use of a linear no-threshold model.

In the case of high-LET radiation if a linear interpolation of the data obtained from relatively low doses is made and the dose response curve bends as shown, the risk for low doses of high-LET radiation will be underestimated. In Fig. 6 it can be seen that the curve for the incidence of Harderian gland tumors as a function of dose of fission neutrons bends over. As the mice in

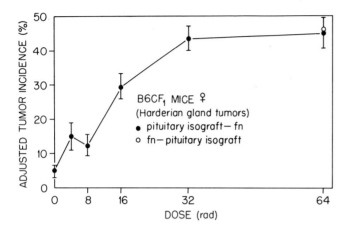

Fig. 6. The adjusted incidence of Harderian gland tumor as a function of dose of Janus fission neutrons in mice with pituitary grafts before irradiation x——x. The incidence of tumors in mice exposed to 64 rad fn and that received pituitary isografts post irradiation is indicated: 0

this experiment had pituitary isografts before irradiation, which we assume maximizes the expression, the bending is probably due to factors influencing the initial events of induction. The reason for the bending over is not known but may reflect cell killing[21]. Another possibility is that with high-LET radiation there is a linear increase as the number of effective targets traversed by a particle increase but as soon as the dose reaches a level at which each effective target has been traversed by a particle the curve saturates. The distinction between cell killing and the saturation effect is difficult and, of course, both may be involved.

Human Risk Estimates. Estimates of risk are expressed in one of two ways, either in absolute or relative terms. For radiation protection, absolute risk estimates are usually used and the absolute risk is expressed as the number of excess cases of cancer assumed to be radiation-induced per unit of time in an exposed population of stated size per unit of dose; for example, 1 case/10^6 persons/year/rad. Such estimates normally assume a linear dose-response relationship for dose levels for which there are no data. The estimate of the total risk to a population exposed also requires knowledge about the period of years over which the excess risk exists. Except for radiation-associated leukemia it is not known for how long an excess risk exists. In the case of solid cancers the excess risk may last to the end of life. In the case of leukemia the risk decreases after 20-25 years after exposure. The risk period is also dependent on the type of tumor and perhaps the age at time of exposure

302

of the person. In persons exposed at older ages (over 50) the risk of
developing a radiation-associated tumor is offset by competing risks. Relative
risk is the ratio between the irradiated population and the risk in the non-
irradiated population and is expressed as a multiple of the natural risk. The
dose that doubles the natural incidence is referred to as the doubling dose.
If the natural incidence determines the susceptibility and the increase in
risk after radiation is proportional to the natural risk then the use of
relative risk would be appropriate. The importance of understanding the
relationship of the natural incidence of a tumor to the response to radiation
is not just a matter of interest in risk estimates but could provide a possible
insight into mechanisms.

The determination of the relationship of the natural incidence with
radiation response would seem amenable to experimental validation. Surprisingly
the question has not been systematically investigated. The data in Table II
show that in the case of the tumors selected it is not possible to eliminate
the possibility that the risk of radiation carcinogenesis is influenced by the
natural incidence. The paucity of cases of chronic lymphocytic leukemia in the
atomic bomb survivors and in the rest of the Japanese population is consistent
with the hypothesis that the natural incidence does influence the response to
radiation. It seems surprising that there has been so little attention to this
problem.

CONCLUSIONS

Experimental radiation carcinogenesis has demonstrated that there are a
considerable number of factors that influence both the initial events that lead

TABLE 2

Tumor Site	Mouse Strain	Relationship of Natural Incidence and Susceptibility	
		Natural Incidence %	Radiation Excess Incidence per rad (%)
Ovarian	RFM	2.4	0.39
Ovarian	BALB/c	6.4	1.2
Mammary Gland	BALB/c	7.0	0.12
Mammary Gland	BCF$_1$	1.2	0.01

to cancer and the expression of those events. It is clear that the dose rate and the LET of the radiation influence the induction of the initial events. The factors that influence the expression, and therefore the actual incidence of cancer, are multiple and include endogenous factors such as hormones. Since estimation of the effects of very low doses of radiation must be based on models rather than direct observation it is clear that we need models that take into account the multistage nature of carcinogenesis. We also need a greater understanding of how the natural incidence of various types of cancer influences the response to radiation.

REFERENCES

1. Harisiadis, L., Miller, R. G., Harisiadas, S. and Hall, E. J. Br. J. Radiol. (in press).

2. Hill, J. (1979) Br. J. Radiol., 52, 2-13.

3. Frigerio, N. A. and R. S. Stone (1976) Carcinogenic and Genetic Hazard from Background Radiation, in Biological and Environmental Effects of Low Level Radiation. Vol. II, pp 385-393, IAEA.

4. Urbach, F. (1974) Ultraviolet Carcinogenesis Experimental Global and Genetic Aspects in Sunlight and Man. (eds.) T. B. Fitzpatrick, M. A. Pathak, L. C. Harber, M. Seiji and A. Kukita, University of Tokyo Press, pp 259-283.

5. Magnus, K. (1977) Int. J. Cancer, 20, 477-485.

6. Lundin, F. E., Jr., Lloyd, J. W., Smith, E. M., Archer, V. E. and Haladay, D. A. (1969) Mortality of Uranium Miners in Relation to Radiation Exposure, Hard-Rock Mining and Cigarette Smoking - 1950 through September 1967. Health Physics, 16, 571-578.

7. Blum, H. F. (1959) Carcinogenesis by Ultraviolet Light, Princeton University Press, Princeton, NJ.

8. Fry, R. J. M., Ley, R. D. and Grube, D. D. (1978) Photosensitized Reactions and Carcinogenesis. Natl. Cancer Inst. Monogr. 50: 39-43.

9. Druckery, H. (1967) Quantitative Aspects of Chemical Carcinogenesis, in Potential Carcinogenic Hazards from Drugs, Evaluation of Risks, UICC Monograph Series (ed.) R. Truhaut. Vol. 7, Springer-Verlag, New York, pp 60-78.

10. Albert, R. E. and Altshuler, B. (1973) Consideration Relating to the Formulation of Limits for the Unavoidable Population Exposure to Environmental Carcinogens, in Radiationnuclid Carcinogenesis. AEC Symposium Series 29, (eds.) C. L. Sanders, R. M. Busch, J. E. Ballou and D. D. Mahlum, pp 233-253.

11. Evans, R. D. (1966) Br. J. Radiol., 39, 881-895.

12. Nelson, N. (1978) Environmental Health Perspectives, 22, 93-95.

13. Ainsworth, E. J. (1977) Dose-Effect Relationships for Life-Shortening, Tumorigenesis and Systematic Injuries in Mice Irradiated with Fission Neutron or ^{60}Co Gamma Radiation. Proceedings of International Radiation Protection Association IVth Intern. Congress, pp 143-151.

14. Grahn, D. (1970) Biological Effects of Protracted Low Dose Radiation Exposure of Man and Animals in Late Effects of Radiation. (eds.) R. J. M. Fry, D. Grahn, M. L. Griem and J. H. Rust. Taylor-Francis Ltd., London.

15. Albert, R. E., Burns, F. and Shore, R. (1978) Comparison of the Incidence and Time Patterns of Radiation-Induced Skin Cancer in Humans and Rats, in Late Effects of Ionizing Radiation, Vol. 2, IAEA, Vienna.

16. Brown, J. M. (1976) Health Physics, 31, 231-245.

17. Ullrich, R. L. and Storer, J. B. (1978) Influences of Dose, Dose Rate and Radiation Quality on Radiation Carcinogenesis and Life Shortening in RFM and BALB/c Mice. in, Late Effects of Ionizing Radiation, Vol. 2, pp IAEA, Vienna.

18. Ullrich, R. L. (1979) Carcinogenesis in Mice after Low Doses and Dose Rates, in Proceedings of 32nd Annual Symposium on Fundamental Cancer Research, Houston, Texas (in press).

19. Upton, A. C., Randolph, M. L. and Conklin, J. W. (1970) Late Effects of Fast Neutrons and Gamma Rays in Mice as Influenced by the Dose Rate of Irradiation. Induction of Neoplasia. Radiat. Res., 41, 467-491.

20. Ullrich, R. L. and Storer, J. B. (1979) Influence of Gamma Ray Irradiation on the Development of Neoplastic Disease. III. Dose Rate Effects. Radiat. Res. (in press).

21. Mole, R. H. (1975) Br. J. Radiol., 48, 157-169

© 1980 Elsevier/North-Holland Biomedical Press
The Scientific Basis of Toxicity Assessment
H. Witschi, editor.

THE NEED TO UNDERSTAND MECHANISMS

W.N. Aldridge, Medical Research Council, Toxicology Unit,
Carshalton,Surrey,England.

As a contributor of the final formal paper in this Symposium I feel
somewhat superfluous.   Over the last four days we have been presented
with experimental results which illustrate the need to understand mechanisms.   I am sure that I could sit down now and the message would be
understood.   However,I have a task before me and shall try to state some
of my personal views about the conduct of research in toxicology.   It
is often the case that in such a general approach precision is lost and
only an expression of pious hope results. I hope to avoid this end product, beginning with some definitions and then illustrating them with
examples which have not been discussed extensively during this symposium,

The emphasis I wish to present is that in the biological sciences
toxicology is a unique example of a science which, if it is to develop,
must be the meeting place of work carried out by scientists trained in a
variety of basic disciplines.   Success requires that the best scientists in these disciplines collaborate on a common problem - none may be
relegated to a subordinate or service role.   As a science requiring
such a multidisciplinary approach it provides a model for us to explore
the administrative arrangements to facilitate progress.   In such a task
we cannot ignore the fact that the structure of Universities, dominated
as they are by their teaching role, often is not conducive to fruitful
multidisciplinary collaboration; the grant-giving bodies also,I believe,
have not yet discovered how to assess, in a predictive sense, the
requirements for and success rating of multidisciplinary grant applications.

Toxicology is the science of toxic substances and toxicity is a
change from the normal in the structure or function of living organisms.
The purpose of this symposium is to generate information which allows
rational decisions about hazards to man.   During the course of this
contribution I hope to show that the exploration of mechanisms provides
information not only useful for this purpose but for other purposes also
- not least the possibility of the design of chemicals active in their

primary purpose but much safer in use and less hazardous to man.

Before proceeding with the selected topic - the need for understanding mechanisms of toxicity - I wish to digress a little and say a little about the development of scientific knowledge. It is often implicitly assumed that the flow of useful information in science is from the basic or pure studies to the practical. This is not by any means the case. Historically the development of particular areas of science has followed from the need and/or desire to understand some natural phenomena. Himsworth in a book entitled "The development and organisation of scientific knowledge" has presented a convincing case that this is so. The usual analogy for the development of knowledge is the tree of knowledge, the trunk being the general science out from which develops via the branches the more specialised sciences. Himsworth considers that this is entirely misleading and presents an analogy which is diametrically opposite. The model he puts forward is that of a vast globe of primitive ignorance, around which there is a whole series of problems prompting men to seek knowledge. In this model these problems provide the specialised information in total contrast to the tree of knowledge analogy. To continue his extension of his "globe concept" I quote from his book:-

> "I have been emboldened to suggest a different
> concept of structure: that of a vast globe of
> ignorance from the surface of which at many
> different places enquiries are being driven
> centrally to deeper levels where they tend
> increasingly to coalesce and to produce sub-
> jects that come to underline, not one, but
> several such penetrations. These penetrations
> I have called provinces of natural knowledge
> and I conceive of each of these forming a
> smooth continuum of interrelated subjects from
> its specialized periphery to the more unspec-
> ialized depths of its penetration. It is
> within the perspective of such provinces that
> the individual scientific subjects find their
> intellectual context and larger significance".
>   Himsworth (1970)[1]

The application of this view to Toxicology is obvious. The drive to understand mechanisms, prompted by the specialised requirements of the assessment of the hazard of a chemical capable of producing a particular change in structure or function, leads to the development of information of value for the solution of many problems. Not least, something which Himsworth goes to great lengths to emphasize, the drive to understand the problem thrown up by practical questions , throws light on hitherto little understood areas of science. In no other science is this more true than in the study of toxicity. Very few toxins are understood in the sense that the relationship between the primary interactions of the chemical with the final clinical condition is clear.

It is vital that support for the understanding of mechanisms of toxicity of many kinds is forthcoming. Although our major worries are in the assessment of hazards arising from chemicals producing chronic toxicity - carcinogenesis, mutagenesis, teratogenesis, central nervous effects and immunological responses - we must not restrict work to these areas. The advance of knowledge of all forms of toxicity provides the climate of thought on which all assessment of safety must depend. The emphasis I would like to make is the encouragement of young scientists with the drive to understand mechanisms - i.e. if people of the right calibre are involved, the understanding will follow. The study of mechanisms conjures up to many the generation of great detail about a topic. This is often necessary to confirm or demolish a hypothesis but it can also be, although involving exacting methodology, very pedestrian in its intellectual content and sometimes purely gap filling. In the study of the interactions of chemicals with biological systems, great emphasis is and should be placed on the definition of molecular inter-actions, but it should not be assumed that advance only arrives by this route. Molecular biology by its success has provided us with many lessons but I suggest that it's main contribution has been to show those of us interested in biological processes the value of precision in the hypotheses we develop. It is the attitude of mind which is important and a topic may be advanced by the appreciation that a series of symptoms in an animal may be separated into several with different structure - response relationships. Such a finding requires patient observation of poisoned animals and no molecular approach - only a discriminating and enquiring mind. Some observations which come to mind have, in my view, great potential for advance in knowledge, not only in toxicology, but also in basic biological science. For example, the new insecticides, the synthetic pyrethroids, may be separated into at least two groups by the different symptomology they produce in mammals[2,3], the multiplicative effect of smoking on brochogenic carcinoma in those exposed to asbestos[4],[5], the demonstration that trimethyltin produces neuronal lesions only in the hippocampus, pyriform cortex and amygdaloid nucleus[7],[8] a long time after the original observation of the behavioural effects produced in rats by this compound. Of course the selection of these examples is highly personal but serves to illustrate that advance in a particular area nearly always depends on some qualitative view of cause and effect. The exploration of the mechanisms involved provide the means of using the information for other purposes and the acceptance of generalising concepts. Before passing to a topic to illustrate the importance of the continual traffic in information and ideas between the practical and the detailed research, and of the benefits which may develop from the knowledge of mechanisms, I wish to provide a simple framework to consider most toxicological problems. In figure 1 is illustrated the whole process from entry of the chemical

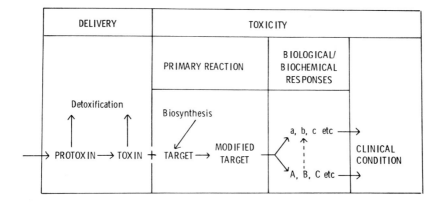

Fig.1. Scheme illustrating different aspects of toxicity

into the final clinical condition. In the first section are all those processes which affect the delivery of the toxic chemical to its site of action. The primary target (enzyme, membrane, macromolecule, receptor etc.) and its reaction with the proximal toxic chemical is the second section. This is followed by the exceedingly complex definition of the many cascades of biochemical/biological responses which flow from this primary interaction. Some of these lead to disease and the final clinical condition. This framework is, of course, a highly simplified view but may serve to focus on certain aspects of toxicity and to emphasize the importance of continual interplay between the beginning and end of the process i.e. entry of the chemical and the clinical condition - on the progress of research into mechanisms. The identification of the primary target is vital for the elucidation of the quantitive importance of factors other than the structure-activity relationships of chemicals for the target.

The anti-esterase compounds (esters of organophosphorus, carbamic and organosulphur acids) have been studied long enough for the value of research into mechanisms to be assessed.

Amongst this class of compound there are an almost infinite series of structures. The quantitative extent of other processes which affect the delivery of the toxin to its site of action are also very varied - for example in the influence of the route of absorption, physical properties of the compound, secretion, excretion, organ distribution, non-specific binding etc . A major determinant of toxicity is the metabolic transformation of this class of chemical; some lead to detoxification but many lead to increased toxicity. It is mainly due to difference in the above processes that selective toxicity arises i.e.high toxicity to insects combined with low toxicity to man. However, these are not the only ways toxicity may be modified. When certain spider mites or houseflies become resistant to organophosphorus compounds changes have taken place in the primary target, acetylcholin-esterase, such that it is much less susceptible to inhibition by a par-ticular organophosphorus compound[9],[11]. The enzyme, in the case of the spider mite so radically changed in its reactivity with organophos-phorus compounds, clearly retains an ability to hydrolyze acetylcholine. Organophosphorus compounds, carbamates and sulphonates are selective reagents for esterases possessing a particular catalytic centre containing serine and react in way analogous to their hydrolysis of substrates (Fig.2).

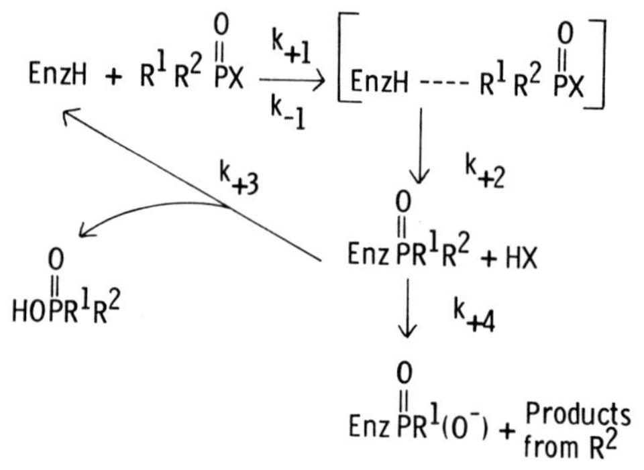

$$\text{EnzH} + R^1R^2\overset{O}{\underset{\ \ }{P}}X \xrightarrow[k_{-1}]{k_{+1}} \left[\text{EnzH} \text{----} R^1R^2\overset{O}{\underset{\ \ }{P}}X \right]$$

$$\downarrow k_{+2}$$

$$\text{Enz}\,\overset{O}{\underset{\ \ }{P}}R^1R^2 + HX$$

$$\downarrow k_{+4}$$

$$\text{Enz}\,\overset{O}{\underset{\ \ }{P}}R^1(O^-) + \begin{array}{l}\text{Products}\\ \text{from } R^2\end{array}$$

with k_{+3} leading to $HO\overset{O}{\underset{\ \ }{P}}R^1R^2$

Fig.2. Reaction of organophosphorus compounds with esterases.

except that the rate of hydrolysis of the acylated enzyme as (k_{+3}) is very slow[12]. Evidence for all the steps shown in Fig.2 is complete and as a direct consequence of the elucidation of the mechanisms of inhibition effective therapeutic agents for poisoning were developed. Acetylcholinesterase can effect a transfer of an acetyl group from one compound to another and in an entirely analogous fashion, phosphorus containing groups to oximes and hydroxamic acids; the best known are pyridine 2-aldoxime methiodide, pyridine 2-aldoxime methylmethane-sulphonate or toxigonon. A phosphorylated oxime is formed. Since these are often very potent inhibitors of acetylcholinesterase, they must break down spontaneously if inhibition of the enzyme is to be prevented.

Poisoning by organophosphorus compounds can be treated or prevented by a variety of means. Prophylaxis by pretreatment with carbamates is effective[13,14]. Thus in this case the reactivation of the unstable carbamylated acetylcholinesterase in the presence of the build-up of acetylcholine produced by the administration of an organophosphorus compound is sufficient to save life. Once phosphorylated the enzyme may be reactivated by therapeutic oximes and, in addition, the toxic effects due to the build-up of acetylcholine may be prevented by treatment with with atropine or scopolamine[15]. The somewhat unexpected benefits from treatment by benzodiazapine derivatives[16] would benefit from further detailed study.

Subsequent to the discovery of the reactivation of phosphorylated cholinesterases by oximes and hydroxamic acids, it was shown by Hobbiger that after incubation the phosphorylated enzyme became unreactivatable- the aging reaction (cf. reaction 4 in Fig.2)[17],[18]. The reaction was shown to occur _in vivo_ as well as _in vitro_. Further work, and an appreciation of the significance of past work, has now shown that at least two mechanisms can bring about this change; which is operative depends upon the esterase and upon the structure of the phosphorus containing group attached to it[19-23]. As will be shown later this understanding is a vital component for progress in the elucidation of the mechanisms in the production of delayed neuropathy by some organo- phosphorus compounds.

The progress of understanding of mechanisms of acute toxicity produced by organophosphorus compounds is an excellent example of the practical value flowing from it. Knowledge of the quantitative contri- bution of different factors allows safer insecticides to be designed, it allows a better assessment of hazard from their use, it allows exposure to be monitored _in vivo_ by their effects on enzymes, it allows rational therapy to be used if accidents occur and it is now allowing an organo- phosphorus compound, metriphonate, to be used with safety for the treatment of parasitic infection with the Schistosome haematobium[24],[25]. It is a salutory fact that even though the potentiation of malathion toxicity in experimental animals by other organophosphorus compounds was known in 1957 and the mechanism was largely understood[26],[27],a serious episode of poisoning of 2800 men by impure commercial malathion occurred in Pakistan in 1976[28],[29].

Some organophosphorus compounds produce a delayed neuropathy often in the central nervous system and so leave a permanent disability. The primary target has been identified and it is now known that this target (an esterase but not a cholinesterase) must be phosphorylated and the phosphorylated enzyme must lose one of the groups attached to the phos- phorus and produce an aged enzyme (cf reaction 4 Fig.2)[30-32]. Inhibi- tion of the enzyme is not sufficient and the group loss is an obligatory step in the genesis of the disease process. Thus, those organophos- phorus compounds (phosphinates),carbamates or sulphonates which inhibit the esterase but the resulting acylated enzyme cannot age, do not cause delayed neuropathy[33],[34]. Indeed inhibition of the esterase in the hen by such compounds protects against subsequent treatment with neurotoxic organophosphorus compounds. What have been the advantages following from this knowledge?. It is now possible in the hen, knowing the structure of the compound, to determine shortly after dosing and before clinical signs the inhibition of the esterase and to predict, in relation to the acutely toxic dose, whether the compound will produce delayed neuropathy in the hen with one or more doses. The almost all or none response detected by neuropathological examination of tissues as long as six weeks after first dosing can be replaced by a quick quantitative enzymic assay. Further it has recently been shown how, prediction of the hazard to man may be based on in vitro studies with hen and human enzymes[35]. It has been routine to test carbamate insecticides in hens for their ability to produced delayed neuropathy. It is clear, now the primary mechanism is known, that carbamates cannot cause this disease and the testing protocol for this group of compounds may be abandoned. In the design of new organophosphorus pesticides a meaningful structure--activity relationships for the production of this type of delayed neuropathy can be used[31]. Of course not only is the knowledge of the mechanism of reaction with the primary target important in this respect, but also the extensive information about the pathways of metabolism of the administered compound often leading to the production in vivo of the proximal toxic chemical. At the moment there is no knowledge of immediate biochemical/biological consequences of the primary interaction. While this ignorance persists there is no hope of therapy by interruption of processes leading to the dying-back lesions in the nerve tracts in the central nervous systems[36]. Perhaps we may acquire some leads from morphology; detailed electron microscopy of the sequential development of the changes in the nervous study is now being carried out for the neuropathies produced by acrylamide,n-hexane and methyl n-butyl ketone and recently for the organophosphorus compounds[37-43]. These studies are not only detecting early morphological changes but are showing that the application of the dying back concept is a simplification since early multifocal lesions can be demonstrated. Mechanistic studies on the toxicity of organophosphorus compounds have been carried out long enough for the benefits to be assessed. For the remainder of my lecture I wish to look further ahead and state a personal view of a need for understanding of mechanisms in other fields.

During the course of this meeting we have heard of the assays for mutagenic potency for chemicals or their metabolites. The development of these tests has been a big step forward. I do not have to point out that the development of these tests depended on previous extensive work on the reaction of mutagenic chemicals with genetic material. We now have tests which allow us to detect those chemicals reacting with genetic material so as to induce mutations. This is a big step forward. By the addition of enzymic systems capable of converting inactive chemicals to reactive products, the procedures have gone some way to take account of the fact that many environmental chemicals are biologically inert until activated by enzymic systems in vivo.
Substantial as these advances are and the stimulus that has been given to look at other cell culture lines to use to detect mutagens, we will be deluding ourselves if we do not accept that these tests do not and may never be suitable for quantitative risk assessment in man. In our approach to risk assessment for carcinogens is the basic premise that carcinogenesis is as an aspect of mutagenesis. Two major problems exist; (1) the measurement of exposure of man in a form which allows us to know the dose received in vivo and (2) the elucidation of early changes in chemical carcinogenesis in animals so that those factors which prove important may be examined in human tissues.

It has been accepted for a long time that exposure of animals or man to organophosphorus compounds can be monitored by measurement of their effect on enzymes whose inhibition causes no toxic consequences. Thus in man inhibition of butyrylcholinesterase in the serum of man indicate the exposure of this enzyme to whatever concentration of organophosphorus compound is circulating. Similar measurements may be made in the rat or guinea pig using another esterase present in serum. The principle has been extended, using recent developments in the sensitive determination of alkylated amino acids, to the measurement of reaction products of alkylating agents and suitable macromolecules. The macromolecule must be readily available and have a reasonable half-life in vivo. Haemoglobin fits these specifications and in a series of papers, excellent studies of the determination of alkylated products in haemoglobin - notably 3-alkylhistidine and alkyl-S-cysteine[44-47]- are given.   These papers have established the principle and methodology involved and have shown that some time after exposure to an acute dose, the integral of the concentration with respect to time may be determined from the amount of alkylated products found in haemoglobin.   Tissue dose has always been a somewhat elusive quantity.   Provided a suitable macromolecule can be found the methods elaborated by Ehrenberg could be used for the assessment in animals of the dose received in a particular tissue.   That this information may be able to be extended to other tissues and other macromolecules seems likely   from   the   ground   work   being   carried   out   in   Henchler's laboratory[48-50].   It seems probable that below high doses of reactive chemicals or intermediates that the relative binding to different tissues is independent of dose and the reaction with critical sites in macromolecules (i.e. primary biochemical lesion) is directly correlated with the binding to non-critical targets[49].

Thus progress is being made in linking measurements made in man and animals so that predictions may be made of tissue dose.   Likewise progress is being made in the identification of the primary chemical lesion. 0^6-alkylation of guanine has shown[51-55] good correlation with the development of tumours and 0^6-alkylguanine has been shown to be mutagenic[56-57].   Other factors such as the ability of tissue enzymes to repair modified DNA, their specificity, the requirement for cell division, immunological reactions are all being explored.   Tissue culture of cells taken from animals treated with carcinogens and the detailed definition of the earliest morphological correlates of tumour formation and the identification of the particular cell type involved are playing an increasing role.   We can now, with developing method-ology, discern the possibility of bridging the gap between the primary chemical attack and cell transformation following detailed morpholog-ical studies to identify the cell concerned[58-60].

The   toxicity   of   trimethyltin   (and   tetramethyltin   which   is dealkylated to trimethyltin in vivo[61,62]) has been known for many years[7,63,64].   The main signs of poisoning in animals are tremors and hyperexcitability.   Rats become very aggressive and stand up in pairs facing each other as if sparring. Two cases of poisoning have been recently reported[65], the symptoms included memory defects, loss of vigilance, insomnia, anorexia, disorientation, mental confusion and generalised epileptic seizures.   In a recent study it has been shown that trimethyltin chloride is very cumulative in rats. The LD_{50} is 12.6mg/kg but symptoms and some deaths are seen after 3 doses of 4mg/kg each dose spaced 7 days apart. A detailed neuropathological study has established that bilateral and symmetrical neuronal alterations are produced only in the hippocampus, pyriform cortex and amygdaloid nucleus. Although the detailed distribution of trimethyltin in the brain is not yet known, the overall concentration associated with the above morphological changes is 1.4µg trimethyltin/g wet. wt. of brain. Why do I consider that these findings should be followed by an attempt to understand the mechanisms involved, even though no-one could pretend that trimethyltin is a serious hazard to man? First, many substances produce damage in the nervous system which is selective to particular areas and cells. Our ability to assess the hazards of exposure to chemicals which damage the nervous system is greatly hampered by lack of knowledge of the selective vulnerability of different cells. By an analysis of the mechanisms involved in the effects of chemicals producing defined responses we will generate information of much value in this field. Until we have some concept of mechanism we cannot intelligently predict structure-activity relationships.

In experiments with rats the survivors appear normal, although their brains had been severely damaged with cell loss in the hippo-campus and each pyriform cortex. One of the problems facing those involved in behavioural studies is to quantify the consequences of cellular deficits produced by exposure to chemicals in utero or during the development of the central nervous system. Treatment of rats with trimethyltin provides an experimental model to examine the behavioural consequences of such a selective cell loss.

For such a complex system as the nervous system I cannot see how meaningful structure-activity relationships can be produced unless we possess knowledge of mechanisms involved. If the information on mechanisms is of a biochemical or molecular nature it is then possible to determine dose-response relationships and to establish whether there is a real threshold dose based on quantitative measurements rather than some functional change in the whole animal.

From my examples it is my opinion that there is a great need to understand mechanisms. If such research is to be successful two

316

factors are very important. The development of a suitable experimental model is crucial in that the examination of the problem then becomes feasible. Often an experimental model can only be developed using a chemical to which man is not exposed; a homologue of an important chemical in general use is often more suitable. For example the effort required for sequential electron microscopy can hardly be justified until an experimental model for carcinogenesis is found which produces from a small number of doses substantially 100% of animals with tumours. The second vital factor is to involve scientists with the drive to understand phenomena rather than to collect facts. To use the analogy so beautifully used by Forscher[67] in a letter to Science entitled "Chaos in the brickyard", we require scientists not only excellent in making bricks but in using them to construct conceptual buildings.

Recruitment of first class scientists from many basic disciplines into the science of toxicology is vital. Unless there are in a sufficient number of centres groups of scientists engaged in understanding of mechanisms of toxicity and capable of conveying to the young that toxicology is an exciting intellectual challenge, the subject will not develop. I sometimes think that the word relevance is the most misused word in the English language, but it is relevant that support, no doubt much less than the sums spent on routine toxicology, must be given to scientists with ideas. Instant solutions cannot be expected but there can be no doubt that as understanding of mechanisms increases, solution to practical problems will appear.

REFERENCES

1. Himsworth, H. (1970) The development and organisation of Scientific knowledge. Heinemann, London, pp 1-180.

2. Verschoyle,R.D.and Barnes,J.M.(1972) Pestic.Biochem.and Physiol 2 308-311.

3. Barnes,J.M & Verschoyle,R.D.(1974). Nature,(Lond.) 248, 711.

4. IARC Monographs on the Evaluation of Carcinogenic risk of chemicals to man. (1977) Asbestos 14, 1-106.

5. Hammond,E.C.and Selikoff,I.J. (1973) in "Biological Effects of Asbestos" Eds Bogorski,P, Gilson,J.C, Timbrell,V. & Wagner,J.C, IARC Lyons,, IARC Scientific Publication No.8 pp 312-317.

7. Stoner, H.B., Barnes, J.M. & Duff, J.I.(1955) British J. Pharmacol 10
    16-25

8. Brown, A.W., Aldridge, W.N., Street, B.W.and Verschoyle, R.D. (1979)
    Amer.J. Path. in the press.

9. Smissaert, H.R.,(1964) Science 143, 129-131.

10 Smissaert, H.R.,Voerman, S.,Oostenbrugge, L and Renooy, N.(1970)
    J. Agric. Food Chem. 18,66-75.

11. Devonshire, A.L. (1975) Biochem.J. 149, 463-469.

12. Aldridge, W.N.,and Reiner,(1972). Enzyme Inhibitors as Substrates.
    Interaction of esterases with esters of organophosphorus and carbamic
    acids. North Holland, Amsterdam pp 1-328.

13. Koster, R. (1946). J. Pharmac. exp. Ther. 88, 39-46.

14. Barnes, J.M. (1974). "Forensic Toxicology". Ed. B. Ballantyne.
    John Wright & Son, Bristol, U.K. p.79-85.

15. Bertram, U., Kasten, A., Lüllmann, H. and Ziegler, A. (1977).
    Experientia. 33. 1196-1197.

16. Lipp, J.A. (1973). Arch. int. Pharmacodynamie 202, 244-251.

17. Hobbiger, F. (1955). Brit. J. Pharmacol. 10, 356-362.

18. Hobbiger, F. (1956). Brit. J. Pharmacol. 11, 295-303.

19. Lee, W. and Turnbull, J.H. (1958). Biochim. & Biophys. Acta. 30,
    655.

20. Lee, W. and Turnbull, J.H. (1961). Experientia. 17, 360-361.

21. Hovanec, J.W. and Lieske, C.N. (1972). Biochemistry. 11, 1051-1056.

22. Aldridge, W.N. (1975) Croat.Chem.Acta.47,215-233.

23. Michel, H.O., Hackley, B.E., Berkowitz, L., List, G., Hackley, E.B.,
    Gillilan, W. and Pankau, M. (1967). Arch. Biochem and Biophys. 121,
    29-34.

24. Plestina, R., Davis, A.,and Bailey, D.R. (1972). Bull. Wld. Hlth.
    Org. 46, 747-759.

25. Holmstedt, B., Nordgren, I., Sandoz, M. and Sundwall, A. (1978).
    Arch. Toxicol. 41, 3-29.

26. Frawley, J.P., Fuyat,.N., Hagan, E.C.. Blake, J.R,
    and Fitzhugh, D.G. (1957) J. Pharmacol. 121, 96-106.

27. Murphy, S.D,and Dubois, K.P. (1957). Proc.Soc. Exp.Biol & Med. 96,
    813-8.

28. Baker, E.L. Zack, M. Miles, J.W. Alderman. L. Warren McW. Dobbin,
    R.D. Miller, S and Teeters, W.R. (1978), Lancet, 31-33.

29. Aldridge, W.N. Miles, J.W., Mount, D.L.,and Verschoyle, R.D.
    (1979) Arch.Toxicol.in the Press.

30. Johnson, M.K.(1975a) Crit.Rev. Toxicol. 3, 289-316.

31. Johnson, M.K.(1975b) Arch Toxicol. 34, 259-288.

32. Clothier, B. and Johnson, M.K. (1979) Biochem. J. 177, 549-558.

33. Johnson, M.K. and Lauwerys R. (1969). Nature (Lond.) 222,1066-1067.

34. Johnson, M.K. (1974). J. Neurochem. 23, 785-789.

35. Lotti, M. and Johnson, M.K. (1978) Arch. Toxicol. 41, 215-221.

36. Cavanagh, J.B. (1973) Crit.Rev.Toxicol. 2, 365-417.

37. Spencer, P.S. and Schaumburg, H.H. (1977a) J. Neuropath Exp.Neurol. 36, 276-299.

38. Spencer, P.S. and Schaumburg, H.H. (1977b) J. Neuropath Exp. Neurol 36, 300-320.

39. Schaumburg, H.H.and Spencer, P.S. (1974) J.Neuropath Exp. Neurol.33 260-284.

40. Spencer, P.S.and Thomas, P.K. (1974) J.Neurocytol 3, 763-783

41. Bouldin, T.W. and Cavanagh, J.B. (1977) Neuropath. Appl.Neurobiol. 3, 493-4.

42. Bouldin, T.W. and Cavanagh, J.B. (1979) Am.J.Pathol.94, 241-252.

43. Bouldin, T.W. and Cavanagh, J.B. (1979) Am.J.Pathol.94, 253-270.

44. Ehrenberg, L. Hiesche, K.D. Osterman-Golkar, S. and Wennberg, I. (1974). Mut.Res. 24, 83-103.

45. Osterman-Golkar, S. Ehrenberg, L. Segerback, D. and Hallstrom, I (1976) Mut.Res. 34. 1-10 .

46. Osterman-Golkan, S. Hultmark. D. Segerback, C.J. Calleman, R. Gothe, R. Ehrenberg, L. and Wachmeister, C.A. (1977) Biochim. Biophys. Res. Comm. 7, 259-266.

47. Segerback, D., Calleman, C.J., Ehrenberg, L., Logroth, G. and Osterman-Golkan, S. (1978). Mut. Res. 49, 71-82.

48. Wieland, E. and Neumann, H.G. (1978). Arch. Toxicol. 40, 17-35.

49. Neumann, H.G. (1979). Abstracts European Society of Toxicology Symposium "Quantitative Aspects of Risk Assessment in Chemical Carcinogenesis". Rome, April 3-6, 1979.

50. Neumann, H.G., Gangler, B.J.M. and Taupp, W. (1978). Proc. 1st Intl. Cong. Toxicol., Toronto 1977.Academic Press,New York p.177-190.

51. Lawley, P.D. and Shah, S. (1973). Chem. Biol. Interactions, 7, 115-120.

52. Goth, R. and Rajewsky, M.F. (1974). Proc. Nat. Acad. Sci., USA. 71, 639-643.

53. Nicholl, J.N., Swann, P.F. and Pegg, A.E. (1977). Chem. Biol. Interactions, 16, 301-308.

54. O'Connor, P.J. Capps, M.J. and Craig, A.W. (1973). Brit. J. Cancer, 27, 153-166.

55. Kleihues, P. (1978). Proc. 1st Intl.Cong. Toxicol., Toronto 1977. Academic Press, New York. p.191-206.

319

56. Loveless, A. (1969). Nature (Lond.) 223, 206–207.

57. Gerchman, L.L. and Ludlum, D.B. (1973). Biochim. Biophys. Acta. <u>308</u>, 310–316.

58. Hard, G.C. and Butler, W.H. (1971a). Cancer Res. 31, 337–347.

59. Hard, G.C. and Butler, W.H. (1971b). Cancer Res. 31, 348–365.

60. Hard, G.C. and Butler, W.H. (1971c). Cancer Res. 31, 366–372.

61. Cremer, J.E. (1958). Biochem. J. 68, 685–692.

62. Cremer, J.E. and Calloway, S. (1961). Brit. J. ind. Med. 18, 277–282.

63. Jolyet, F. and Cahours, A. (1969). CR Acad. Sci. Paris 68, 1276–1280.

64. Barnes, J.M. and Stoner, H.B. (1958). Brit. J. Ind. Med., 15, 15–22.

65. Fortemps, E., Amand, G., Bomboir, A., Lauwerys, R. and Laterre, E.C. (1978). Int. Arch. Occup. Environ. Hlth., 41, 1–6.

66. Brown, A.W. Aldridge, W.N. and Street, B.W. (1979). Proc. Brit. Neuropath. Soc. July, 1978, Neuropath. Appl. Neurobiol. In the press.

67. Forscher, B.K. (1963). Science 142, 339.

© 1980 Elsevier/North-Holland Biomedical Press
The Scientific Basis of Toxicity Assessment
H. Witschi, editor.

CONCLUDING REMARKS - SYMPOSIUM ON THE SCIENTIFIC BASIS OF TOXICITY ASSESSMENT.

W. N. ALDRIDGE

Medical Research Council Toxicology Research Unit, England

In this Symposium we have been presented with scientific work by leading experts which have illustrated the extraordinary range of activities which toxicology covers. It is an almost open-ended commitment with respect to the kind of organisms, the type of chemical and the many biological responses they bring about. The organizing committee and particularly their chairman, Peter Witschi, are to be congratulated in the choice of subjects. This has no doubt allowed many to see unsuspected connections between rather diverse areas.

We have seen during the course of the meeting the use of the increasingly sophisticated technology in the exploration of those processes affecting the delivery of the toxic chemical to its site of action. It seems to me that problems arising in this area can now be solved. It is in the definition of the primary interactions of the chemical responsible for toxicity that we require more understanding, e.g., we must know what is done to what cell leads to the manifestations of toxicity. Advance in such understanding requires collaborative work by scientists from many basic disciplines and will require much creative thinking. Only as more mechanisms of toxicity are unravelled can we expect to consider on a rational basis species differences, structure-activity relationships, dose-response and whether a threshold exists. All of these are absolute requirements for risk assessment.

I would like to mention two actions which will require efforts by research scientists in their educative role. Although we all regret serious chemical accidents there is no doubt that they will continue to happen. When they do it is vital that we learn as much as we can about toxicity in man. Analysts, clinicians and experimental biologists, all experts in the relevant field, must be on the spot before other interested parties restrict access or the flow of information. It is important as research scientists to point out the paramount importance of information about toxicity in man.

There is also in industry a very large number of chemicals which have been rejected due to untoward or unexpected toxicity. We should explain to those in industry that access to these chemicals may provide the experimental models which will make possible the solution of mechanisms of toxicity. If such chemicals could be released as soon as it is economically possible, or if we can be more persuasive before then, it would be a great advantage. As one

example only, we should not forget the enormous stimulus to research brought
about by the discovery of chemicals capable of inducing one-shot carcinogenesis.

   Although we may as scientists have to reply to questions from the lay public
that we do not know, we cannot evade the challenge when society tells us to
find out. I think the present successes in the science of toxicology,
exemplified by work presented in this Symposium, means that we can convince
able young scientists (perhaps I should say those young-in-heart and then
everyone can be happy) that research in toxicology is an exciting challenge --
exciting because of its intellectual content and exciting because it involves
the solution of problems of concern to society. If we can interest able
scientists that this is so then the future is bright and the understanding of
mechanisms of toxicity will advance. Toxicity assessment will then have a
sound scientific basis.

AUTHOR INDEX

SUBJECT INDEX

A

Acetylcholinesterase 309

Acid phosphatase 216

Acrylamide 312

Aerobic bacteria 265

Aflatoxin B1 213

Ah-locus 226

Air pollutants 31

δ-ALA synthetase 215, 225

Alkyl-S-cysteine 314

Ames test 47, 61

Aminopyrine dimethylase 214

Anaerobic bacteria 264

Anesthesia, theories of 171

Anthracycline antibiotics 172

Annelida 257

Anti-esterase compounds 309

Anti-inflammatory drugs 213

Army worm (Spodoptera eridonia) 258

Arsenic 211

Arthropoda 257

Aryl hydrocarbon hydroxylase (AHH) 225

Atherosclerosis 177

Atropine 310

Avoidance tests 95

Azobenzene 232

B

Bacterial systems 48

BALB/3T3 cells 62, 63

Bay region theory 137

Behavior, definition 91

Behavioral teratology 93

Behavioral tests 92, 93, 95

Behavioral toxicology 92

Benzo(a)pyrene:B(a)P 123, 129, 135

Benzo(a)pyrene, metabolites 132, 133, 134, 135, 225

Benzo(e)pyrene 135, 136

Benzo(e)pyrene metabolites 136

Benzphetamine 242

Biological transport 26

Bioaccumulation 114, 121

Bird lungs 144

Botulism 287

Butyrylcholinesterase 313

C

Cadmium 218

Calcium, interacellular 212

Cambrium 263

D-Camphor 263

Carbamate esters 309, 312

Carbon disulfide 242

Carbon-sulfur bond 249

CCl_4 151, 203, 208

Cardiomyopathy 167

Cardiotoxic drugs and chemicals 168

Cardiotoxicity assessment 167

Cell death 201

C3H mice 294

C3H/10T1/2 cells 62, 63, 65

Chick embryo 225

CHO cells 52, 159

Chilopoda 257

Chloracne 224

Chlorodimeform 169

Chlorinated hydrocarbons 69

Chlorpromazine 205

Cholestasis 204

Chordata 257

Circular dichroism 205

Clara cells 148, 150

CNS 94

326